Gerhard Wolfrum (Ed.)

The Power of Brainspotting. An International Anthology

Gerhard Wolfrum (Ed.)

The Power of Brainspotting. An International Anthology

With a preface by David Grand

Asanger Verlag • Kröning

Layout: Wolfgang Wohlers, einsatz.berlin
Druck: PBtisk, a.s., Czech Republic

Bibliographische Informationen der Deutschen Nationalbibliothek:
Die Deutsche Nationalbibliothek verzeichnet diese Publikation in der Deutschen Nationalbibliographie; detaillierte bibliographische Daten sind im Internet über http://dnb.d-nb.de abrufbar.

ISBN 978-3-89334-630-1

Editorial for the Brainspotting-Anthology "The Power of Brainspotting"

For me it is a great joy and honor to present this anthology containing articles about the power of the brainspotting procedure to interested specialists – even more so as I, a relatively "young" brainspotting trainer – not young in age but young with respect to the brainspotting community – have succeeded in recruiting so many highly qualified brainspotting trainers as contributors. To some extent, they have already been familiar with this exceptional treatment much longer than I have, and they have vastly more experience. I am very pleased that they took the trouble to present so thoroughly the fundamental importance of the treatment principles that David Grand developed and the fields where brainspotting can be implemented.

Our Spanish brainspotting colleague *Mario Salvador* discusses the basic concept of "attunement" – attuned to the patient not only at the relationship level but also at the physiological level, a concept, as far as I know, which does not exist anywhere else in psychotherapy. He describes in great detail how important it is to establish this "double" relationship. Only then is it possible for the brain to activate "the healing bubble". In a further article he describes the preparatory steps with which brainspotting can be implemented in cases of complex trauma. The author explains a model of ego fragmentation inspired by the structural dissociation approach and the primary emotional systems, especially the ones wired for survival. It reveals a model of dissociation and ego splits related to the threshold of the windows of tolerance in order to refer to hypoaroused parts and hyperaroused parts.

Our Brasilian colleague *Andrè Mauricio Monteiro* describes which possibilities multifocal brainspotting offers in therapy work with patients suffering from fragmentation. At the same time he emphasizes the importance of work within a window of tolerance, which he connects with Stephen Porges's polyvagal theory, and his social engagement system. A detailed case example describes the therapeutic approach of entropy as a set of dispersive forces which hinder the internal efforts of this system of parts from integrating the self. This explains how multifocal brainspotting addresses this entropic configuration of the system of parts and provides dissociative clients the opportunity to explore the interdependent dynamics of inner parts in relation to the self in a way that preserves this internal complexity.

Cynthia Schwartzberg from Altlanta, Georgia, (USA) discusses brainspotting as a grounding model and observes the importance of grounding from an energy point of view, as recovery of homeostasis and coherence. Along with case examples she illustrates the basic principles of brainspotting and how, in light of grounding in the here and now, gains in tolerance can be found through which ups and downs released by feelings and experiences can be endured better. In this way the inherent powers of self-healing can help the client progress from the previously existing dysregulation to a better regulation of his stress processing systems. She emphasizes that we humans are survivors, and this process can take our clients a long way within a grounded, supportive container that allows the unexpected to happen.

Susan Pinco from New York – to whom I personally owe my first steps into the brainspotting procedure – points out the importance of the uncertainty principle in the brainspotting process, of patiently waiting during therapy with clients. She tries to debunk the myth of the talking cure. Contradicting all verbally oriented psychotherapy treatments, she emphasizes the necessity of silence, the willingness of the therapist to put up with the process of coming to terms with things and to wait – without knowing what will happen and above all without needing to steer or control the process. Allowing this trust in the therapy process, as you know, is especially difficult for many psychotherapists because they prefer to have everything under control. In her second article she also describes how very differentiated therapy must be managed when working with patients suffering from complex trauma. By means of various case descriptions with victims of September 11, with ego state patients, as well as with patients with dissociative identity disorder it becomes clear which preparatory groundwork has to be carried out, how important it is to find, hold, and adapt a suitable framework, which roles the core elements of brainspotting play: Dual attunement, framing and focus, the principle of no assumptions and following the head of the comet in order to understand and thereby to deal with whether you are confronted with „apparent normal part(s)" or „alters". She describes the behavior of the therapist as crucial, that the client has powers of self-healing available and that alters and symptoms have a communicative function and that the therapist accompanies this process in a safe framework and only intervenes in moderation.

Reflecting on her personal experiences, *Deborah Antinori* from New Jersey discusses the importance of dealing with experiences of grief and loss as a result of existential trauma with the help of brainspotting. She describes how the feelings, thoughts, basic assumptions about ourselves and the basic assumptions about the world, both located in the subcortical centers, can be shaken up through such experiences and how purposeful coherences can be detected in therapy with brainspotting. Combined with comprehensive specialist knowledge of the participating structures of the brain and taking into account Panksepp's panic and grief system, she explains how mourners can be helped by activating the limbic system – the home of all human interpersonal bonding experiences – and with the help of an attuned therapist can reach a safe bonding experience in a new homeostasis and can let go of previously suppressed feelings.

On the basis of many examples of this treatment, the New York trainer *Martha Jacoby* and my Vienna colleague and cooperation partner *Monika Baumann* and *Mark Grixti,* a brainspotting trainer and clinical psychologist currently living in England, show the characteristic features of work with children and teenagers and the diverse possibilities for a creative use of brainspotting. Both women authors point out the necessity of much more flexible methods when treating these younger clients, the importance of letting brainspotting just happen instead of forcing it and of paying attention to a more developmentally adequate use of the method. Examples of treatment illustrate what is meant. Case descriptions again make it clear that the brainspotting therapist must patiently follow the tail of the comet of the young patients even when confronted with regressive behavior. These descriptions also show how the therapist can observe that, in the sense of the "double effect", an activating point can shift into a resource point.

Mark Grixti emphasizes the validity of the most important basic principles of brainspotting in treating younger clients. More from the theoretical side and also with respect to the development of affect regulation, he examines the underestimated significance of unconscious right brain-to-right brain communication that becomes immediately important with children and teenagers, also because their brain structures aren't yet matured but rather still developing. He compares this intersubjectivity to a wifi connection, which, depending on the quality of the bond or relationship, can be allowed or neglected and points out the effects in terms of limbic transference and reverse transference. Many case examples illustrate his observations.

Santiago Brand, a neuroscientist living in Columbia, complains that there are still far too few research findings or empirical studies about the brainspotting procedure. From his neuroscientific point of view, he points out how the specific methods of EEG brain mapping in combination with biofeedback and neurofeedback and the brainspotting procdure could help patients deal with traumatic experiences better. He comments in detail on the first empirical results of a pilot study begun together with Deborah Antinori and Susan Pinco (both authors also appearing in this book) in February, 2018. It seems to confirm the previously established hypotheses for activating powers of self-healing, better self-regulation supported by brainspotting („from dysregulation to regulation"), and better homeostasis between the activating sympathicotonic and damping parasympathic systems.

A former collegiate baseball pitcher and high school football and basketball player and now clinical psychologist, *Calder Kaufmann,* currently living in Detroit, Michigan, (USA) very creatively examines the practical aspects of applying brainspotting to sports psychology, also referring to his own sports experiences. He is disappointed by the more superficial and cognitive treatments, with mental and skills training, offered to athletes with performance problems. In contrast, he understands the mostly underestimated sports injuries as experiences of trauma which leave their traces in the body's memory when so-called „yips", „alligator arms", or „whiplash" not only become visible but also can be very obstructive in athletic events. He tries to understand them in terms of a reconceptualizing, as a conversion disease, that is to say, a somatoform, structural dissociation – disturbances in the cognitive consciousness generally inaccessible brain-body system. He therefore argues the case for treatment on the basis of clinical experience and seems to be very successful using brainspotting.

Christine Ranck, the colleague also living in New York, describes how brainspotting is not only applicable in the clinical realm but also in the creative realm of artists, in the world of music and the theater, where many struggle with stage fright. Incidentally she also performs with her own band in public and therefore contributes a great deal of personal experience as a brainspotting trainer. She compares the unusual processes of therapy with holographic processes in which every part contains the whole, emphasizes the importance of intuition, and over and over again demonstrates the statement by David Grand: „There is no healing without creativity, and there is no creativity without healing". She is especially impressive in describing how an actor can be supported in becoming Othello and also how he can return from the role as well as showing how spontaneous creativity can get under your skin and save your own life.

Altogether, therefore, a colorful bouquet of very informative chapters on the implementation of this unusual method of treatment, which is why the title „The Power of Brainspotting" is in no way an exaggeration. In another context (in the editorial to issue 3/2017 Brainspotting in TRAUMA) I spoke about a paradigm shift. I would like to thank the "inventor" and developer of brainspotting, Dr. David Grand, very much for taking the time to write a preface for this anthology in order to describe and explain the technique once again at a meta level. Thank you so very much, and I wish all interested readers much enjoyment and many new insights.

Gerhard Wolfrum, July, 2018

Preface

This book implicitly poses the question "What is the power of Brainspotting?" There is no single answer to this query. Brainspotting is developed on an articulated foundation with a set of fundamental principles. It is accurate to assert that the integration of all of the articulated aspects of Brainspotting generates its power. Throughout the evolution of Brainspotting, I have repeatedly shifted my position about its core foundation and fundamental principles. Initially I believed that the relevant eye position, or Brainspot, was the essential element of the modality. That made sense, on one level, as the discovery and development of Brainspotting started with the profound eye wobble and freeze, of the ice skater, leading to the ten minutes of intense processing.

In that regard, Brainspotting was a highly technical therapy based on locating relevant eye positions through reflexes (Outside Window), eye positions matched with heightened somatic activation (Inside Window), and spontaneous gaze (Gazespotting). In gaining more experience with the modality, I recognized the relational primacy of Brainspotting. At that juncture I labeled this interpersonal aspect as Clinical Brainspotting. This brought more of my attention to the paired attunement of both the relational and the brain-body components of Brainspotting. I labeled this phenomenon Dual Attunenment, playing off of the pre-existing designation of dual attention, which was associated with other models.

With my further study of neurobiology, I learned that the brain is comprised of between one to four quadrillion synaptic connections, numbers that are virtually infinite. This startling revelation of the incalculable and unknowable complexity of the human brain challenged the notions I had been taught since professional school and subsequent trainings. I had been taught, along with all other students, that therapists must know comprehensive information about the client in order to help them in any organized way. This entails extensive history taking leading to diagnostic formulation leading to strategic treatment planning.

But it became apparent to me that we, as therapists, sit in front of clients possessing an essentially unknowable system. I called this the Uncertainty Principle (knowing wink to Werner Heisenberg) which posits that therapists cannot possibly know the inner workings of the neurobiological client system directly in front of them. Facing this reality challenges the therapist's wish and need to have some control over the process unfolding inside the client. But facing and accepting the infinite, unknowable reality is ultimately liberating for the therapist.

The Uncertainty Principle ultimately led me to develop the metaphor of "getting into the tail of the comet", which implies the necessity for the therapist to follow the clients wherever they go in their process. This demands absolute trust from the therapist for their client's process. Emanating from the Uncertainty Principle is the enhanced attunement of the client and the converse that any measure of certainty on the therapist's part as impeding attunement. So, if therapists accept that they are facing an unknowable system, then what actually can they do? The Brainspotting answer is to "frame it".

I wrote earlier that Brainspotting therapists mindfully use the Dual Attunenment of relational and neurobiological presence with their clients. This implied the concept of the frame which is designated in Brainspotting as the Dual Attunenment Frame. We posit that the therapist, mindfully applying relational attunement simultaneous to neurological attunement (awareness of body activation with attendant relevant eye positions), creates a frame for the clients which focuses both their experience and neurobiology. This yields focused mindfulness processing which facilitates internally derived change in the client's infinitely complex system. This ultimately reveals the power of Brainspotting.

The frame is designed to be in the moment, flexible, formed and held according to the client's needs. If sufficient, the basic frame can be held throughout the session yielding optimal healing for the client. In situations of greater complexity, based on attuned following of the client's process, the frame can be reconfigured. This happens both in the moment and throughout the session. There is an infinite number of frames, which matches the infinite nature of the human nervous system. A few examples are the somatic frame, the affective frame, the developmental frame, the parts frame, the child therapy frame and the performance-creativity frame.

This book provides chapters written by Brainspotting experts from around the world. Each author is writing from the expertise that they have integrated into the Brainspotting model. These chapters are rich and informative and creatively expand the foundational model. I encourage you to encounter and engage with each chapter as a frame unto itself. In other words, each chapter posits and elaborates a specific framed approach that enhances and expands Brainspotting. I hope and expect you will find this to be an intriguing and informative journey.

David Grand
United States, June 2018

Brainspotting, Attunement, and Presence in the Therapeutic Relationship

Mario C. Salvador

Each life is a work of art, created by all the available means
Pierre Janet (mentioned in van der Kolk 2015, p 125)

From Interpersonal to Intrapersonal Attunement

A core principle that defines Brainspotting (BSP) is the principle of "dual attunement" which implies that neurological attunement that can be found with the location of the "relevant eye position" or "brainspot" must be used within the frame of an attuned therapeutic relationship with the client's experience.

Even if the attunement and the presence of the therapist are common to all psychotherapy approaches, in Brainspotting they have a predominant and key position that will allow the neurological attunement that can be reached with eye position as a neurological access point to have its powerful effects on reprocessing the experience.

According to the researchers Lambert & Barley (2002) and Lambert & Simon (2008), 30 % of what affects the results of psychotherapy may be attributed to what they call common factors, such as the qualities of the therapist (presence and empathy) and the therapeutic relationship. Many years of research confirm that the most important ingredient in effective therapy, regardless of the paradigm or the therapy model, is the empathetic capacity of the therapist (Hutterer & Liss, 2006; mentioned in Badenoch, 2008). Frequently, when we ask our clients what has helped them in the therapeutic session, they refer to the fact that their therapeutic process would not have been so healing without the active presence of the therapist.

Every human being has the desire to be understood; it is a basic hunger that creates a secure attachment. When we feel understood, we experience somebody external to us seeing confirming, and giving validity to our experience in all its phenomenological dimensions (cognitions, affections, fantasies, behaviours ...). This contributes to consolidating the experience of feeling accepted just the way we are.

In a therapeutic relationship, attuned with the client's experience the client can start lowering his defences towards the outside world and the others, as well as the defences towards his own painful experience. Thus he is able to deepen his own experience in a more fulfilling internal contact in order to be able to know it, to be interested in it, and accept it. These are the requirements for reprocessing. Ultimately, it is through a deeply attuned therapeutic relationship that we convey that we are fully oriented towards the other, in order to know and to help his more rejected and dissociated experiences emerge, so that they may be seen and recognised as the intelligent and desperate attempt to survive in painful conditions. The last goal of attunement is to enable the client to enter into a deeper contact with his intra-personal world, with his own experiential aspects that he had to marginalise or set aside from his consciousness and from the relationships with others in order to protect himself from criticism, rejection, an even abuse, ultimately, preparing and directing the client's mind towards a self-study and self-observing mode.

I subscribe to the powerful self-healing capacities of the brain and our inner system. But to be able to wake up and access the self-healing capacities, the brain must loosen its survival, defensive systems. This is more likely to happen when the therapist seems available in the therapeutic relationship and is involved in understanding and supporting the client's experience the way it is.

Attunement and Therapeutic Relationship

Daniel Siegel in his book T*he Mindful Therapist* defines attunement in a sublime way in the following quote:

"Attunement is how we focus our attention on others and take their essence into our own inner world ... The physical side of interpersonal attunement involves the perception of signals from others that reveal their internal world: sensing not just their words but also their nonverbal patterns of energy and information flow. These signals are the familiar primarily right-hemisphere sent and received elements of eye contact, facial expression and tone of voice, posture, and the timing and intensity of response. The subjective side of attunement is the authentic sense of connection, of seeing someone deeply, of taking in the essence of that other person in that moment. When others sense our attunement with them, they experience "feeling felt" by us... Attunement requires presence, but is a process of focused attention and clear perception." (Siegel, 2010, p. 34)

Likewise, Allan Schore has inspired us to consider the emerging interactions between the right hemisphere of the therapist and the right hemisphere of the patient as a dance that usually happens below our consciousness, and provides the essential basis of healing. Thinking in this regard in therapy takes us to the unavoidable conclusion that the mental health of the therapist is the cornerstone of his capacity to be an agent promoting the neurological integration of the patient's experience. Subsequently, the ability to embrace and handle one's own internal and continuously emerging consciousness is the primary responsibility of the therapist. What the therapist does are not techniques but a way of 'being', since the attuned contact of the right hemisphere to the right hemisphere is the main road of the neurological change (Schore, 2003b)

It is common for some people, and maybe also for many therapists, to think that they know what is happening to the client, based on the fact that they have had similar experiences or that they have accompanied other similar processes; then they slide into saying to the client "I understand you". But the experience of "being understood" is exclusively relational. One feels understood when he senses the other being present and interested in his experience, when he feels that the other one is involved in what is happening and curious to know and understand. Therefore, feeling understood is something that happens during the process of how the therapist and the client co-construct the relationship at that time, of how the therapist formulates his inquiries about the phenomenological experience that the client manifests, and essentially depends on the therapist's manner of being and on how present he is. As Siegel said, the therapist must be sensitive to the entire narrative of the client beyond the words, particularly sensitive to the language arising from the right hemisphere (intonation, gestures, facial expressions, physiological reactions, postures and emotional tone, which I will call 'emotional markers'), and sensitive to all signs of more intimate and deeper, more physical, subcortical, and unconscious aspects of the story. This is how the therapist is able to grasp the essence of the client at that moment, the living story that is arising in him at the present moment in the face of the therapist as he exposes his problem and activates his pragmatic strategies that were shaped at some point to survive something painful.

Thus, feeling understood and in contact involves more than someone knowing the logical, rational meanings of our words. It involves having them know how we feel about those words and sensing that they share or reverberate with how we feel (Erskine et al., 1999).

Attunement begins with empathy; it is the relational quality within which interpersonal contact thrives. And it goes beyond empathy, because it involves the deeply personal response to the listener as well as the intent of the speaker (Stern, 1985). It is about the "in between", the space where two people meet in a kind of shared awareness (Tustin, 1986; Bettelheim, 1967, quoted in Erskine p. 12).

On the other hand, attunement is a two-part process. The therapist who is attuned to the client must first be aware of the client's perceptions, feelings, desires, or meanings. Maintaining such awareness, the therapist must also communicate to the client that he is aware, does understand, and is willing to shape his responses accordingly (Erskine et al, 1999). One way for the therapist to convey awareness is through his process of inquiry and becoming involved in the client's experience through his acknowledgement, validation, and normalization (we'll talk about this later).

The therapeutic relationship as a secure frame for exploration: Attunement, presence, and the healing bubble.

About attunement

Every client brings to the relationship with the therapist a long story of being in relationships with his significant people; this is normally a story full of misunderstandings, frustrations, and frequently pain and trauma. Thus, the brain is programmed with a "being in a relationship" mode that activates the "relationship strategies" shaped by his early bonding. In traumatised patients this "being in a relationship" mode activates survival responses (relational strategies that carry stories with an emotional burden) of "defending from" or "avoiding". Clients come to therapy with attachment relational strategies (that Bowlby called internal working models) of anticipating relational failures or experienced attacks in their previous relationships with caretakers and educators. The figure of the therapist involves both the hope of finding a new relationship in which to heal and develop and the trigger of the memories of the painful failures in the prior relationships; this is the nature of the transference. Transference implies that the therapist acts as a screen onto which the traumatic stories of former relationships can be projected. Therefore, a first important task in the therapeutic relationship is to create safety and help the patient to differentiate between his transferred reactions of the past and sensing himself in a new safe relationship with someone present in the here and now.

Our brain has two basic ways of functioning: growth or survival. The human brain is the most gifted and capable of learning, creating, and transforming. It has developed brain areas not present in other mammals, especially the prefrontal cortex. It can develop its maximum creative and optimal performance capacities when it feels safe. As wisely explained by the polyvagal theory of Stephen Porges, in mammals safety is essentially provided by the relationships with their fellow beings; our neuroception notices subcortically whether the other one is safe or dangerous. Therefore, the first basic task that must be accomplished in the therapeutic relationship is forming a safe environment. This is created mainly by adopting an attitude of radical acceptance of the experience of the other as it is, by initiating interventions that neither imply preconceptions of the client's experience, nor judgements, nor definitions. Only in this radical acceptance, can the defence system of the client grasp that the relationship is safe and that the client can relax; this is the basis for attunement in a relationship.

The relational attunement has several purposes:

1. *Building a new relational context of safety and involvement with the other* that will help differentiate between this new relationship (someone present, available, and safe) and the previous relational schemeloaded with pain, frustration, and/or trauma.
2. Helping the client to *access deeper areas of his inner experience* and to keep in touch with them.
3. *Co-constructing the therapeutic space as a healing space* in which the therapist is counted on as guide, an external emotional regulator, and a co-constructor of a framework that acts to support of the pain coming from the experiences; I will call this space the "healing bubble".
4. Encouraging the client to *be present in his own experience.* Through interpersonal attunement and the radical acceptance of any experience, we enable the patient to enter into an attitude of attunement and presence in his own experience, placing him in a state of mindfulness and self-compassion that will help him take ownership of his experience.

In the interpersonal framework of safety, the client's system can loosen the defences and access the self-healing mode. When the survival systems no longer need to be active in responding to a perception of external danger, the brain can turn its attention to itself and simply listen and compassionately embrace the experience as such. In accordance with the polyvagal theory of Stephen Porges, the neuronal pathways of support and social engagement are shared with the neuronal pathways that support health, growth, and healing.

In the process of attunement, the therapist simply follows the natural process of the client where it flows. Only feeling safe and stable in the therapeutic relationship can allow the client to go towards places that scare him, to dissolve his denial, and, if necessary, to access the traumatic memories or foundational memories to recover his lost parts of himself (Guntrip, 1971; quoted in Erskine 1999 p. 49).

On the other hand, attunement must occur on several levels. Expanding on them would exceed the possibilities of this chapter but I want to mention some of them.

Some levels of attunement:

On the *cognitive level.* This refers to what the client is thinking and the content of his expressions; it implies attending to the logic of the patient, the process of linking concepts together, the kind of reasoning by the client to try to create meaning. Not only what he thinks matters, but also how he is thinking it. The therapist must be thoughtful and listen to the underlying meaning in the words, to the elements organising the experience that they have forged linguistically. These are windows of entry to the deepest experience. For example when the client expresses conclusions such as "*there is no room for me*", "*nothing to give to me*", "*they never wait for me*", "*why cry, if nothing is achieved*", ... These expressions are access doors to an old story; the therapist must ask himself and ask things such as "*when was it true that crying was not useful at all?*", "*how, who, and when do others not wait for him?*", ... Using the same words as the client reinforces attunement.

Affective level. Here we must be sensitive both in the intensity and in the quality of the emotion. The client who feels scared needs the therapist to provide safety; when he feels sad, the quality of the attuned response of the therapist is compassion and nourishment. If what the client manifests is rage or anger, he expects the therapist to listen and take him seriously; and if what he feels is joy, the response in resonance is to share it in a playful way.

Development level. Frequently, during the session, the client goes from a subjective experience associated more with his recent experience but at some point there is a connection and access to older developmental stages. The therapist must be sensitive and respond to the level of development in which the client is living at that moment. He must learn to develop a double view and the capacity to produce a language for the child that is being reactivated in the client as well as a language to sustain his observer's awareness. Expressions such as "listen to what that 5 year old child who was being beaten by his father needs to express and needs from you to know", "allow him to express everything that is kept in these physical sensations", "ask the child what he needs from you now", aim at maintaining "the dual awareness" of an observer in the adult person who now listens with empathy and presence to the observed one the child part that is manifesting itself and which crystallised a way of feeling, thinking, and acting. With this, the therapist controls the processing, and a new internal relationship of the client engaging with his own experience in an accepting way and without judgement comes about. This promotes the reprocessing and the reclaiming of that which had been divided or denied

Attunement with the development level manifests itself especially in the choice of words, the tone of voice, the facial expressions, and the gestures he uses. This is the language of the right hemisphere, and they are the physiological elements that awaken the social engagement system that the polyvagal theory of Porges so wisely describes. When the therapist is attentive to the non-verbal codes of the client, he can find the formulas to help the client connect with his own experience more deeply.

Attunement emphazises the therapeutic relationship and allows the client to experience the therapist as someone who is there and in contact, and who acknowledges, validates, and normalises the experience as a survival resource determined by the subcortical intelligence. As the therapist shows that he is attuned with the thought processes, the affections, the rhythm, and the developmental level, the client starts to trust. With trust, survival defences are loosened and the system enters the growth and healing mode. We continue to train and prepare the brain of the client to orient itself towards an internal view as the environment is safe and supportive.

About presence

Just as inquiry (which we will talk about further on) is a trainable capability with practice and learning, as well as attunement (even though this one is determined by the attitude and emotional capacity of the therapist), *presence* requires capability of course, but it is more of an attitude issue, of knowing how to be a person and how to be part of a the relationship. Attunement and inquiry are about what the therapist does, presence is seen as how the therapist is as a person and as part of the relationship . How we are therapeutically means being fully present, fully in contact, an ordinary person with needs and shortcomings and all the background that makes him a real person, while he is still a therapist who is with and for the client (Buber, 1958; quoted in Erskine 1999 p. 83). At the same time, presence is a requirement for achieving attunement.

It is in the relationship with someone who can offer a full and safe attitude of presence that the other one can find the courage to look at his inner world, daring to know what he does not want and cannot look at in the loneliness of pain, because he feels supported by someone who is there for him. Then, his brain can direct its attention and self-healing processes towards the inner or intra-personal world, towards himself. The kind, compassionate presence of the therapist without any agenda sows and supports a frame in which the patient can see himself with the same compassion and kindness and become friends with his own experience. Experiencing the contact with his own experience the individual can reclaim what was always his, by accepting and listening to the long buried, denied, and/or rejected story, of 'owning' and 'living' his experience but at the same time standing out from it and transforming it adaptively.

Therapeutic presence (Geller & Greenberg, 2012) is defined as bringing in our whole self when meeting with the patient, and being fully present at that moment on multiple levels: physical, emotional, cognitive, and spiritual. Presence implies (1) being fully in touch with ourselves at the moment, while we remain (2) open, receptive and immersed in what is emerging at the moment, with (3) an extensive sense of spaciousness and expansion of consciousness and perception. This rooted, immersed, and expanded consciousness is accompanied by (4) the intention of being with and for the patient, at the service of the healing process. The internal status of receptivity implies a full opening to the multidimensional inner world of the patient, including his verbal and body expressions, as well as a full opening to the therapist's own body experience, to that which he is experiencing at the moment, in order to access the knowledge, professional capacities, and the wisdom embodied in it.

D. Siegel (2007/2010) says about presence: "Presence is the bare attention to the wide receptiveness of the mind (Siegel, 2007/2010, . 160 Spanish Ed.)" ...

"it is the state of mind that occurs with all the dimensions of the reflective function; it is the quality of our disposition to receive whatever the other brings, to feel our own involvement in the interaction and to be conscious of our own conscience ... we see ourselves in the eyes of the other, and when this reflex is well attuned, we feel our real us (2007/2010, p. 250 Spanish Ed.)".

In a way similar to the practice of Zen Buddhism, it is only when we empty ourselves of self-concepts, that the crystalline clarity of the nature of the other's being can really be seen. When we empty ourselves of our own concerns, concepts, judgements, and needs, we create an inner, clean space that can be filled and struck by the experience of the other. Presence means leaving aside our own needs, our susceptibility, and our own wounds and being able to touch the pain and the disowned parts of the other. If we are filled with ourselves, there is no space for the other; there is no healing (Hycner & Jacobs, 1995, p. 49). From here we create a space for the divine and spiritual nature to surface (Hycner, 1993).

The therapist who is present and involved perceives the client's experience and resonates with it; this resonance is an unconscious communication between the two of them, which mixed with attunement leads the way to the inquiry process (Bollas, 1987; quoted in Erskine 1999 p. 85).

As therapists, we must prepare our minds to sustain the full experience of the other; this becomes the most important aspect of the therapist's training.

When we wish for the other's experience to change, we usually develop a subtle resistance to what it really is, to what it is right now, to what can be called 'unconditional presence': the ability to find the experience in a complete and direct way, without having it filtered by concepts of what it should be or by an action plan.

The inquiry, the attunement, and the presence are the aspects with which the therapeutic relationship is built; with these three a real and intimate relationship is built, a relationship in which there is support, interest, and care for the other, and a relationship that prepares the framework of the dual attunement principle in Brainspotting.

Principles which need to be present and attuned

1. *Uncertainty.* Being attuned requires the assumption that we do not know anything about the experience of the other. Even when we believe we have shared an experience or have seen it before in someone else, it is always unique and unrepeatable. Each person's experience is intrinsically constituted by the prior experience that the individual has had with the world and his own method of perceiving it, and it is always different from that of any other human being. The therapist must feel comfortable experiencing the uncertainty of not knowing and therefore being open to perceive the unique meaning of the other's experience. On the other hand, assuming the uncertainty not knowing makes it possible to leave the space free and clean from any assumption and any concept about the other, makes it possible for the other's experience to occupy this space which can be defined as it rises and is witnessed both by "the loving observer" of the client and by the present, compassionate therapist, accepting things as they are and as they come. In this experience-awakening process, the own experience can be completed, modified and consolidated in a new adaptive meaning.
2. *Non violence.* It is a principle that completes the previous one. Ron Kurtz elegantly explained the philosophy and principles of no violence in therapy. Everything which is imposed on the client or on his experience and which does not belong to him is violence. Judgements, plans, advice, any kind of exclusions, the arrogance of both therapists and individuals who think they know what is best for the other or what should happen to him, all of these are types of violence and each of them provokes defences in the other person. But including, empowering, and showing respect, enables the others to have the space to do what they want and to be what they want, without the need to change (Kurtz, 1990, page 103 Spanish Ed.).

If the therapist, or someone else, needs to help the client to feel competent, or imposes his idea of what helping means, he blocks the client and his possibility of discovering in his own experience what his pain expresses and what he needs or what is useful for him in order to have a full and happy life.

Ron Kurtz, in his book Body-Centered Psycotherapy (1990), expresses it masterfully:

"If a therapist raises questions in order to obtain more information for himself, interrupting the patient many times, that is violence".

"Violence is being caught up too much in oneself and in the one´s own agenda to really heal the other" (p. 31 of the Spanish edition)

There are two factors that help the therapist be present and attuned with the experience of the client:

a) The therapist must *give up any intention of changing the thoughts, beliefs, feelings, or behaviours of the client.* This implies that the therapist must be in a place of full presence, with interest, curiosity, and empathy to support the client's experience both happening and going deep. The therapist must be patient and impartial in order for the change and the transformation to both emerge and rise from the impulse and 'momentum' of the client. I say to my students "*do not need anything from your clients*" referring to the fact that the therapist must not need for his client to change or be cured; the cure will arrive by itself. Most of our patients and most of us come from parental relationships where their wishes and needs were projected on us, and for survival reasons we had to adapt to them. The therapeutic relationship must be empty of the therapist's wishes.
b) The *attention of the therapist must be completely available* in order to offer responses of optimal attunement. The mind and attention of the therapist must be completely on what is happening right now with his client, and on what is happening between him and the client. This includes what is happening in the therapist himself, as a reaction or response to the client.

Additionally, to create the experience of mutuality, of being together in the task, we need to have some internal basis that supports a mutual, continued connection (Badenoch, 2008):

– The therapist must *make deep compromises in order to enter the internal world of the patient, whatever the pain is.* This will depend on the level of consciousness and healing that the therapist has from his own pain. If the therapist blocks his own pain areas, he will not be able to accompany the those of the patient.

The therapist needs to *feel comfortable in providing comfort to the client.* The support and comforting can be communicated in several ways: in the gaze, the posture, the rhythm of breathing, the moist eyes, the tone of voice, or simply through a deep internal feeling of being, of trusting, and of having hope. The patient his internal child still looks for the source of hope and sustenance in someone external, therefore the therapist must feel comfortable passing through, sometimes, a period of necessary emotional dependence of the internal child of the patient. Deep healing and good therapy must help the patient to locate his centre of identity in a dimension of himself which can be a stable provider of self-support, understanding, welfare, and self-healing. The sense of one's self will no longer depend on how others treat us circumstantially; instead it will be based on a solid internal feeling of value.

A third essential basis is the capacity of the therapist to *follow and accompany the internal movements of the patient.* The therapist must 'listen' not only to what the patient describes in his verbal narrative, but also and mainly to what he describes with his entire body, even more in the subtlest physiological manifestations. This body and its physiological narrative are the ones that tell the story of the pain that was rejected for a long time, that he tried to forget or deny in order to survive, but which fights constantly to emerge to the surface and reveal its truth to someone who will embrace it and validate it. The therapist's mind 'free from itself' prepares a kind of internal sanctuary to receive the painful story of the patient. When the therapist is empty of himself, then images can be created about the internal world of the patient that allow the therapist to prepare responses that fit in attunement with the internal reality of the patient. This promotes the patient's internal experience of being deeply understood, the loosening of the patient's defences, and the emergence of deeper and more vulnerable material, which, when coming to light, can experience the transforming power of being expressed and being gathered.

– Finally, the therapist *must embrace the person of the patient in its totality,* not only his cognitive and emotional aspects, but also his spiritual side and respective concerns. These concerns may or may not be assigned to a particular religion, or they may simply reflect a deep search for a sense and purpose in life.

In the words of David Grand, developer of Brainspotting, the patient is the head of the comet; his brain follows the path that the experience needs to follow in order to to be transformed. The therapist is only the tail of the comet and follows the head wherever it goes (Grand, 2013 p. 59). This analogy tries to express how the therapist must follow the experience of the patient as it is, accompany it, and help the process to be held inside the ' window of tolerance '. If we help the experience to be expressed in a safe framework, it will take a transforming path.

About the relational frame: The healing bubble.

Within the frame of the safe therapeutic relationship a relational framework is created which establishes a supportive environment as Winnicott said (1992). Bion (1962) uses the term "*containment*" to describe how the primary caretaker provides a psychological environment that promotes the self-regulatory capacities of the child. Through 'containment' and 'the supportive environment' a mother can hold her child, both literally and in her mind, in such a way that it shows her recognition of the physiological and affective states and also her capacity to manage them effectively. The same way the therapist offers the necessary control and support for the client to be able to process his intense emotions. The orbitofrontal cortex is responsible for capturing the quality of what is happening in the interpersonal world of the client, and when "reading" the physiological state of calmness and presence of the therapist, it may likewise influence the emotional regulation of the subcortical brain and help with self-regulation.

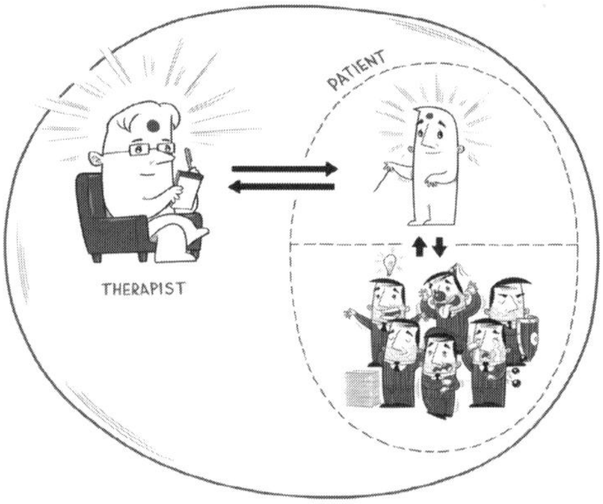

fig. 1

I call this relationship-based frame "the healing bubble" (fig. 1) of the therapeutic space. In this "healing bubble" the patient's subcortical brain no longer needs to stay on top of nor to be in charge of survival, because, since the patient does not perceive the other the therapist as someone potentially dangerous or threatening, he can now simply maintain calmness (social parasympathetic activation in terms of Porges) and the curious and respectful introspective view.

In this healing bubble, the therapist once the attuned relationship and a state of clean presence are established, without agendas or demands supports the relational frame for the client to be able to awaken the capacity for his brain's self-healing to turn on towards itself: to observe the world he experiences or the different parts of his personality. Now the "experiential self" can tell the truth about its story, long retained in the body in its language of sensations, images, emotions, and limiting beliefs. The task of the therapist is to help the client to keep himself in his own loving observer, from which he can receive and embrace his own experience as it is. I call the loving observer the 'Essential Self', as it is the dimension of the self that has always been present in each of us even before having had any experience and has always been there beyond any experience that we have lived through. The Essential Self is immutable; it does not have concepts, and its nature is essentially not judgemental. It is present and compassionate. As long as the therapist stays in his Essential Self, he supports the capacity of the client to remain in his own Essential Self. Now the therapist no longer needs to use inquiry to bring the client back to the interpersonal field. Instead he must promote and invite the client to observe, be present, and to relate with the story that reveals itself from his Essential Self, in order to be able to reappropriate it again and inhabit it in a new and transformed way. This way a new friendly and loving internal attachment of the client to his own experience and/or to different ego states implied in survival, is created and sustained (see chapter of this book focused on the ego states).

The interventions of the therapist in this reprocessing phase must be formulas that help maintain the contact and the internal relationship, without adding anything: *"embrace what these tears express and observe what they say", "invite this sensation to offer you what it has", "focus your attention on this and let's see what it brings to you or where it takes you to", ...*

When the experience can be expressed bottom-up, as it was registered in its own implicit and procedural nature without concepts it manifests itself in its analogical nature, without barriers, as it was once experienced, and reveals the truth that had to be repressed for so long a time. In this process the experience that was disowned, repudiated, refused, and dissociated can reveal itself, develop itself until completion, finish, transform, and consolidate in a new way.

To be with and in connection with our sensations and emotions and 'to listen' to the recorded story in our bodies allows that which had been trapped and encapsulated to now be awakened and start its path towards transformation.

Silence as a support of presence in the healing bubble

Creating a silent space is the necessary complement to sustaining the internal view and the relationship of the Essential Self and the Experiential Ego. Once the therapist has created and formulated the frame, has helped the patient to connect and activate his own experience, and has invited the Essential Self of the patient to emerge, he has to create and support the silence so that the patient's brain may direct its view towards the internal world and use its capacities of regulation and healing. This silence is a structured silence, as it has a task and a direction, and is accompanied by the presence of the therapist. The structured silence is the condition through which the experience reveals itself, expresses what it has experienced in the context in which it was experienced while it is observed and accepted in an intimate and compassionate internal relationship. The structured and effective silence contains an explicit organisation (it is offered at a proper moment), contains an explicit task (it is focused towards something), and includes an invitation both to experiment and to observe some meaningful aspect of the subject that is being treated.

Diana Fosha (2008), mentioning Gendlin, states that by helping our clients to work in silence, we expand their ability to be with their emotions, and to start to trust that "each painful feeling is potential energy towards a more real way of being if we give it room to move towards what is true. It knows the direction ... as surely as you know how to adjust a picture that is crooked ... there is no possibility for you to move it into a mistaken position. There is a sense of what is correct". Processing intense emotions until their completion describes a *'transformation arc'* (Fosha, 2005); this goes from a) the defences against something, and the anxiety and shame about something, the sense of being both creatures and divine beings, towards b) the experience of what is sensed in the body, the subcortical, and up to c) the divine; this is what I call the Essential Self, where through a sense of what is sacred and effective, we become more deeply human and we turn into the best of ourselves.

Active Methods of Attunement and the Therapist's Involvement: The inquiry, the involvement, and the frame.

As stated by Siegel in the previous quote, attunement demands presence but it is also a process of focused attention and clear perception. In other words, for attunement to happen, the listener (therapist, caregiver, friend, ...) must be in a state of presence (be available), but must also initiate actions that convey and confirm that he understands and is involved. In this section I will develop the active processes of attunement: the inquiry (being a detective), the focused observation and the access to the entry doors of the deep experience of the client, the formulation of the frame, the involvement of the therapist, and the attitude of the therapist who is there in presence.

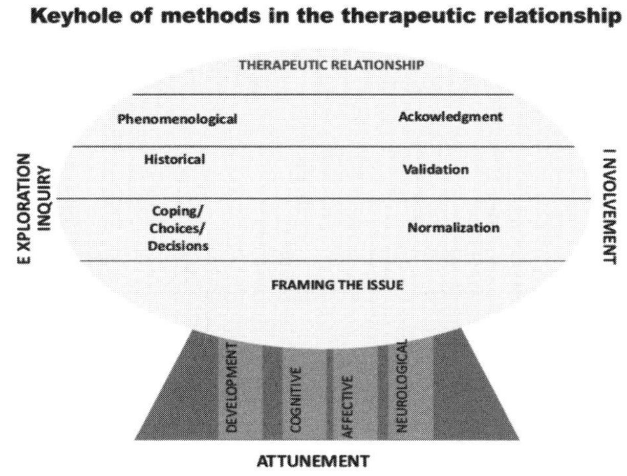

fig 2. Adapted from Erskine et al., 1999

In the chart above we include the active methods based on the inquiry of the experience as well as the interventions based on the way to be oneself and the way to be in the relationship of the therapist (the involvement), and the frame that the therapist formulates and maintains to ease the reprocessing. Attunement and presence must wrap up and back up any of the interventions. Both must take place during all the processes; one supports the other. Whatever the intervention of the therapist is, it cannot be effective if it is not attuned to what the client is living through and does not come from a state of presence.

The therapist as a detective: The Inquiry.

Part of the active work of the therapist is to work out a precise investigation of the experience and difficulties to which the client refers. The therapist "does detective work" to help the client's brain clarify the nature of the difficulty, find its roots and the context in which it was adaptive in order to expand the frame that exposes the organising scheme of the painful and limiting experience.

In hands of the therapist, inquiry is a powerful tool for driving the healing process. It is through respectful inquiry that the therapist helps the client's brain to dig deeply into the nature of the problem, searching for its root, and the impulse towards its resolution. Inquiry motivates the brain to turn towards itself when directed towards the intrapsychic process and to awaken the reflection or the meta-reflection capacity: the brain that observes itself. It is through attuned inquiry in a therapeutic relationship that we help the client's mind adopt a self-study approach. This is a way to awaken the client's state of mindfulness or full presence in his own experience, without judgement, without expectations or suppositions or definitions about the experience. The ultimate goal of inquiry is to help the client to enter into a more intimate and friendly contact with his own experience, and develop a sense of natural curiosity to know and accept himself.

The goal of the inquiry is not to obtain information but to promote thereflection and internal viewing process themselves and in perspective towards the intrapsychic phenomenological-experiential world of the client, as our life system on automatic pilot trains us to work in a usually more reactive way towards the external world, and there is no time for the meta-reflective process. It essentially focuses on the internal meaning of the story more than on the external details. In a focused and consistent way it explores what is beneath the details and beyond the external and the social aspects.

The function of this inquiry must be:

Co-construct the experience of being understood in which we can experience the fact that there is someone present and available who shows interest and genuine curiosity in understanding our subjective experience and who honours the wisdom of our subcortical brain to help us survive. One of the core beliefs of any traumatic experience is "*I'm alone; there is no one there for me. No one understands me*". The fact that now in a new and present relational scheme there is someone who is there for the client, creates a new experience that activates an alternative neuronal network to that of the trauma. Our task is to maintain this experience simultaneously with the other one, so that as Hebb (1949) stated "*neurones that fire together wire together*".

Help the client to enter into a more intimate and deeper contact with his own experience and to find the aspects that limit his current behaviour, that is, being able to access the historical context in which the scheme of the "sensation-emotion-belief-action" was set up in order to survive a painful situation. In this task, the dorsolateral prefrontal cortex (DLPFC) and the hippocampus are involved neurologically to locate the context and the original meaning in which the organising scheme of the experience was established and in which it was conducive for surviving an adverse situation. Being able to access the context also helps to create a distance and a differentiation between present and past. Additionally, knowing that whatever is happening already took place and had come to an end, makes most of the experiences tolerable (van der Kolk, 2015, p. 75). As we know, the nature of traumatic experiences is that they remain registered timelessly and out of context. Therefore helping to find and locate the context where the survival mechanisms were formed is an essential task in order to help create a dual awareness: A self that observes an ego that suffered during the past from the perspective of today.

Support the emotional regulation of the client. Our orbitofrontal cortex, among many other functions, is in charge of what happens in the interpersonal world and is directly involved in emotional regulation. As Schore states (1994), regulation starts being biologically interactive and then becomes biologically autonomous. The therapeutic relationship in attunement and in contact with the experience acts as a frame containing the emotional intensity of the patient's experience, the patient then feeling that he is not alone in the horror. This way he is able to keep his prefrontal cortex active and maintain his self-regulation in order to make an efficient processing of the old experience easier. To associate intense internal sensations with the sense of safety, comfort and one's own domain [that is provided by the present and calm presence of another person] is the basis of self-regulation, self-relaxation, and self-care (van der Kolk, 2015, page 127). As David Grand[1] states, an important part of therapy work is to help the client's brain to go from deregulation to regulation. Attunement promotes the experience of being connected and invites the deregulated brain to enter into attunement with the regulated brain of the therapist. From the perspective of interpersonal neurobiology, when explaining how our social lives contribute to our welfare, it considers neural integration to be the result of having established attuned relationships (Siegel, 2007 p. 55 Spanish Ed.)

Methodology of the inquiry

Asking questions and conducting extensive interventions that stimulate and support this kind of internal search, respecting the intelligence and the courage with which the client has built his defences, is the essence of a good inquiry (Erskine et al. 1999). Effective inquiry helps the person obtain his unique responses by inviting him to look at places and in ways he had never considered (or dared to) by himself. On the other hand, the goal of the inquiry is not for the therapist to obtain a response, but rather it is essentially for the client to find it, reappropriate and inhabit the parts of his experience that he had dissociated, refused, or repudiated. The answer is more for the client than for the therapist, even if the therapist also learns from the responses and helps in organising and working out the frame that the client's brain will use to hold the reprocessing phase.

As the inquiry advances, the therapist increases his level of attunement with the client's process and the client will feel deeply understood by someone who is involved

[1] Workshops of Brainspotting training Phases 1, 2 and 3

and interested. One of the reasons the inquiry itself is part of the healing is that it establishes an authentic relationship between the therapist and the client; this provides the safe context in which the client can discover, know, and heal himself. In fact, the therapeutic relationship can and often should be open to inquiry itself, as this new relationship stimulates the activation of a new neurological network in the client, the one of being accompanied by someone safe, present, and interested. Helping the client compare the new relational scheme, experienced in the relationship with the therapist with the old and traumatic relational scheme, when there was no one present or the one present was the source of threat, is a powerful means for helping to integrate new material in the old schemes (Hebb ′s principle).

In the attuned inquiry, the therapist has no hidden agenda; he is open to what surfaces naturally. Each intervention on the part of the therapist will be based on the response that the client has given to the previous one. This way it is a co-constructed and unpredictable process.

Inquiry (see fig. 2) starts with researching the *phenomenological* experience of the client with respect to the difficulties and circumstances in which he lives. The aims of the inquiry can be not only cognitive aspects (beliefs, fantasies, expectations, hopes, ...), but also emotions and physiological reactions that carry the living story that is being manifested now. It is especially relevant for the therapist to observe and track the physiological experience that is being manifested in the client as it contains the signs of the living history : subtle physical reactions, changes in the colour of the skin, a new pattern of breathing, important postures, ... The therapist must be subtle, kind, and elegant in methods of inquiring. He keeps an open mind without preconceived concepts, pointing out what he observes without attributing meanings or interpretations *("your tightening fist seems to be expressing something", "when you said 'it does not matter' there were tears in your eyes, listen to what they are expressing",* etc.). This way, the therapist simply helps the the client's processes of attention to include in his observation field aspects of the narrative that surface but that are not yet in the area of the conscious listening.

At some point during the research of how the client experiences his own circumstances we can establish a bridge or *connection to the past,* of how, where, and with whom the client started to feel what he is feeling or to forge his painful belief. The appropriate and attuned timing for this may come up at the manifestation of an 'emotional marker' of the traumatic experience; these are 'entry windows' to the 'core material'. These 'emotional markers' can be painful and limiting beliefs (ex. *"my father always told me that I'm not worth anything", "no one ever waited for me", "in my family we never talked",* ...), gestures that are expressed as patterns or habits (a shoulder that lifts itself chronically, a body that submits, a hand that grabs the chair, ...) or spontaneous physiological reactions. All these are windows of entry to the past; they are emotionally active bridges for reaching the founding experiences of the organising scheme, the early scenes that forged the way of feeling and perceiving.

Many *survival mechanisms and decisions taken* to go ahead with life may come to light in the historical inquiry *("I have to be self-sufficient", "it's better not to feel nor need", "I will not trust again", "there is no love for me in the world").* During this inquiry the original context and the extraordinary way in which the child, teenager, or adult of the client had to behave in a painful situation will be manifested. In this process the organising scheme he experienced will be shaped and clarified (belief-emotion-decisions-somatic experience). At the same time, we help the client locate himself in his observing, loving, and comprehensive dimension of how as that child, teenager, or youth he managed to survive.

Presence in action

For its part, presence is manifested actively through three basic interventions:

Acknowledgment. This shows the client that we are aware of his thinking process, his feelings, and needs, that these are seen and we care for them. The therapist becomes present when recognising the experience of the client: "*we are both here, shoulder to shoulder*". The way a therapist shows that he is aware of the client's experiential aspect can be simply pointing out something, such as "*I can see that this hurts you", or "I see your tears";* or other times a comment such as: "*This is sad" or a sympathetic "Wow!"* after something painful (see the transcript of the therapy extract below), or with a non-verbal expression or gesture. This pointing out something only acts as if the client's attention focus needs to be on what has been pointed out. It is a way to increase the client's observation and the client's focus through curiosity.

Validation. It is an essential kind of acknowledgment. It involves acknowledging importance or that the client's experience is something important (Wolf, 1988; Kohut, 1977; in Erskine page 91). It goes beyond looking to unveil the underlying purpose of what is manifested, the reason or the cause behind the behaviour, or the belief that justifies the feelings. Validation tells the client that we take him seriously. It also helps the client to be interested in the reasons and purposes of his experience. It is particularly useful when defences or parts that he is afraid to express, to trust, or to feel are expressed. With validation we explain that there is an adaptive reason *("there is a reason for not feeling, what are you afraid might happen if you feel?"; or "not trusting is a way of pro-*

tecting yourself from other people harming you, what do you consider harmful about the other person?", or in the therapy extract below "*let's see a little more how it is to be in that depression").* With validation we invite the client to focus, give time, and create a space for the experience to be expressed as it is being observed.

Normalisation. The majority of clients come to therapy with a deep feelings of inadequacy and of shame for how they are or how they manage their lives. The goal of normalisation is to counter the feelings of self-denigration and convey to the client that his behaviours and feelings made sense and that they were normal in a context that was abnormal, that that was the intelligent method that the child or vulnerable adult discovered in a painful situation. All clients are normal individuals who had to deal with abnormal difficulties. Sometimes this message can be communicated with psycho-educational information about how the brain responds when faced with threatening situations *("become paralysed and having no words is how our old brain protects us from attracting the attention of those who threatens us and helps us avoid worse harm")* or a "*this was very intelligent for a child only 5 years old*".

With the use of acknowledgment, validation, and normalisation, the therapist actively manifests his presence and involvement and enhances the attunement with the client.

The Frame, "The Lens to Look into the Deep Brain"

An essential role of the therapist to promote a deep healing process is formulating a framework that provides a structure to the brain in which to contain the process. The frame must be formulated based on caring listening to the 'organising schemes' and the 'emotional markers' that the therapist hears in his open and selective listening. To clarify for the reader we will first define the concepts that I am using.

In social theory, the frame is an interpretation scheme, a collection of events and stereotypes that the individuals use to understand and respond to events. In other words, it allows the person to interpret reality and react accordingly; these are therefore psychological structures that allow the subject to give meaning to the world. I accept the proposal of the psychoanalyst José Blegler who defines the frame as a group of signs, which he calls the non-process, and faced with this, co-existing, would be the process, which would be that which is mobile and can be variable. The frame as constant support will operate as a background on which the figure will emerge, that is to say everything that has to do with what is mobile, what is variable, and the process.

Basically, the function of the frame is organising and being at the service of the processing; this function is one of support and containment just as the signs that a mother gives for the growth of her child should be (of care, of protection), which allow the child's self to develop as it is, as the mother shelters and contains, but also sets the boundaries, contains, and limits the intense emotions that could appear during the process. The frame is offered as a framework that provides psychological safety.

The "organisers" constitute underlying schemes that organise (in the sense in which we talk about organisers in embryology) the behaviour of a group. For example, they steer the choices and the decisions. In embryology, an organiser directs development, which stimulates the differentiation of the tissues depending on it. Likewise, a first organiser provides the appropriate conditions for a second organiser to emerge in a tissue that has the potential for it. In the field of psychology René Spitz (1954; 1957) uses the term "organiser" as an analogy to its embryology background and defines it as the result of full integration, that is to say, the formation of a new psychic structure on a more complex level. For example, the patient can organise his experience in particular experiences with a common denominator of impotence, abandonment, distress, ... or organise them around his hope or resources for coming out of a situation, for example a freedom and tranquillity resource. This way these organisers can classify and categorize those experiences that share a similar emotional quality.

I use the term "emotional marker" based on the concept of the somatic marker (Damasio, 1994), which proposes that decision-making is a process guided by emotional signs related to homeostasis, emotions, and feelings. The emotional markers in this model refer to these signs of core material: the phenomenological experience that took place in the previous experiences that lead to the development of the limiting decisions, beliefs, and conclusions, and the associated physical sensations and painful emotions. In the narration of the patient the therapist may hear these markers that that not only determine the patient's way of perceiving but also drive his decisions and actions in dealing with his current situation. We can hear the old story's reminiscences in beliefs such as "*it's useless to cry*", "*no one is present for me*", etc. (which talk about a context in which this was once real and what conclusions the individual has arrived at to deal with that situation). We can also observe gesture patterns (for example covering the legs with the skirt repeatedly as marker of when someone touched the client sexually in the past), behavioural patterns such as isolating himself and not asking. We can observe the markers of physiological reactions that contain the somatic narrative of what has been experienced in the past, or even the language that reveals differentiated parts or ego states (ex. "*a part of me is scared of...*").

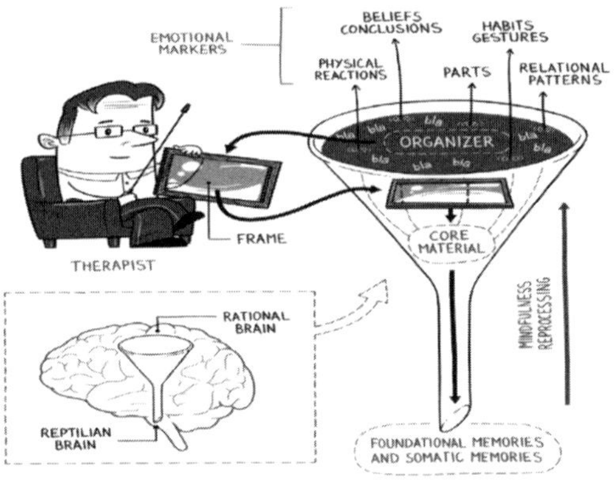

Fig. 3

In the model on fig. 3, the frame refers to how the therapist, at some point in the inquiry process, can detect the organising scheme that constitutes the way of perceiving, thinking, and feeling that the client experiences in his circumstances or current situation. In the therapy extract below, the experience of not having had a mother who was good enough was what brought her actions together to make her determined to 'be a good mother' ("organiser"). In the verbal and nonverbal narrative, the client expresses her way of perceiving and experiencing a problem. This has a lot of nuances and words that describe what she is going through (her *"bla, bla, bla")*. Sometimes the *"bla, bla, bla"* also is a distraction from the most painful material, and in any case, it is the explanation that the conscious mind and the rational brain have given for the problem. The therapist must develop a very open listening behaviour, attentive but selective to detect the 'organisers', or the 'relational schemes' around which the patterns of perception-emotion-somatic experience-behaviour are to be found. These organisers are constituted in the early relational experiences that were sources of pain and/or trauma. At some point in the narrative of the problem, aspects of the old material in the deep and subcortical system of the client (emotional markers) will surface. They will appear among the contents of the narration. These emerging "markers" reveal 'aspects of the core material' and they can act as 'entry windows' to the deep experience. We can listen to conclusions such as the *"no one cares for me ", "there is no room for me"* -in the therapy extract below-, *"it's useless to cry"*, ... The emerging 'markers' that give intensity to the narrative are manifestations of the old story still alive in the subcortical brain and the body of the client. The therapist, by observing and pointing out these emotional markers, helps the client's brain to focus and to look for the context of the early story (therapy extract: *"when I was born, my mother was depressed, stressed, and she had nothing to give")* not yet updated, and access the 'core material' that influences the way of behaving in the current context (the struggle to be a good mother). The therapist when detecting these 'emotional markers' and 'organisers' can offer a 'frame' (therapist: *"it seems that being a good mother is the most important thing in your life")* through which the client can look at a deeper level. Then her brain can place itself in a self-study and compassionate self-observation mode (mindfulness) and hold and focus the internal view of the painful experience in a self-regulation state in which it is possible to reprocess and to heal. The frame acts therefore as the 'eyehole' or 'window' through which the brain of the client can focus and go more deeply (acting as a funnel that reduces its focus to become more and more concentrated) and access the core material, the founding experiences, and the historic context. At the same time it acts as support and containment for the processing, in a way that the person keeps observing (structured silence) what comes from the subcortical and somatic world (bottom-up reprocessing). Now the client can remain in a dual awareness state more easily (the self that observes and the observed ego) in which the subcortical brain and the body tell the truth which was hidden for so long.

In developing an appropriate frame, we make it easy for the brain to reprocess the 'core material' that makes up the experience (limiting conclusions, beliefs, emotions that respond to the frustrated needs, the somatic experience that accompanics it, and the survival decisions). Now the client is capable of accepting and processing the story that his body is telling in the language of his sensations, emotions, images, conclusions, and decisions about the way he survived. This is the process that creates a space for self-healing (that I've called 'the healing bubble'). The space in which the non-digested story awakes and starts to be told in a sequential mode: start, development of the plot, outcome, and resolution. This story goes from the contact and the story of the defences towards accessing and unburdening the painful story of our vulnerable nature and until the story reaches the emergence and experience of our natural qualities such as joy, creativity, love, freedom, spontaneity, courage, … . It is in this telling the buried story and unburdening the client that the transformation process that drives the reprocessing occurs: the story now received and accepted by the dimension of the observing self (Essential Self) that takes ownership and lives its own experience in a new way.

Therapy Extract: The Implementation

Let's listen to a part of therapy with Constanza, who started treatment for her feeling of guilt about "not being the good mother she would like to be". In the time prior to this transcription she exposes her experience of much pain during the birth of her two sons and her subsequent depression.

T: *What was happening in your life or how was your life when your second son was born.* The therapist recognises the pain, but decides to take the client to the context prior to the birth of the second son)

Cl: *Good, it was good. When he was born?*

T: *Yes.*

Cl: *Well I had a very hard post-partum period with the second son. A very hard delivery and post-partum time.*

T: *What made it hard?* (Phenomenological inquiry. The therapist shows interest in knowing more about the experience)

Cl: *A lot of pain. A lot of pain during the delivery. Enduring so much pain for the idea of natural childbirth, of delivering at home. A lot of pain. The first one was also like that.*

T: *The first one was also like that?* (Repeating the question is an elegant way of saying "tell me more about this", without overexerting the interrogation).

Cl: *The first one was a very painful delivery, with enduring very much, that ended in an emergency C-section and after the 2nd one I had a lot of pain, I was worn-out and very physically shattered and with 2 little children. A new-born and another one... I also breastfed both of them, at the same time.*

T: W*ow! And how was it to be so tired, with a lot of pain and having two children that still need you so much?* (Exclamation is a way of attuning and validating the intensity of the experience. After this we continue inviting the client to tell more about the phenomenological experience).

Cl: *Hard, hard because ever since the second one grew up, I have felt like this* (she extends her arms and balances them) *as pulled apart. As ... by each of them ... with really a difficulty in integrating everything. And I still feel like this. I keep feeling that both of them are only reclaiming me for themselves, or something like that, you see?*

T: *As if each of them pulls you from the opposite side.* (This intervention expresses the involvement of the therapist which again gives back acknowledgment and validation of the experience. The intervention condenses the experience "I see how hard this is and there is something important in your experience")

Cl: *Helpless, not being able to provide them with what they want, what they need.*

T: *And I have the feeling that this touches a matter that is very important to you.* (The therapist takes advantage of something that had come up at the beginning of the session, the client's worry about being a good mother. This intervention tries to focus on the frame about how important it is to be a good mother and the helplessness as 'organisers' of the experience. At the same time, this way of asking does not suggest any content; it only emphasises the importance of 'being a good mother' as the 'organiser scheme of the experience see fig. 2. The seed of focusing 'on being a good mother' as the founding root experience is planted).

Cl: *Yes.* (The "yes" from the client confirms the fact that the intervention of the therapist is an appropriate frame).

T: *Wanting to be... I heard you suffered to have two natural deliveries and I understand this as the desire to be the best mother and to give them the best possible experience.* (Here the therapist again acknowledges and validates the effort and suffering of having a natural delivery as the desire for 'being a good mother'; it is a confirmation. 'To be the best mother' establishes a *frame* to focus more on the search. Interventions tighten the funnel of the experience to help deepen and refine the focus)

Cl: (She nods her head)

T: *Therefore your frustration arises at least from that time. Wanting to give them that experience, different and natural, that you finally could not.* (Attunement here is expressed in the acknowledgment – "I see it" and the validation –"I see that it is important" of the effort as the attempt to be a good mother; at the same time the seed of maybe this attempt comes from some time ago -*"arises at least from that time"*- is planted; the emotional bridge to the old experience is stimulated – the client can float back).

Cl: *Yes, now I don't feel so much like that anymore. It is as if I have been able to think it over and not blame myself, at least a little bit. But yes there was something about Why can't I?*

T: *And what was your answer to that question?* (The therapist in this intervention drives at being conscious about the survival conclusions and decisions adopted by the client).

Cl: *I had no answer* (she starts to cry). (The emotion is itself the answer)

T: *We have to stop with this issue because now I can see your suffering.* (This intervention contains acknowledgment "I see your pain" and validation "and it is important". The therapist with this intervention proposes giving time, focus, and deeper listening to the story the tears express; the funnel is tightened -fig. 2).

Cu: *Yes, when he was born I didn't feel good. I felt depressed for a while, I learnt what a post-partum depression is- I did not feel depressed for a long time, but yes at the beginning yes until my physical pain ended. But then, the intensity of the experience with the two little ones has been very stressful and it still is. And in part I still feel that I am depressed because of that.* (This answer reveals that the offered frame of "being a good mother" has had a high and personal price for the client).

T: *Let's look at it...* (With this expression you communicate 'there is something of great importance in this, let's stay here and give it some time. It is a way of inviting the client to tighten the focus, close the funnel)

Cu: (She cries. Signal that the therapist's intervention is effective)

T: *It's good that you show your emotions, you do not need to suppress them. Let's listen to them where they need to be listened to.* (Once again the therapist validates the emotions manifesting implicitly that they are important and that they have a story to tell, while he/she manifests his/her attitude of being present and interested and welcomes the observer of the client).

Cu: (She cries)

T: *Let's have a look at what happens to you when you have that depression. How is it to be in this depression?* (This validation gives space to focusing more on the experience of being depressed and to tightening the framework of the experience by putting our view lower in the funnel to access the core material -fig. 3).

Cl: *Well, fatigue, and like it's impossible to take care of myself. There is no room for me. (Here the oldest root of the organiser schema is revealed: "there is no room for me";* the client is reaching the *core material.* This painful belief is a survival conclusion and an 'entry window' to the deepest and oldest experience)

T: *Listen to that conclusion: 'There is no room for me'. Hang on to it and listen to what else it contains...* (Now inquiry is used as a marker to make client able to look at the entire importance of this old conclusion in a more focused way: part of the *core material.* Observe that in the formulas used by the therapist, he repeatedly addresses both the observing self and the ego to keep the experience "listen to that conclusion". Let's have a look at where the marker and the offered framework take us).

Cl: *There is no room for me. For my needs, for some of my needs.*

T: *It sounds like a very old conclusion in your life: 'there is no room for me'. Because others occupy that space. When you resonate with that emotion I feel that you are connected to even deeper emotions.* (Now the inquiry tries to jump from the most current phenomenological experiences to *the historical root, the founding memories* that made up the organising scheme of the experience. In terms of attunement it is the right time to create the emotional bridge to the past; here we have an 'entrance window' to an old story. It is the right time as until now the client had expressed her current experience).

Cl: *Yes, yes... well, I go to my childhood and to the parallels with my mother's experience when I was born. She was depressed, stressed, and had nothing to give.* (Inquiry is successful and the client enters in her early founding experience)

T: *Wow! Nothing to give!* (This indication and validation communicate the importance of the pain for the child)

Cl: *Not much, not much.*

From here, the client accesses the childhood memory of her mother also being very depressed when she was born, and how she had to develop a hardness defence of "living with very little". In the extract we can see how the interventions of the therapist are directed towards the client's entering into a deeper contact with her own experience, so that she can know it, express it, and invite deeper emotions to tell the story that was encapsulated. All the interventions aim towards directing the research to its internal process. During the process, the therapist invites the client to stay on her intense emotions so that they can express part of the story they have. We can also observe how each intervention of the therapist is based on the response that the client just gave. This is the way to keep attuned, no new paths are opened but we just invite the client to deepen her search and to enter in contact with what was silenced. The involvement of the therapist is constantly shown through the genuine interest – manifesting both the exclamations that show the importance of something – as well as the interventions of validation and acknowledgment.

In this extract, we see how the inquiry has gone from exploration and consciousness about the psychological phenomena (sensations, emotions, cognitions) experienced in the current context, which are manifesting during the session and are connected with the experience of trying to be 'a good mother' and 'the helplessness' (organisers), until reaching the historical context, where the client relived the neglect from her own mother because she also was depressed (founding memory or root). Also, during the research process, the survival decisions are explained: "*there is no room for my needs; there is nothing to give*" (and further on "I have to be tough, so that I don't need"); this is the *core material* that needs to be reprocessed now. We see how as long as the therapist is present and involved, he can prepare his interventions in accordance with the material that has awakened; he only waits for it and accepts it in attunement. During the inquiry, also the capacity of the client to be present in her own experience is trained self-study mode , of observing the experiences, knowing them, accepting them … . Interpersonal contact is the bridge to internal contact (Orange, Atwood & Stolorow, 1997; Bollas, 1979; mentioned in Erskine, 1999), gradually in this way building an internal bond between the observing self of the patient and its experiential ego.

During this session time, the organiser scheme of the experience 'being a good mother' has been manifested (fig. 3). The founding experience "*as a newly born child who had no available or nurturing mother*" made up the organiser scheme of how to perceive and sense the mother-son relationship that then created her determination to 'being a good mother'. With all this we have an optimal frame and the necessary activation to move on to the reprocessing phase with Brainspotting and to promote a transforming healing. Now the client has discovered the original context from which her experience comes, and she has developed an observing attitude that will help the reprocessing in mindfulness supported by the neurological attunement of the relevant eye position and the 'brainspot' and a consolidated relational attunement.

Bibliography

Badenoch, B. (2008). Being a Brain-Wise Therapist. A Practical Guide to Interpersonal Neurobiology. W. W. Norton & Company: New York.

Bleger, J.. Psicoanálisis del encuadre psicoanalítico. In: Bleger,José. Simbiosis y ambigüedad: estudio psicoanalítico. Buenos Aires: Paidós, 1967. p.237-50. (Biblioteca de Psiquiatría, Psicopatología y Psicosomática, 42). Lo: B615s, 1967

Damasio, A. R. (2004). *El error de Descartes.* Barcelona: Crítica. (Orig. 1994).

Erskine, R.G., Moursund, J.P., & Trautmann, R.L. (1999). *Beyond Empathy: A Therapy of Contact in Relationship.* Brunner/Mazel, Philadelphia, PA.

Geller, S.M. & Greenberg, L.S. (2012). *Therapeutic Presence. A Mindful Approach To Effective Therapy.* Published by American Psychological Association: Washington.

Grand. D. (2013). Brainspotting: The Revolutionary New Therapy for Rapid and Effective Change.

Hebb, D.O. (1949). T*he Organization of Behavior*. Wiley, ed., New York.

Hutterer, J. & Liss, M. (2006). Cognitive Develpment, Memory, Trauma, Treatment: An Integration of Psychoanalytic and Behavioral Concepts in Light of Current Neuroscience Research. *Journal of the American Academy of Psychoanalysis and Dynamic Psychiatric Annals,* 374, 236-241.

Kurtz, R. (1990). *Body-Centered Psychotherapy: The Hakomi Method.* Mendicino: LifeRhythm.

Lambert, M.J. & Barley, D.E. (2002). *Research Summary on the Therapeutic Relationship and Psychotherapy Outcome.* In J.C. Norcross (Ed.), Psychotherapy Relationships That Work: Therapist Contributions and Responsiveness to Patients (pp.17-32). New York, NY: Oxford University Press.

Lambert, M.J. & Simon, W. (2008). The Therapeutic Relationship: Central and Essentials in Psychotherapy Outcome. In S.F. Hick & T. Bien (Eds.), *Mindfulness and Therapeutic Relationship* (pp. 19-33). New York, NY: Guilford Press.

Siegel, D. J. (2007). The Mindful Brain. Norton & Company. New York. London.

Siegel, D. J. (2010). The Mindful Therapist: A Clinician's Guide to Mindsight and Neural Integration (Norton Series on Interpersonal Neurobiology). WW Norton & Company

Spitz, R.A. (1957). No y sí: sobre la génesis de comunicación humana. Nueva York: Prensa de Universidades Internacional.

Stern, D. N. (1985). *The Interpersonal World of the Infant: A View from Psychoanalysis and Developmental Psychology*. Karnac Books

Van der Kolk (2014). *The Body Keeps the Score: Brain, Mind and Body in the Healing of Trauma.* Viking Penguin.

Brainspotting and Grounding

Cynthia Schwartzberg

> *"In a totally healthy organism, energy flowing into and out of the person could move freely as circumstances permit, in something of the way that a rose gives off perfume and takes in sunlight throughout its petals."*
> John Pierrakos (1987)

We Are Energy Beings

We, as human beings, are made of energy and have electrical currents flowing throughout our brains, hearts, and entire body. Our brain fires enough electricity to light up a 15- to 20-watt bulb. Our heart generates 40 to 60 times more amps than our brain. When our body is sufficiently charged, we're grounded.

When the energy breaches the point of containment in a safe way, we become flooded with feelings and sensations that are overwhelming – within ourselves as well as within relationships. The currents between human beings are strong and influence our state of being. For example, some people come away from interactions with others feeling drained or confused, whereas others feel charged up and happy.

The electrical current in the body pulsates among states of charge, discharge, and containment. It's much like the breath – we breathe in and our lungs expand, we breathe out and our lungs contract, and there's a pause between the inhalation and the exhalation called stasis.

This cycle mimics the ebb and flow of life, which shows up in multiple situations including in the flow of a treatment session and overall treatment plan. There are times in which the work has more charge and times when there's more discharge or containment. Said another way, there are times when we feel a sense of expansion, contraction, or a state of stasis. When things are in harmony, there's a healthy relationship between all three states. There's a balance all the way to the cellular level that allows for any number of actions to take place.

This process is primarily subcortical, and yet, we often get caught up in our emotional reaction to the outcome. Let's say we have an inspiration to move our hand. A series of electrical impulses is required for that movement to take place. With sufficient electrical charge, the action is accomplished. If the charge is insufficient, the movement may begin but isn't completed. If there's too much charge, the movement doesn't go according to plan.

Our brain and body are involved in a constant flow between our internal and external environment. Our senses experience the environment, our nerves send signals to our brain, and our brain interprets the experience – all in a nanosecond. This ebb and flow supports our life and interactions. If we find ourselves so out of balance that we can't get back to homeostasis, we often reach out for help. We need support to ground.

The Importance of Grounding

Grounding is a state of being present in the here and now. When we're grounded, we can better tolerate the ups and downs resulting from our emotions and experiences. We have a sense of our body in the present moment. We're neither too tense nor too relaxed. We're neither hovering above the ground nor collapsed into it. Grounding is a healthy tension of presence and vitality. We can feel our backbone, our heartbeat, and our breath. We feel our connection to the earth. We're in relationship with gravity. When we're grounded, we're connected to our birthright of existing and possessing a sense of purpose.

"Grounding is concerned with what happens when energy flows out towards the surface of the body and the quality of contact it finds there" (Boadella, 1978). Because various forms of grounding have gone wrong for so many people, therapeutic work involves re-contacting the ground (Nabb, 1999).

Our feet, hands, eyes, and skin are key points for feeling grounded. When we're ungrounded, we tend to be less aware of these points in relation to our environment. We can feel floaty, awkward, disconnected, out of sorts, or absent-minded. When we're ungrounded, we may slip more into fantasy regarding our self, our life, our past associations, and the people around us. We tend to overthink and to lose touch with our feelings. Our sense of self and our relationships is different when we're centered. The difference is profound.

Grounding helps us find balance in the very pulse of our being, in the increases and decreases of electrical currents. This rhythm of expansion, contraction, and pause provides a tangible way for us to stay within our window of tolerance. Every movement has a cycle. The pulse of life moves through every fiber of our being.

One of the aspects of grounding is the principle of balancing the charge, discharge, and containment of current in our bodies. The sole goal of grounding is to help our clients go from dysregulation to regulation. Grounding is immensely helpful in trauma therapy, because it feels empowering instead of re-traumatizing.

Brainspotting as a Grounding Process

Brainspotting (BSP) is a grounding process. All its components support going from dysregulation to regulation in a contained process attuned to the innate wisdom of the body to heal itself. Brainspotting goes beyond grounding because it helps clients locate, focus, and process unprocessed traumatic experience in the subcortex. When an individual has long-standing chronic stress or has experienced trauma, their body is flooded with cortisol and adrenalin. The individual no longer integrates and processes implicit memory. Implicit memory stays frozen in time. To unlock this memory and allow the individual to heal, we need to work with both the body and the brain.

Let's look at the various components of Brainspotting, how they support and enhance grounding for the client and therapist, and how grounding is used before, during, and after a session.

Phenomenology as it Applies to Brainspotting

The original Brainspotting-derivative definition of phenomenology can be summed up as "open observation without forming assumptions." This has since developed into the Uncertainty Principle.

The Uncertainty Principle

The uncertainty principle refers to the process of a standard in which it's impossible to gauge correctly both the placement and the momentum of a particle at a particular point in time. It stems from the fact that the act of gauging will itself impede upon the system being gauged in unpredictable ways (https://psychologydictionary.org/uncertainty-principle/). In other words, the uncertainty principle, in a therapy venue, means we can't gauge what's correct for a client based on the direction the work is going or what we may know from their past. Neither can we gauge the client based on our professional studies. We can't truly know what's right for the person sitting in front of us.

This may sound ungrounding; yet you, as the clinician, can't know what's really happening in another person's mind. You may have theories and ideas, but whenever you start to entertain those thoughts during a session, your focus is taken away from the client. You're rushing ahead and losing the ground of discovery in the moment. We'll examine how to reconnect to your grounding when this occurs. A client's process is unpredictable and, to be fully grounded, we need to stay in the present. What better way to do this than to be there without assumptions or references that relate to something that isn't happening?

"No Assumptions" Model

As stated above, when we make assumptions about another, we become ungrounded. We shift our attention from the present moment to our thoughts and are no longer focusing on what's happening in front of us. When we think we know what's right for our client or feel the impulse to give them advice, we're ungrounded. It's our role, as clinicians, to become aware of how and when we do this so we can reground ourselves. (See below for ways to reconnect during sessions.)

If I sit with a client and trust they're doing exactly what they need to do, I witness them with deep attunement. I track their movements and respond to them. If I embrace uncertainty and don't have assumptions, it's much easier to track the individual and stay present to whatever is emerging in the process. I may not know the details, the story, or the people involved, but I'm aware that something is occurring and their reflexive movement is signaling to me this possibility.

"Lyons-Ruth (2000) discusses affective exchanges as "implicit relational knowledge" within the therapeutic relationship. She observes that most relational transactions rely on these non-verbal cues. Scaer (2005) describes these implicit communication patterns within the therapist-client relationship when he states: "Many features of social interaction are nonverbal consisting of subtle variations of facial expression that set the tone for the content of the interaction. Body postures and movement patterns of the therapist ... Tone and volume of voice, patterns and speed of verbal communication, and eye contact also contain elements of subliminal communication and contribute to the unconscious establishment of a safe, healing environment" (pp. 167–168)

And it is in these non-verbal communications that our clients are attuned to us as we are to them. These right brain/mind/body nonverbal communications go both ways, The therapists' non-verbal movements are unconsciously experienced and registered by the client, as the therapist continues to track the clients movements without assumptions. The regulation of the therapists within themselves enhances and supports the client's regulation.

These biological communications are the regulation of right brain/mind/body states. Shaw (2004): discusses: Psychotherapy is an inherently embodied process ... we need to take our bodily reactions much more seriously than we have so far because ... the body is "the very basis of human subjectivity" (p. 271).

Every moment of our life, the cells of our bodies are working to bring us to a state of equilibrium. Our cells can heal themselves and repair damage (http://tummy-calm.com/self-healing.html). The body is constantly scanning itself to activate this healing and repair cycle. The BSP process helps turn the scanner on our self through awareness and curiosity. We do this deliberately when we ask the clients where they feel activated or most grounded in their bodies.

I remember a time when I was sitting with a client who was working on issues around money, and she started to speak about the loss of her brother. My mind immediately jumped ahead in thought. In BSP, we'd say I fell out of the tail of the comet. Having my internal scanner on, I redirected my thoughts back to the present, increased my attention to the client by consciously gazing at her, and listened more deeply to her process even in the silence. My presence to the unknown gave support to her as she spoke of how things had shifted since the loss of her brother and her family's perspective on that loss. Staying present as she worked toward her discovery, I witnessed her take a deep breath and report that something had just shifted. Neither one of us needed to know *what* had shifted only *that* it shifted. Her work continued, and she felt freer and lighter around her tight beliefs in relation to money.

Assumption is defined as: A thing that's accepted as true or as certain to happen, without proof (https://www.google.com/search?q=assumption+definition&ie=utf-8&oe=utf-8&client=firefox-b-1-ab). Think about that for a moment and how it applies to a session. If my perception is based on an interpretation of the person before me, I'm influencing the outcome. The Rosenthal-Jacobson study addresses this. This study supports the hypothesis that reality can be positively or negatively influenced by the expectations of others, which is called the observer-expectancy effect. Rosenthal argued that biased expectancies could affect reality and create self-fulfilling prophecies. (https://en.wikipedia.org/wiki/Pygmalion_effect).

Understanding how we influence outcomes emphasizes to me the value and importance of my awareness and turning my inner scanner/supervisor onto myself, as well, during a session. I ask myself what consciousness I'm bringing to the session, how can I support myself in staying grounded, and how am I perceiving my client.

This leads us to another phenomenon of BSP: *I don't know what it is, but I know that it is.* (Grand, Brainspotting Phase 1 training slide). I may not be able to know what's going on inside a client, as in the above example, but I do know that something is, and I trust that knowing. I also know the body has an amazing capacity to heal itself, and I trust in that. Sitting and trusting our client's process is extremely grounding.

Dan Siegel, MD, a clinical professor of psychiatry at the UCLA School of Medicine and Executive Director of the Mindsight Institute states, "We are hard-wired to perceive the mind of another being." He speaks about the importance of understanding mirror neurons and attunement: "When we attune with others, we allow our own internal state to shift, to come to resonate with the inner world of another. This resonance is at the heart of the important sense of 'feeling felt' that emerges in close relationships. Children need attunement to feel secure and to develop well, and throughout our lives we need attunement to feel close and connected" (http://cultureofempathy.com/References/Experts/Daniel-Siegel.htm). Bringing this understanding into the session room, I realize that how I connect directly impacts the healing of my client.

Case Study in Brainspotting and Grounding

Brainspotting is based on the attuned presence of the therapist in relation to the client. When I think something isn't working, I go back to the relationship. How can I strengthen my attunement to my client? What am I missing? What are they really telling me? What's my agenda? Am I assessing the therapy through a lens of expectations? How are my blind spots limiting the work?

An example of this is a young man whom I saw for anxiety and depression. He was unable to work and had become extremely disorganized. Another therapist, whom he saw for healing work, referred him. The other therapist ended the work, sensing there hadn't been enough movement. It wasn't long before I began to question my work with this client as well and why there was so little movement. I found myself thinking, "This is the worst work I've ever done."

I gather that while you're reading this, you've figured out I became quite ungrounded. I got focused on what was wrong and on the experience of the other therapist. I also got caught up with how to give the client what he wanted. He wanted me to take his pain away. That wasn't possible for me to do, and no technique was working. Has this ever happened to you?

We all have those clients who shake us to our own core wounding. I think of them as my Buddhas from whom I learn and grow. With some deep soul-searching, some self-spotting and supervision, I shifted my approach with this client. I deepened my trust in the process. I deepened my trust in him and let go of teamwork with the other therapist. During the teamwork process, I noticed old patterns of mine were playing out, and I lost the connection with the client. I share this because I believe we all come across situations that test us, and the way to ground in-session includes doing our work outside of session.

I looked closer at other things as well including, what's movement? The deeper question seemed to be, what defines movement? The client felt he was gaining a lot from being with me. I heard this differently as I got more grounded in the work. I took his statement as my clue to realize the value he placed on the relationship and how to harness that in the work.

I started to work differently. In BSP Phase One training, when nothing is working, we turn to the Brainspotting Resource Model. The client wasn't able to find a spot that was calming enough to pair it with an eye position, so we took a different approach to the work. I put emphasis on the attunement that Dan Siegel described above and also on the Rosenthal-Jacobson study, which meant I supported his strengths and emphasized how much I valued him. In my presence and reflections, I focused on intentionally believing in him. Slowly, we worked with a gaze spot for short durations of time. This seemed to correspond to the work we'd been doing on his different self-parts and other relationships.

Another point I want to address in this case regarding grounding and BSP is the use of techniques. We typically wait before we use an intervention and, with grounding, we also want to wait and see what's needed and what the clients are able to calibrate on their own. Is the person inside *the window of tolerance* and, if not, how do we assess whether to offer an intervention and/or wait for the innate wisdom of their body to shift?

As we spoke of earlier, there's a rhythm to each session, and there's a rhythm to interventions. The skilled clinician tracks their client's movement and behavior to know when to intervene and when to wait. Again, we need to ask, Is this technique for me or the client? David Grand, PhD, often says, "When I think I need to do something, I wait, and when I think I really need to, I wait some more." Why? Because we don't want to interrupt the client's natural self-regulation. Sometimes these interruptions can be wounding.

Think about the development of self-regulation in humans and how it gets interrupted. A newborn needs to learn to self-regulate. It needs to discover its natural rhythm and cycles, its life pulse. Supporting this process is "not always easy, however. It requires the ability to read and understand the baby's needs and the knowledge, energy, and resources to respond in ways that are helpful. Providing the experiences that allow children to take over and self-regulate in one aspect of their lives after another is a very general description of the job of parents, teachers, and protectors of children that extends throughout early childhood and into the adolescent years. The first step in the earliest days of children's lives is to establish regulatory connections with them and then gradually shift the responsibility of regulation over to them in the day-to-day domains of sleeping, waking, and soothing" (https://www.ncbi.nlm.nih.gov/books/NBK225568/).

Many of our clients come to us due to dysregulation and having had poor support to help them learn their internal processes of regulation. No matter what the technique is and for whom it may have worked in the past, this doesn't mean it will work for the client sitting in front of you.

As Dr. Grand states, "A resource is only a resource if it works as a resource." Regarding grounding as a technique it works optimally when the granular isocortex (prefrontal cortex) is bypassed and the agranular isocortex (vmPFC, OFC, and the ACG) and allocortex (specifically the insula and hippocampus) are engaged. Accordingly the agranular isocortex and allocortex are directly involved in subcortical and somatic regulation, whereas the granular isocortex is not. Thus, the concepts and practices of grounding need to be aligned with access to the agranular isocortex and allocortex for them to be maximally effective (del Monte, D., 2016, 2017).

And, as with the case study just mentioned, there's much more needed than matching a grounded body position with an eye position and using a technique. With that client, the entire work shifted to framing the relationship and the grounding moments in the relationship.

Clients like this young man remind me of the grace of BSP. It's in the space beyond technique that we find the essence of grounding: presence and mindfulness.

Let's now turn to key components of the BSP session, starting with the frame.

Key Components of the Brainspotting Process

The Frame

BSP uses the concept of the dual attunement frame. We frame the work relationally and neurobiologically. When we add in grounding, we're providing the dysregulated client with a frame for regulating neurobiolgically and experientially. In essence, grounding during a session is a grounding frame within the dual attunement frame.

Dr. Grand has shared how he did this with a survivor of the Orlando shootings. The man had worked previously with a Brainspotting therapist and felt hesitant to return to BSP. There was a diagnostic question of whether the shooting became a re-traumatization of more complex PTSD issues and how this client could be helped in 90 minutes. David began the session by asking the man where he felt most grounded in his body. The client responded that he felt most grounded in his feet on the floor, his hands gripping the chair, and the biolateral sounds. Once they decided on a gaze spot, he reported feeling overwhelmed. David told the patient he was going to count to five and, at five, the man was to return his focus to the grounding spot of being in the chair with his hands gripping the arms and his feet on the ground.

The man went through different aspects of the shooting as he focused on his gaze spot, and David counted out loud to five or 10 (but never more than 10 seconds). He continued to check the client's SUDS throughout the process. At the end of each count, the man returned his awareness to the grounding spots. As the process moved on, at one point the man noted that he was looking at a tambourine. David asked him to describe it. As the client processed different aspects of the shooting while focusing on the gaze spot, David continued counting and checking the SUDS. David chopped the process into five- and 10-second increments and used the SUDS. At the end of each count, he instructed the client to leave his thoughts on the gaze spot and return his awareness to grounding in the chair.

I've done this with clients. I use the clock and say, "Go with that for 30 seconds. I'll let you know when 30 seconds is up." Watching the time or counting both contain grounding elements. In the face of trauma, there's unpredictability. Counting or clock-watching and calling off time offers predictability in the face of the trauma. It's in the here and now, concrete, reliable, and within the relationship. The therapist becomes someone the client can depend on to help bring a stop to the emotional turmoil. In addition, "researchers have identified populations of neurons that code time with extreme precision in the primate brain. These neurons are found in two interconnected brain regions, the prefrontal cortex and the striatum, both of which are known to play critical roles in learning, movement, and thought control" (https://www.sciencedaily.com/releases/2009/10/091019162921.htm).

Another aspect of counting is the client hears something other than the sounds of the trauma. The sound of the therapist's voice can be highly grounding when we're mindful of our intonation. Dr. Porges says we need what he calls "the social engagement system ... in which we listen to intonation in voice and use facial engagement. When a person has vocal intonation, an expressive face, and eyes open when we talk to them, this expressive individual is also contracting middle ear muscles that facilitate the extraction of human voice from background sounds" (http://attachmentdisorderhealing.com/porges-polyvagal3/).

For this client, the background noise of the biolateral sound and counting added to the grounding of the present versus him becoming overwhelmed by sounds of the traumatic event – gunfire.

Framing a session on the client's sense of feeling disconnected and using the dual attunement frame to integrate grounding is demonstrated in another clinical example. This client described feeling outside herself when with others. We spoke of disconnection and anxiety and framed the process on her sense of separation. I had her look at my hands and asked, "If this hand is you (indicating my right hand), are you saying that with others you feel here?" I moved my right hand far away from the left. She said yes, and we processed from there. It was a double spotting: Looking at one hand, the other, and the space in between and noticing what happens. Toward the end of the session, I slowly moved my hands closer together. She started to feel calmer and more connected. She spontaneously and with great surprise stated, "I feel grounded!" After the session, she reported using this technique on a regular basis with her own hands to help her reconnect.

BioLateral Sound

"Blowing of the wind, sea waves, birds singing are more than audible sounds; they have the ability to interact with the emotions and mood of a human being and create feelings. Music is the human effort to express emotions. It has the ability to influence mood, to remind us of a certain moment, to create feelings. Music contributes to communication and conveys information with semantic and emotional elements. These elements indicate the involvement of the central nervous system through processes of integration and interpretation together with the peripheral auditory processing" (https://www.ncbi.nlm.nih.gov/pmc/articles/PMC400748/).

Psychoacoustics and psychophysics research informs us that music lights up all areas of the brain. One key area we look at in Brainspotting is the superior colliculus. It's here where we get support for the importance of integrating sensory information including auditory information. Biolateral music taps into the primitive structures of our brain that are related to motivation, reward, and emotion. These structures are also involved with self-regulation, which "consists of several stages, and individuals must function as contributors to their own motivation, behavior, and development within a network of reciprocally interacting influences" (https://en.wikipedia.org/wiki/Self-regulation_theory).

Music crosses the barrier between the right and left hemispheres of the brain, thus supporting the integration of the two. Including sound in the clinical set-up is highly grounding, as we saw in the case discussed above.

I want to return to the emphasis on BSP as a grounding process as we continue to go through its different components. In all these components, we're working subcortically as we integrate the different senses. Above, we spoke about the sense of hearing. We'll now move to vision and then to the sense of touch. All three are located in the superior colliculus and are key in self-regulation.

Focused Mindfulness

Brainspotting is based on the premise that "where you look affects how you feel." We harness this in the work and use it for locating relevant eye positions that are then used for mindful focusing. Let's break down the parts of focused mindfulness, as there are many grounding components built into this piece of the session. We'll look at both the mindfulness and the process of vision.

We'll begin by focusing on the eyes and how central they are for grounding and attachment. When we find a relevant eye position that matches with a reflex, a felt sense, or intuitive gazing, the focused visual containment obtains access to the visual layer in the superior colliculus – which, we believe, is a form of visual grounding as defined by the aspects of attunement and maintaining focus.

The eyes contain 200 million working parts and have the most quickly responsive muscles in the body. They help us orient in our environment and connect to our brain to allow us to determine what we're looking at. In this sense, we see with our brain *and* our eyes. Signals sent from our eyes are processed deep in our brain. The brain then reflexively and intuitively redirects where we look. "Eyes are one of the first organs to develop in utero at five weeks. The embryo's growth takes place from the head down, and, at this time, the head is grotesquely large compared to the rest of the body. Only much later does the body catch up. ... Optical stimulation, more than other senses, produces changes in electroencephalographic rhythms" (https://books.google.com/books?id=XEzJAwAAQBAJ&pg=PA34&lpg=PA34&dq=gazing+in+mother%27s+eyes&source=bl&ots=89Bks6i-bA&sig=wh37tVvyRTScVMEBey5m_hRUAZo&hl=en&sa=X&ved=0ahUKEwi5ydzAyLDYAhWkzIMKHX5KDQEQ6AEIXzAM#v=onepage&q=gazing%20in%20mother's%20eyes&f=false).

Relevant eye positions are then harnessed for processing. Having a specific point of focus supports grounding because it stabilizes our attention. According to *Hatha Yoga Pradipika* (a classic Sanskrit manual on hatha yoga), "Trataka (gazing at an object during meditation) eradicates all eye diseases, fatigue, and sloth, and closes the doorway creating these problems." In addition to improving concentration and memory, trataka cleanses both the eyes and the cerebral cortex, balances the nervous system, and relieves depression, anxiety, and insomnia. Another yogic text, the *Gheranda Samhita,* states that this practice cultivates clairvoyance and inner vision (https://yogainternational.com/article/view/candlelight-insight-trataka).

Think about the process of bonding or attachment in human beings. As an infant and caregiver gaze into one another's eyes, a strong attachment is formed. "Researchers found that infants' brainwaves were more synchronized to the adult's when the adult's gaze met theirs and the babies also made more vocalizations when in snyc" (http://www.telegraph.co.uk/science/2017/11/29/mothers-babies-brainwaves-snychronise-gaze-scientists-find/). From the moment of birth, the infant begins searching for its mother's gaze. It's as if we're hard-wired by evolution to seek out our mother's eyes. As stated in Mary Ayers' book: *Mother-Infant Attachment and Psychoanalysis: The Eyes of Shame,* "Finding her [the mother's] eyes gazing back is the infant's primordial desire ... Eye-to-eye contact is reciprocal ... and unlike the other tasks of raising a baby and senses involved, is a part of every phase of interaction. Touch, holding, breastfeeding, all engage the eyes" (https://books.google.com/books?id=XEzJAwAAQBAJ&pg= PA 34&lpg=PA34&dq=gazing+in+mother%27s+eyes&source=bl&ots=89Bks6i-bA&sig= wh37tVvyRTScVMEBey5m_hRUAZo&hl=en&sa=X&ved=0ahUKEwi5ydzAyLDYAhWkzIMKHX5KDQEQ6AEIXzAM#v=onepage&q=gazing%20in%20mother's%20eyes&f=false).

Referring to our earlier discussion on rhythm and pulsation, the eyes and attachment are integral parts of grounding that help the individual develop an internal rhythm. They're also part of the dual attunement process. Our clients are very aware of us looking at them and supporting the internal movement of their neurobiology. As we witness them, they feel held and supported.

This became clear to me one day while working with a client. At the end of the session, the client reported, "I was watching you watch me." Here was a client struggling with his sense of self, trusting himself, and grounding in life. He was often observant of my actions and would remark on my state of being. Whether it was a projection or not, what I got from this was how important my attunement to a client's neurobiology is for healing to happen. This is a primary component of the container we work in.

This process of gazing and witnessing with no agenda supports homeostasis, as stated by Robert Scaer (2011): "Brainspotting is based on the profound attunement of the therapist with the patient, finding a somatic cue, and extinguishing it by down-regulating the amygdala. It isn't just PNS (Parasympathetic Nervous System) activation that is facilitated, it is homeostasis" (https://brainspotting.pro/).

He also brings to light the importance of intimate attunement, stating, "The attunement activates the mirror neurons between the cingulate and the OFC (Orbital Frontal Cortex), creating an empathic environment and inhibits the amygdala. This sacred, face-to-face, empathic attunement is a critical environment for trauma therapy to work, just as it is in maternal-infant bonding, and this state of presence is essential for healing" (Scaer, 2001).

This fine attunement includes those sessions in which we become the pointer and the resource spot. I have one client who doesn't like headphones or a pointer and wants

BSP. In some sessions, I integrate a gaze spot around the issue being presented but not always. In sessions in which we're framing the issue, she develops a connection to her body-felt sense and processes by looking at me as her spot. And there are times when she pendulates in and out of the processing by being with her feelings and then talking about other people and trying to problem-solve. It's all part of the frame, tracking, and resourcing. She's made great movement and is finding a deeper sense of self.

Asking clients to sit and witness their own thoughts and body-felt sense turns on other aspects of the brain-body connection. It helps clients start to objectively identify something rather than be identified with it. I often teach my clients that as soon as we can identify something, we're less identified with it. We gain some space and distance from it, which also helps us perceive it differently. The past and the present gain separation as clients move to being able to distinguish "then" from "now" when we ask where they feel most activated. This awareness is a type of grounding that arises, most likely, from gaining direct access to the tactile layer in the superior colliculus, so it's possibly a form of subcortical grounding.

Another type of grounding in relation to the body-felt sense is when we ask a client where they feel most grounded, calm, and connected in the body. In both approaches – activation or resource model – the inner scanner locates a body sensation connected to the present. We build a bridge through awareness and felt sense between the past and the present.

When clients have trouble locating a spot, this can indicate anything from needing body-felt sense awareness (they'd never thought of themselves in those words before) to dissociation to anything in between. We can help them by suggesting they bring their attention to the backs of their legs as they sit, to their feet on the floor, to their hands on the arms of the chair, or maybe the placement of one hand on top of the other or their hand on their thigh. Whatever you suggest, have it be something that connects a body sensation to the environment so the client can begin to feel themselves in present time and space. This supports the hippocampus coming back on board. And, as mentioned, integrating the sense of touch works with the tactile layer of the superior colliculus.

Choosing to use the resource model can be extremely grounding. With a resource model of BSP, you use an area of perceived groundedness in the body and find an eye position that matches this, which further enhances the groundedness.

The following is an example of working with grounding and touch during a session: I treated a client who had a panic attack triggered by a work-related event that grew into a tremor throughout her body which she couldn't stop. She described the panic as a fear of authority and associated it with her mother's punitive nature. We decided that her frame should be directed to grounding her limbic-system activity. I educated her about the brain and its different regions and structures, specifically the limbic system, in an attempt to ground her conceptually. Together, we located a gaze spot connected to her limbic brain activity. She began to process and, at a certain point, I guided her to walk over to the spot, touch it, and describe it. As instructed, the client walked slowly toward the spot along the z-axis. As she was touching the spot, I asked her to describe it to me to ground her in touch and detailed description. I asked her to detail the texture, the temperature, and the shape she felt on the spot. All my questions were intended to support grounding her in the present and engaging her neocortex. Once she did this, she slowly returned to her seat and gazed again at the spot, exploring the z-axis from a greater distance. The SUDs, which had started at 8.0, had receded to a 0.5 level. Following that session, the client reported the tremor had ceased. Touching the gaze spot appeared to trigger her sensory cortex, parietal, and temporal lobes and, accordingly, helped to integrate brain and body processes.

Accessing the three-dimensional z-axis appears to be a highly effective way of increasing the grounding experience. In this case, it was used to work with seeing close and far and then actively experiencing the body movement along the z-axis. By adding the physical movement to the process, the client was able to have a body-felt sense of motion in the here and now and connect to her rhythm of movement.

As stated at the beginning of this chapter, the inspiration to move triggers a series of electric currents. When the charge is too high, the SNS become overactivated. Think flight, fright, or freeze. When we have the ability to flee, run, move, or fight, we can release the overactivity. When we're frozen, there's no movement and therefore we're unable to return to regulation.

Having this client walk across the room reinforced her capacity to move and discharge, which supported the process toward regulation. "The long-term, alarming, debilitating, and often bizarre symptoms of PTSD develop when we cannot complete the process of moving in, through and out of the 'immobility' or 'freezing' state. However, we can thaw by initiating and encouraging our innate drive to return to a state of dynamic equilibrium." (Levine, 1997, p. 19) "When we are unable to liberate these powerful forces, we become victims of trauma... The result, sadly, is that many of us become riddled with fear and anxiety and are never fully able to feel at home with ourselves or the world" (Levine, p. 21).

Sometimes during session, people will begin to tremor or shake. One person I worked with would regularly respond to this situation by saying, "I'm sorry. I don't know what's happening." She'd then start to laugh spontaneously and her whole face would light up. As the work continued, the laughter and jerky body movements were less dramatic, partially because the traumas we were working with had been released through the unprocessed movements. I once heard the tremors and releasing in relation to opening up the body and grounding being compared to a car being tuned up: At first there's a lot of rattling, but eventually you get a nice hum.

Regarding the use of the z-axis, what we know from research is, "The use of oculo-cardiac convergence visual therapy for somatic intervention in the event of anginal pain, panic disorders, and vagally mediated stomach and breathing problems, perhaps even globus hystericus, is an interesting and novel prospect of using OCR stimulation as a simple vagal maneuver for managing these symptoms of sympathetic activation. It appears capable of providing a quick palliation to these distressing symptoms in many situations" (https://www.researchgate.net/publication/216064110_Treatment_of_Panic_Attack_With_Vergence_Therapy_and_unexpected_visual-vagus_connection). Incorporating the z-axis is a highly effective way of increasing grounding. It can be used as part of the set-up, brought in during the session, or added toward the end.

I want to mention a few more things about this case. Here was a woman who was able to understand the history of her symptoms but couldn't resolve them. She needed to get to the agranular level for change to happen. Her neocortex couldn't override her instinctual defense response. As Levine (1997) states: "The neo-cortex is not powerful enough to override the instinctual defense response to threat and danger – the fight, flee, or freeze responses. In this respect, we human beings are still inextricably bound to our animal heritage. Animals, however, do not have a highly evolved neo-cortex to interfere with the natural return to normal functioning through some form of discharge. In human beings, trauma occurs as a result of the initiation of an instinctual cycle that is not allowed to finish. When the neo-cortex overrides the instinctual responses that would indicate the completion of this cycle..." (Levine, p. 100-101, *Waking the Tiger: Healing Trauma)* (https://www.cheap-health-revolution.com/peter-a-levine-5.html).

Another example of using movement during a session to reinforce grounding is when we reflect on the movement that's happening in the client. In a session with a client who suffered from panic attacks, I introduced movement by changing the focus of sharing to the present by pendulating off the activation, setting up another resource spot, and through physical movement. Each was used to strengthen the grounding and help the client proceed to regulation.

At the beginning of this session, the client kept speaking about her father – how he was and how this made her behave in a certain way. The focus was diverted from the details of the times this happened to the felt sense she experienced as she spoke. Sticking to the historical story around her father seemed to cause her to feel disconnected. Inquiring more about what, specifically, she was referring to while she was speaking – in an almost automatic-pilot manner – helped ground her in what she was speaking about.

It also helped her slow down her thoughts, which helped her focus on what, specifically, disturbed her.

During the work, she had some moments in which she reported a floaty feeling. I made a clinical decision to suggest she return to her body's resource spot, which had been determined as part of the set-up process. With other clients, I often wait longer to do this, but, in this case, I could tell she wasn't feeling grounded enough to continue. The work progressed, and then she came to another point where she wasn't able to calm down, even when focusing on the resource spot.

I chose to inquire about her relationship to God, as she's a religious woman and turns to her faith often. I introduced her attachment to God as another spot to focus on. This seemed to help her feel more grounded. Her body began to demonstrate a lot of reflex movement. I called her attention to it by saying, "I notice your foot is tapping." The process soon led to her physically releasing a lot of movements. I offered her a pillow to use as she released. I watched her shake off the frozen trauma state. She felt surprised, relieved, and calm. I believe it was because she'd felt sufficiently grounded through the process that this occurred.

As I continued to work with her, she was able to delay her emotional responses, bring reason into her actions, and think more clearly. Toward the end of our work she shared an incident in which someone who's been an authority and bully figure asked her to do something unethical. In the past, she would have been frightened and compliant. This time, she was able to remain calm, think things out, speak with others, and plan her response in a way that allowed her to act ethically. She was pleased with herself and gained self-respect from her actions. She also realized how much she's grown and shifted out of her fear response. Brainspotting helped her recondition traumatic, conditioned responses through releasing her body sensations and slowing her thinking process.

The last client I want to mention is an individual who spontaneously moved at the end of the session. He had a sense of being finished, yet there was more time. He asked to take a break. When he stood up, he started to stretch. I offered him a tennis ball to roll around under the bottom of his foot. My sense was a lot got released in the session, but his body needed more movement for grounding and integration. I gave him space to move around the room. When he stretched, the spontaneous movements began. During these movements, he reported different parts of himself were starting to integrate. He reported feeling more grounded and a huge weight was released. He felt much calmer.

Self-observation is a form of meditation. Meditation has been around for thousands of years, and research is starting to show the health benefits of this practice. A research review published in *JAMA Internal Medicine* in January 2014 listed relieving anxiety, pain, and depression as some of these beneficial effects. Meditation works on the sympathetic nervous system and therefore can lower blood pressure and enhance creativity and a sense of peacefulness – all of which are grounding and regulating (https://hms.harvard.edu/sites/default/files/assets/Harvard%20Now%20and%20Zen%20Reading%20Materials.pdf).

The Benefits of Brainspotting to Assist Clinicians in Grounding Themselves

I'd like to turn our discussion to the therapist's grounding. Two key elements of BSP that address this are: Staying in the tail of the comet and W.A.I.T. (Why Am I Talking?). "We cannot touch the core of the sufferer unless we reach out from our own core." (Pierrakos, 1987, p. 201)

One day, a colleague and I were exploring using BSP with a neurofeedback machine to track the process. This was a single case study we did prior to starting research. At one point in the session, when I reflected something to the client with the intention of giving support, the computer indicated a disruption. The neurofeedback program showed that the client went straight from her subcortex to her neocortex. This was a great lesson in W.A.I.T. In that moment, my reason for talking was, as stated, to be supportive and reflexive.

One can ask more questions in this W.A.I.T. inquiry such as: Who am I talking for? What happens if I don't know what's going on? In that moment with this client, my unconsciously falling out of the tail of the comet took me back to graduate school and professional conditioning. How often do we act from professional conditioning, and how often does that eject us out of the tail of the comet?

I was using my reflexive skills to let the client know I was present with her. Did she need me to say anything, or could she sense my presence and my attunement to her neurobiology, just as the client mentioned previously did when he stated he was watching me watch him? Had I really been present, with all my conditioning left at the door, I'd have been able to observe with deeper curiosity and less need to check in and know how she was doing. I guess that's why we call our work a "practice." That day, I was offered another opportunity to learn and grow as a clinician.

I was also given a new understanding of self-reflection and grounding. When I'm functioning from conditioning, I'm ungrounded. I'm out of attunement and not in the present moment. Pausing and becoming curious about why I'm using an intervention and who it's for is a way to stay present and grounded during the session.

We each have our ways of catching ourselves before we fall out of the tail of the comet. Some of us get more verbal while others may intervene too quickly with a grounding exercise thinking the client can't tolerate their feelings, when it's actually us who can't tolerate what's happening in the moment. Turning our inner scanner on ourselves and finding a grounding spot is key for clinicians to stay grounded during a session.

Common grounding spots are feet, hands, or the dantien (the spot on the abdomen two inches below the belly button). Sometimes, I bring my awareness to my sit bones, sense my back against the chair, or feel one part of my body in contact with another. I also notice my body posture and may lean in a little more or bring my awareness to my eyes and enhance my focus on the client. Also, taking note to review later on my need to attend to what got triggered is helpful. I believe the self-reflection and commitment to attend to it afterwards grounds the triggered part of me.

And, referring to what we said earlier about the electric currents flowing between us, we can think of the importance of the dual, attuned relationship in terms of working on our own sense of grounding. As we help ourselves become more attuned, in and out of session, we can be more present and not respond from conditioned learning. Our clients will experience us differently as we deepen our state of compassion and empathy.

Schore (2014) proposes that repeated experience of somatic attunement in the therapeutic relationship facilitates neurogrowth in the subcortical and cortical regions of the right brain, thus enhancing the client's ability to self-regulate and tolerate stress. Others, have written about the unconscious somatic responses between the client and therapist. "Patient and analyst mutually regulate each other's behaviors, enactments, and states of consciousness such that each gets under the other's skin, each reaches into the other's guts, each is breathed in and absorbed by the other ... The analyst must be attuned to the nonverbal, the affective ... to his or her bodily responses." (Aron, L ,1998) Within this interactive psychobiological regulation, the client learns to regulate internal experiences and receives help for internal change. Brainspotting is a Daul Attunement process working at these deeper levels of the process.

In the example of my client with money issues, my attuned presence and returning to the tail of the comet allowed the processing to continue because I resumed a calm, grounded state that supported the field of her healing. In BSP Phase One, we speak about the primary resource being the therapist's empathic, attuned presence – a calm, grounded, connected presence. As we therapists continue to do our work to stay present and develop ourselves, we can further develop our intuitive presence. This is where all possibility exists.

The HeathMath Institute is doing research on this and has found that "intuition may play an important role in social cognition, decision-making and creativity. When addressing life situations, people often default to familiar patterns of thoughts, feelings and actions in both the decision-making process and how they see others. Rather than responding to situations from habitual patterns that are not necessarily healthy or constructive, those situations could be more effectively addressed with new and creative solutions. These solutions can take into consideration the available inner resources that are congruent with one's deeper intuition and core values. In other words, we can learn to intentionally align with and access our intuitive intelligence, which can provide moment-to-moment guidance and empower what HeartMath calls heart-based living -reliance, in all things, on the wisdom, intelligence and qualities of the heart" (https://www.heartmath.org/research/science-of-the-heart/intuition-research/).

Additional Thoughts on Developing Grounding Processes

I'd like to suggest that the grounding exercises/experiences you offer to clients be based on different parts of the brain to further strengthen the work. As we mentioned with regard to music, a process that engages the right and left brain is key for integration. It strengthens the corpus callosum and supports an overall increase in mental health. "The right and left sides of the brain focus on different skills which, when combined, enable individuals to be rational and spontaneous, analytical and creative" (https://www.livestrong.com/article/111852-left-right-brain-exercises/).

Toward the end of a session, to help with integration, I'll have the client move an arm and the opposite leg while sitting or walking. As they move, I urge them to go slowly and focus on the movement. Any form of movement that supports this left brain-right brain integration can be used before, during, or after a session.

Trauma survivors often unconsciously hold their breath or breathe shallowly. This deprives the brain of oxygen, which can make anxiety more intense. Having a client stop and focus on deepening and slowing their breathing brings them back to the moment. One way to do this in a session is, when you notice your client taking a deep breath, questioning them about whether they noticed this change in breathing – was it spontaneous or conscious? I believe this helps emphasize to them the organic capacity of the body to do exactly what it needs. Also, by bringing awareness to the breath, we're connecting conscious thoughts with an unconscious movement, and this is grounding.

There are many types of breathing techniques you can integrate when and if appropriate. The key with any technique is to know why we're using it and how it's supporting the work, as discussed previously.

Deep breathing can connect us to our sense of smell, which is one of our primary senses. Integrating our senses and awareness into the moment has many grounding benefits. We've addressed the eyes, ears, and skin (touch), and now we'll speak to smell and taste as they relate to grounding.

Some clinicians incorporate aromatherapy in their work and find it helps clients to ground. I often notice smell coming up naturally during a session when, all of the sudden, a client comments about an odor as if their mind is in the past. They may comment that they realize they're experiencing this in the past, and this helps ground them in the present and in the room. This is similar to a client "all of the sudden" noticing biolateral music with great surprise.

Observing and describing can also support the integration between the right and left hemispheres of the brain as well as the bottom-up and top-down areas. When we describe an object, our mind switches focus from emotion to thinking – with grounding as a result. I may use this during a session when someone is highly dysregulated and ask them to find and describe an object in the room. This process brings their attention back to the here and now.

A similar technique involving taste can be used at the beginning of the process of helping someone learn mindfulness skills by having the client suck on a raisin or a piece of candy and describe it.

I'd like to conclude by mentioning that grounding supports survival and thriving. As we move through traumas, we discover aspects of ourselves that have been hidden or untapped. We also have the opportunity to use BSP for enhancement. Being grounded and present in our lives opens up all kinds of possibilities. And, as we've seen from the benefits of meditation, the practice of presence strengthens our minds. "Meditators showed significantly larger volumes of the right hippocampus. Both orbito-frontal and hippocampal regions have been implicated in emotional regulation and response control. Thus, larger volumes in these regions might account for meditators' singular abilities and habits to cultivate positive emotions, retain emotional stability, and engage in mindful behavior. We further suggest that these regional alterations in brain structures constitute part of the underlying neurological correlate of long-term meditation independent of a specific style and practice" (https://www.ncbi.nlm.nih.gov/m/pubmed/19280691/).

To summarize, we have looked at different aspects of the Brainspotting model and how it is a grounding model. We addressed the components of Brainspotting, case examples of grounding within the session for the client and the therapist, and given some grounding processes for both the client and the therapist. In BSP, we're looking for long-lasting change for our clients. We human beings are survivors, and this process can take our clients a long way within a grounded, supportive container that allows the unexpected to happen.

The immense energies that create the symptoms of trauma, when properly engaged and mobilized, can transform the trauma and propel us into new heights of healing, mastery and even wisdom. Peter Levine (1997): *Waking the Tiger*

References

Aron, L. (1998) The Clinical Body and the Reflex Mind. In L. Aron & F. Sommer Anderson (Eds.), Relational Perspectives on the Body (pp. 3-37) Hillside, NJ: Analytic Press.

From http://icpla.edu/wp-content/uploads/2014/03/Aron-L-Ch.-1-The-Clinical-Body-and-the-Refecxive-Mind-pp-3-37.pdf

Ayers, M. Y. (2003, November 13): Mother-Infant Attachment and Psychoanalysis.

Retrieved March 27, 2018, from https://books.google.com/books?id=XEzJAwAAQBAJ&pg=PA34&lpg=PA34&dq=gazing in mother's eyes&source=bl&ots=89Bks6i-bA&sig=wh37tVvyRTScVMEBey5m_hRUAZo&hl=en&sa=X&ved=0ahUKEwi5ydzAyLDYAhWkz-IMKHX5KDQEQ6AEIXzAM#v=onepage&q=gazing in mother's eyes&f=false

Bloom, Sophie. (2017, August 14): Left & Right Brain Exercises. Retrieved March 27, 2018, from https://www.livestrong.com/article/111852-left-right-brain-exercises/

Boadella, D. (1978): "Steps to Transfiguration: Birth moments in Human Experience," Self and Society, 6 (7), pg. 245.

Bowen, M. (2018, January): Treatment of Panic Attack With Vergence Therapy: And unexpected visual-vagus connection. Retrieved March 27, 2018, from https://www.researchgate.net/publication/216064110_Treatment_of_Panic_Attack_With_Vergence_Therapy_and_unexpected_visual-vagus_connection

Brancucci, A., Lucci, G., Mazzatenta, A., & Tommasi, L. (2009, April 12): Asymmetries of the human social brain in the visual, auditory and chemical modalities. Retrieved March 27, 2018, from http://rstb.royalsocietypublishing.org/content/364/1519/895

Google. (n.d.). Retrieved March 27, 2018, from https://www.google.com/search?q=define assumption&enablesearch=true

Google. (n.d.). Retrieved March 27, 2018, from https://www.google.com/search?q=assumption definition&ie=utf-8&oe=utf-8&client=firefox-b-1-ab.

delMonte, D., (2016, 2017): Stress Trauma and Pain in Brain and Body Neurobiology for Trauma and Brainspotting Therapists. 2-day seminar Amsterdam, NL – video post-seminar, at www.lecurio.de

Iakovides, S. A., Iliadou, V. T., Bizeli, V. T., Kaprinis, S. G., Fountoulakis, K. N., &

Kaprinis, G. S. (2004): Psychophysiology and psychoacoustics of music: Perception of complex sound in normal subjects and psychiatric patients. Retrieved March 27, 2018, from https://www.ncbi.nlm.nih.gov/pmc/articles/PMC400748/

Knapton, S. (2017, November 29): Mothers and babies brainwaves snychronise when they gaze at each other, scientists find . Retrieved March 27, 2018, from http://www.telegraph.co.uk/science/2017/11/29/mothers-babies-brainwaves-snychronise-gaze-scientists-find/

Levine, P.A. (1997): Waking the Tiger: Healing Trauma. Berkeley: North Atlantic Books.

Luders, E., Toga, A. W., Lepore, N., & Gaser, C. (2009, April 15): The underlying anatomical correlates of long-term meditation: Larger hippocampal and frontal volumes of gray matter. Retrieved March 27, 2018, from https://www.ncbi.nlm.nih.gov/pubmed/19280691/

Lyons-Ruth, K. (2000): "I sense that you sense that I sense...": Sander's recognition process and the specificity of relational moves in the psychotherapeutic setting. Infant Mental Health Journal, 21, 85–98.

Massachusetts Institute of Technology. (2009, October 23): Time-keeping Brain Neurons Discovered. Retrieved March 27, 2018, from https://www.sciencedaily.com/releases/2009/10/091019162921.htm

Meares, R. (2005): The metaphor of play: Origin and breakdown of personal being (3rd ed.). London: Routledge.

Nabb, J. (1999): Core Energertic Concepts of Grounding, Southwest Center for Core Energetics, pamphlet, p. 2.

National Research Council (US) and Institute of Medicine (US) Committee on Integrating the Science of Early Childhood Development. (1970, January 01). Acquiring Self-Regulation. Retrieved March 27, 2018, from https://www.ncbi.nlm.nih.gov/books/NBK225568/

Nugent, & M.S., Pam. (2015, July 13): What is UNCERTAINTY PRINCIPLE? definition of UNCERTAINTY PRINCIPLE (Psychology Dictionary). Retrieved March 27, 2018, from https://psychologydictionary.org/uncertainty-principle/

Ogden, P., Pain, C., Minton, K., & Fisher, J. (2005): Including the body in mainstream psychotherapy for traumatized individuals. Psychologist-Psychoanalyst, 25(4), 22.

Pierrakos, J. (1987): Core Energetics: Developing the Capacity to Love and Heal. Mendocino: Life Rhythm Publications. pg. 23.

Podgorny, N. (2013, May 07): Candlelight Insight: Trataka. Retrieved March 27, 2018, from https://yogainternational.com/article/view/candlelight-insight-trataka

Porges, S. (2014, October 3): Social Engagement Heals. Retrieved March 27, 2018, from http://attachmentdisorderhealing.com/porges-polyvagal3/

Pygmalion effect. (2018, March 19): Retrieved March 27, 2018, from https://en.wikipedia.org/wiki/Pygmalion_effect

Scaer, R. (2001): The Body Bears the Burden, New York, NY: Routledge

Scaer, R. (2005): The Trauma Spectrum: Hidden Wounds and human Resiliency, New York, NY: Norton.

Schore, A. (2014): "The Right Brain in Dominant in Psychotherapy." American Psychological Association, Psychotherapy, 2014, 51 (3), pgs. 388-397.

Self-regulation theory. (2018, February 28): Retrieved March 27, 2018, from https://en.wikipedia.org/wiki/Self-regulation_theory

Shaw, R. (2004): The embodied psychotherapist: An exploration of the therapists' somatic phenomena within the therapeutic encounter. Psychotherapy Research, 14, 271–288.

Siegel, D., MD, & Rutsch, E. (n.d.): Dialogues on How to Build a Culture of Empathy. Retrieved March 27, 2018, from http://cultureofempathy.com/References/Experts/Daniel-Siegel.htm

The Human Body's Ability to Self-Heal. (n.d.): Retrieved March 27, 2018, from https://www.tummycalm.com/self-healing.html

Wei, M., MD, JD. (2015, November 18): Now and Zen: How mindfulness can change your brain and improve your health. Retrieved March 27, 2018, from https://hms.harvard.edu/sites/default/files/assets/Harvard Now and Zen Reading Materials.pdf

WAIT… Why Am I Talking
An Exploration of the Role of Silence in Brainspotting Therapy

Susan Pinco

This chapter explores the role of silence both in Brainspotting and in the healing of psychological trauma. The reader is invited to experience silence and to consider their relationship to it.

As I look around at the emerging Brainspotting community I notice a sense of joy that feels as it if is emerging from the center of my chest, radiating out, expressing itself in the drawing back of my lips and the attendant puffing out of my cheeks when I smile; it is a smile that I know lights up my eyes.

You, the reader, may wonder why I have started this chapter on Brainspotting and Silence in this way. I'm curious if you would be willing to take a moment and notice what happens when you wonder about this, because in so doing, you are taking the first step into the process of Brainspotting.

Expanding this moment, you can notice the rate at which you are breathing: the depth of your inhalations, and the length of your exhalations. You can do this without making any effort to change anything. And, as you continue to read my words, you might become aware of any thoughts that are forming inside your mind. Pausing a bit longer you might become aware of what you feel as you move your eyes across the page. Checking inside yourself you can notice the subtle differences between looking to the left, to the center and to the right of the page. You might be aware of the ways that your eyes blink more in one position than in another, and how your face spontaneously moves when your eyes change position. Pausing even longer, you may be aware of smells, of sensations, of images, none of which are available to you when you are in conversation. Here we stand together on the threshold between interpersonal and intrapersonal exploration. This is a vital land, where you, accompanied by a dually attuned therapist, a caring and supportive presence, can meet what is encoded in your viscera, in your brain, in a way that potentiates and makes possible the healthy rewiring of your system. In fact, by helping ourselves and our clients/patients work in silence, we expand the capacity to experience emotions, and to begin to trust that, just as Eugene Gendlin so eloquently said; "Every bad feeling is potential energy toward a more right way of being if you give it space to move toward rightness.. It knows the direction… just as surely as you know which way to move a crooked picture.. there is absolutely no chance that you will move it in the wrong direction. The sense of what is wrong carries with it… a sense of what is right" (Fosha 2011 quoting Gendlin 1957)

In the beginning

Years ago, when I first began thinking about a subject for my PhD studies, I would often sit down with my mentor, David Grand, and explore possible topics. Because I was so immersed in the work of Brainspotting (BSP), recognized the extraordinary power of BSP to facilitate transformation and healing, and because one of the essential elements of Brainspotting is sitting in silence and noticing what happens, I decided that what I wanted to do was debunk the myth of the talking cure. And, recognizing that I might be "biting off more than the thesis committee would be willing to chew", David and I amended the title to "Is It The Talking That Cures? A look at the role of Silence and Words in the Therapeutic Process."

The introduction to my thesis began with the following; "My conviction that silence plays a pivotal role in psychological healing evolved from the seeds of my meditation practice, which began in 1993. The sunlight and nutrience that enabled this concept to grow emanated from my mentorship with Dr. Richard Moss (1996-present), who synthesizes the work of modern psychology, Eastern Practices and energy medicine. Watching myself and my clients heal, and working first with EMDR and later with Brainspotting, both of which I studied under the mentorship of Dr. David Grand, caused this seedling to germinate and propelled me to continue exploring how silence facilitates healing.

Once I began to pursue this topic in earnest, I found that the literature was rife with oblique references to the fertile ground of silence. While relatively few clinical texts speak to silence directly, I have been gratified to find that the emerging literature and practice, particularly in the area of neuropsychology, alludes to the phenomenon of silence and its pivotal role in healing.

As I took my dissertation topic into my work with clients/patients, I came to notice that there is always a pause before a new-found realization is articulated, and that clients often were at a loss for words as these realizations began to surface. I found the first indications that something had happened in the subtle changes in posture, muscle tone, expression and respiration.

I also noticed that as I encouraged the pendulation between verbalizations and silent observation of sensations, emotions, involuntary body movements, images and thoughts, my clients became less anxious, more present and better able to address core issues. For those of you who are not familiar with the term, pendulation refers to the practice of moving back and forth between material that is triggering and material, experiences or sensations that can serve as a grounding resource (Grand 2002-2008; Leitch 2007, Levine 2005).

Those clients who were not comfortable with working in the silence seemed to remain stuck in recitations of issues. Further, many clients/patients who needed to talk and whose speech was often pressured were able to begin to quiet as we focused on generating a sense of containment in session. This containment and focus on the body appeared to permit them to experience a profound sense of being seen, understood, accepted and soothed. This observation suggests that while the words exchanged between therapist and client(s)/patients(s) provide the scaffolding of the relationship, they can at times impede deeper work. Despite the fact that the role of words/narrative and associated left brain activities have been extensively explored, it is only through recent studies of the brain that we are coming to recognize the fact that the left brain alone cannot touch the heart of most "psychological" symptoms which are stored in right brain (Doidge 2003; Levine et al 1997; Lapides 2007; Ogden 2000, 2006, 2007; Schore 2003, 2005; Siegel 1999, 2004, 2006). This research appears to indicate that when the left brain/prefrontal and frontal cortices (language and logic) are "lit up" when viewed via a number of brain imaging procedures, the right brain's activity is dampened or greatly reduced (Mayberg et al. 1999; Oh and Choi 2007; Rauch, Whalen, et al. 2000; Rauch, van der Kolk 1996). Extending these findings, it is interesting to note that research suggests that the imaginal use of words may not use the same areas of the brain as speech does (Doidge 2003; Kosslyn et al. 2003; Waterworth 2002).

Since the locus of most psychological issues is related to right-brained functions (emotion, somatic sensing, etc.) one may intuit that the right brain must play a dominant role in accessing and healing these issues. Nonetheless, traditional talk therapy engages the client via a heavily left-brained process, conversation, verbal exploration and free association. Further, until recently, it largely ignored a key component of affective experience, the body" (Pinco 2008).

Recent research, some of which is presented in other sections of this book, suggests that transformation occurs from the bottom up, i.e., there is a shift in feeling and in experience which can then lead to an increased ability to articulate a new understanding. You will note, that I used the qualifier "can" in the sentence above, as for some individuals there is no new narrative, only an altered sense of well-being, and connection to self.

In the last 10 years, since the publication of my dissertation, Brainspotting has evolved in the most delicious way. It now clearly articulates and invites the conscious utilization of silence, recognizing its unique role in facilitating the rewiring of the neural networks that hold our stuck patterns so that our systems can move to health and transformance.

Brainspotting trainings state, restate, and state again that what is central to being a seasoned and effective Brainspotting therapist is the ability to WAIT (i.e., to ask oneself, "Why Am I Talking") before speaking. The reasons behind this are manifold. Speaking causes the focus to be on the interpersonal relationship rather than the intrapersonal relationship, meaning that the client shifts their focus from inside to outside of themselves when they speak. It also interrupts the trajectory of their client/patient's thought and experience while also slowing down the process. It is noteworthy that the body, brain stem and midbrain/limbic system process information approximately 200 times faster than the neo-cortex.

Unlike most other treatment modalities, where an extensive oral history is elicited, Brainspotting therapists often jump right in, working with what is most palpable for the client/patient in the moment, recognizing that how they engage during the session will provide an understanding of their history in ways that are not possible when information is filtered through the neocortex. This lack of highly structured protocols frees the clinician to "follow the head of the comet", tracking each client's trajectory rather than leading the process. Brainspotting has, in fact, rewritten the rule book. While most schools of clinical practice still teach some form of highly interactive processes, Brainspotting invites the therapist to simply observe, conveying presence in a host of nonverbal, yet powerful ways. As Dr. Grand says, Brainspotting therapists are not less active (because they are not talking); they are merely active in a different way. This being *with,* rather than *doing,* is often difficult for clinicians who are new to Brainspotting. As a result, I often share a study that Francine Lapides referenced in her online training course in 2008 when I teach Brainspotting. In this study researchers looked at the brain activity of two groups of young children who were playing in the presence of a parent. In one group the parent was reading; in the other the parent was watching their children as they played but did not speak with them. What was so striking is that the group whose parent was watching them had significantly more brain activity than the group whose parent was reading. The quality of our attention really does matter.

An attuned Brainspotting therapist will notice subtle changes in posture, movement, breathing, skin tone, facial expression and so much more. This dual awareness of both the physiological and the psychological is conveyed with attention rather than words. And, this attunement begins the moment a client walks into our office. Often we invite our clients/patients to take a few moments to orient themselves to the room, to what it is like to sit with us: allowing themselves to arrive just as I did at the beginning of this chapter.

While working in silence potentiates healing, there are often steps that must be taken before both the therapist and the client/patient feel comfortable working in this manner. For the therapist, it is often their own experience as they go through the training that convinces them of the power of working with minimal words. For those of you who may not have taken the training, you can get a taste of what I am talking about by pausing now and thinking about something you are irritated, upset or triggered by, noticing how activating that issue is for you on a scale of 0–10 with 0 being not at all and 10 being intolerable. Then, talk about the issue for 2–3 minutes with a friend or trusted colleague. If no one is available, you can choose an object in the room and imagine that it is a caring friend. You might place the object in just the right place for you. Don't worry, you will find the right place simply by moving it around and pausing to see how each location feels. Then, talk.

After talking, pause, and notice how activated you feel around the issue. Then, with the friend or the object, find the visual focal point or Brainspot that corresponds with what is activating you. Sit for 2–3 minutes and just notice what is happening inside yourself. What did you learn? What questions do you have? If you'd like to share them you can write to me at: SusanPinco@Coherentself.com or you can share them with the Brainspotting community at www.brainspotting-germany.de or www.brainspotting.com

For some clients/patients, there is often a need to connect, to get to know and trust the therapist before exploring the territory of silence. For these individuals there is often a sense that in order for the therapist to help them, the therapist must know the whole story. For others, there is a belief that being a good client/patient means talking. For some it may be an effort to work and rework what has happened so that it can become intelligible, thereby reducing anxiety. It can also be part of an effort to connect; to be seen, felt and heard. Unfortunately by speaking they are activating the neo-cortex and in so doing they are limiting access to the limbic system which generates the very feelings they are trying to transform.

Slowing down, so that dual attunement can occur; focusing on what is felt both emotionally and in the physical body without engaging the story while orienting "towards" through body posture and eye focus appears to:

- Undo the unbearable aloneness that was evident when the "trauma" occurred. This attunement implicitly conveys a "valuing" of the patient and serves to down-regulate the Central Nervous System (CNS), making physical stillness possible. This stillness appears to permit the containment (i.e., holding) of whatever becomes triggered in the process;

- Create the possibility of our clients/patients feeling compassionately held both by our attention as well as their own, perhaps for the first time in their lives;

  - Develop the capacity for mindfulness, through focusing on the body while watching what comes up without attachment. This is something that is taught implicitly and modeled in the Brainspotting process, and which has been linking to resilience and health;

- Permit the limbic system to be activated within its limits of tolerance, thereby fostering an amazing associative process that occurs at lightning speed as neural nets fire and begin to realign and reform. This process is interrupted and or slowed down when speech is added to the process. Furthermore, the process appears to be enhanced through body position and visual orientation.

This "no assumptions" model encourages both practitioners as well as patients to just *be* with the experience in a way that circumvents old assumptions and stories and creates a fertile ground for transformation.

While other modalities including mindfulness, Focusing, EMDR, and Somatic Experiencing (SE) utilize some of these elements, what is unique is the way Brainspotting explicitly combines these elements to create a process that potentiates emotional, physical and spiritual healing to occur.

In fact, Brainspotting is more than a technique or an approach. It is a stance, a way of being that transforms the therapist/client/patient relationship. This stance is evident from the first to the last clinical encounter. It is apparent in the way that the therapist engages and invites curiosity without judgement and with a good deal of silence. With or without an articulated visual focal point, Brainspotting emerges and determines the trajectory of the sessions.

Speaking more concretely, I will share a few first sessions with new clients. In the first case, "M" contacted me because she was told that Brainspotting would really help her. I greeted her in the waiting room, invited her into my office, and asked her to select where she would like to sit. I then chose a seat nearby, checking to see if our proximity felt ok or if she wanted me to move closer or further away. She said "you are fine". We then smiled at each other again and I invited her to take a moment and let herself just slow down and take in the room. She nodded and looked around the room, then looked at me took, a deep breath. I said, "Good breath?" and she nodded. I then asked how she had come to call me and what she was hoping to achieve in our work together. She replied to both questions, shared a bit of history and as we talked I invited pauses and encouraged her to notice what was happening inside. As she became more expressive I asked her to tell me how distressed she was on a scale of 0-10, with 0 being not at all and

10 being intolerable. She indicated that she was at a 7. I then asked if she would like to do some Brainspotting with this issue and she said yes. I then invited her to scan her body and see what lead her to assign a SUDs (Subject Units of Distress) level of 7 to this activation. She indicated that there was tension in her throat and chest. I nodded and then, taking out my pointer, worked with her to locate the visual focal point that brought her sensations and the associated issue into focus. I held the pointer to the left of me, in front of me and to the right. Once we identified the general area we then zeroed in on the exact spot then checked to see if the sensation was stronger above and below the point. Once we had the spot, we sat together in silence for approximately 5 minutes, at which point "M" checked in with me to let me know what was happening. We then continued in silence for the remainder of the session with her checking in spontaneously from time to time. At the end of the session there was evident relief and the SUDs had fallen to a 2.

What is noteworthy about "M" is that she had a background in mindfulness meditation and didn't need to ease herself into silent processing and self-observation. She also didn't need a lot of direction or reassurance about the process.

In another first session, "G" came to me as family members had experienced Brainspotting and found it very helpful. "G" is an extremely intelligent young man who is highly analytic and epitomizes the term "buttoned down". He was clear about his issues and the role his internal critic was playing. He also epitomizes what I call "ABF" (Anything But Feeling). This is true for both positive and negative feelings. Initially he didn't want to "do Brainspotting" so we talked, and as we talked I frequently encouraged him to just notice what was happening in his body; both the sense of "no feeling" and those areas of relative comfort. Over time we came to welcome the space between the words which permitted him to begin to slow down and to become curious about his internal critic. Over a number of months we have moved from implicitly using Gazespotting to explicitly using Brainspotting, and the sense of calm that he is able to achieve in session is remarkable.

Finally, I will share a first session with a middle-aged man, "Z", who didn't request or know about Brainspotting. "Z" came in wanting to talk about what he was struggling with. He needed me to know his history and to find answers to questions like, "Am I this way because of that", and "why am I still like this after years of therapy". "Z" did not like it when I would use a pause in his speech to invite him to notice what was happening inside. He had to "get it out". With "Z" I followed his need to verbalize, as well as all the micro-details which he shared with me: the pacing of his breathing, the changes in his facial expressions and coloring, the ebb and flow of his body's movements. While we didn't use the pointer or overtly to "do Brainspotting" in the first session, we did begin to lay the foundation, utilizing many of the key elements of Brainspotting. As we have continued to work together "Z" still needs to share what has been difficult outside session and what he is most proud of in the past week prior to our focusing on a particular issue. When he feels heard, he readily assigns a SUDs to his activation, locates where he feels it in his body and locates a Brainspot with exacting attention. Today, as always, this man who used to question the efficacy of Brainspotting, despite reporting significant changes between sessions, knows exactly where the pointer should be and comes ready to work. In fact, he had me move it four times, in inch increments, so that it would be in exactly the right spot. Further, he is able to sit in silence, trusting that his system was reorganizing itself, checking in from time to time for validation and help in refocusing.

As you can see, regardless of where people start out, most individuals can and do respond in dramatic ways to the stance and practice of a Brainspotting therapist. That being said, not all individuals can tolerate or benefit from prolonged silence in session. This is particularly true for people with complex trauma. Today, I had the honor of seeing "A", whom I will talk more about in the chapter on Brainspotting and Complex Trauma. We have not worked together for a number of years, and she recently reached out to me to resume treatment. After letting me know what has been happening in her life, "A" became silent, and looked off to her left, with a 1000-mile stare. I sat with her, checking in from time to time, curious about what was happening inside. She began to talk about her persistent negative sense of herself and her fear that she would overwhelm me. Unlike with the other clients/patients I have described here, I was much more verbal, orienting her to the present, maintaining our connection, reframing her comments. For her, a session with a great deal of silence, structured around a visual focal point other than my eyes or her own Gazespot, would have been too activating and triggering.

As you will find, there are many types of silence in clinical sessions. There are times it occurs when all talking ceases spontaneously as the client searches for a word, withdraws into themselves or is simply being present to what is inside of themselves. There are times when silence is indicative of an individual's refusal to speak, to share information, to be known. There are also the times when silence is the natural culmination of a process such as the client being lead in an imaginal or hypnotic state. And, there is the type found in Brainspotting sessions, where there is the implicit understanding that the therapist is journeying with the client/patient to places and spaces inside of them that will organize and reorganize, permitting the unconscious and preconscious material to be met, depotentiated and defused, reducing reactivity and increasing the capacity for connection and transformance.

When thinking about how you will utilize silence in your sessions it is important to consider a few things regarding your clients/patients:

1. imaginal strengths
2. need to connect verbally
3. intellectualizing
4. positive affect tolerance
5. level of dissociation

People who are very concrete or who tend to intellectualize may have a hard time embracing Brainspotting in general and silence in particular. It will take time for them to build up trust in you and in the process. This is where the clinical skills that you have developed over the years will be important. With time, and with your modeling curiosity, even the most concrete individuals can come to experience the power of process.

For those who need to connect verbally, you can welcome their words, and at appropriate points tell them that you really want to hear what is moving in them, and, that you would like for them to just take a nice, deep, easy breath and notice what they are feeling as they share with you. You can acknowledge that it is often hard to slow down and really feel, and that you want them to go at just the right pace for them. You might also ask if they feel that you are understanding them; what they see in your face; how they imagine you are feeling as you are listening to them. These questions can be used the way you might add spices to a dish that you are cooking; slowly, and one at a time so that you can determine their impact. As always, less is more. You want to be responsive to the client/patient, but you also want to model curiosity, compassion and the use of silence.

This reminds me of a wonderful exercise we did at a meditation retreat I attended. It was called "stickey". We were asked to pair up with someone else in the group. Then one person was assigned to have their eyes open while the other closed their eyes. The person with their eyes closed extended their left hand, palm down. The person with their eyes open put their index finger on the back of their partner's hand. We were then instructed to move about the room, the person with their eyes open was to "lead". I have put the word "lead" in quotes as we quickly found out that if the leader was not exquisitely attuned to the "follower" then the pair would become disconnected. In fact, at times it was difficult to determine who was leading and who was following. It is that type of connection that you will discover as you work in silence with Brainspotting.

As noted above, an individual's ability to tolerate positive affect will also impact their ability to work in silence. The greater the tolerance, the greater the capacity to work effectively in the realm of silence. Remarkably, most people who come into our consulting rooms have difficulty tolerating positive affect. Their early wounding has left them with the beliefs and assumptions that they don't deserve good things; that if something good happens something bad will follow. Many are on a positive affect starvation diet. While this does not prevent them from engaging in silence, it can and does limit their ability to heal. Curiosity about how they can begin to expand their capacity to take in good things creates a cornerstone on which to build their new foundations.

Finally, the level of dissociation and degree of complex trauma can and does impact where someone is in the Brainspotting window of tolerance and their ability to work in silence without fragmenting or going into flashback. More will be said about this in another chapter.

For the moment you might want to ponder: how do I know if someone is dissociative, has DID (Dissociative Identity Disorder) or Complex Trauma? If you haven't had advanced training in working with complex trauma and dissociation you probably won't know the answer to this, and I would highly recommend that find some courses and locate someone who can supervise you, as I am certain that if you aren't already working with someone who struggles with these challenges, you will.

I have had the honor of working with a number of people who are DID and have survived unimaginable trauma, often inflicted by people who should have been protecting them. Love was often intermingled with terror, shame, self-hatred and rage. These individuals often switch from one isolated part of themselves to another. In one moment they might be a 50-year-old professional, in the next a 7-year-old child who may or may not know about the 50-year-old but definitely doesn't feel as if they are the same person. For these individuals, orienting to the present moment, meeting flashbacks with insistent calm and reorientation, working with fragmented parts (which will be discussed in another chapter), providing a safe enough connection, consistent caring and a refusal to condemn is the critical first step in healing.

For one client, who switched frequently in session, I recorded myself reading children's books so that she could listen to me between sessions. For another, who switched more outside of session, we imagined the smell of his grandmother's cookies and the look on her face as she greeted him at her door. These were experiences he could carry within himself and offer his triggered parts as needed. For the woman I described above, the brainspot was my eyes, and the sensation of her hand in mine, when she chose to connect to me that way. These are things that she now tells me have carried her through the last two years when it was too painful for her to come in and see me. For the gentleman, the Brainspot was just to the left of center. For both, my voice was a constant reminder of the present moment, an anchor that kept them tethered in the now.

Deeper processing with Brainspotting requires an ability to be in more than one place at the same time; to be just enough in the past so that it is experienced in a tolerable but not overwhelming manner; and in the present, as a caring observer. This is not something at people with complex trauma can do initially. As skills are developed in this area and flashbacks become memories, these individuals will be able to utilize more aspects of Brainspotting and its attendant silence to facilitate healing.

In closing I want to encourage you to play with silence, notice your response to it when you are home alone, when you are walking on the street, when you are interacting with family and friends. What do you feel when you allow yourself to just be present with what is happening inside of you, in the space around you and in the space between yourself and another? How does silence impact the level of connection within yourself, with your environment, with others? What compels you to speak, what are you feeling just before you form words? How will this knowledge impact how you work with your clients? How will it affect the habits you have developed over the course of your professional career? How will it affect your beliefs?

And remember: modulating the amount of silence in your consulting room is a bit like adjusting the "temperature" of the session. You can do this just as you would bath water so that it is just right for the person you are sitting with in that particular moment in time.

[1] In the US we were a taught that it is most respectful to the people we work with to refer to them as clients. Teaching abroad has alerted me the fact that many people in other countries feel that this monetarizes the relationship and makes it feel too much like a business arrangement. With that in mind, I have used both. Please feel free to simply see the one word that resonates for you.

Bibliography

Del Monte, Damir (Lovric), (2016-2018): Numerous conversations and lectures. http://www.damirdelmonte.de/en/home.html

Doidge, Norman, (2003): The Brain that Changes Itself. Viking.

Fosha, Diana, (2011): Lecture on Neurophysiology of Healing NYC

Fosha, Diana, Siegel, Daniel J. and Solomon, Marion, (2009): The Healing Power of Emotion: Affective Neuroscience, Development & Clinical Practice. *Norton Series on Interpersonal Neurobiology.*

Gabbard, Glen O., (2000): A Neurobiologically Informed Perspective On Psychotherapy. *British Journal of Psychiatry, 177.*

Gendlin, E.T., (1957): A Descriptive Introduction to Experiencing. Counseling Center Discussion Papers, 3 (25). *The University of Chicago (Special Collections: Archival Monographs).*

Grand, David, (2002-2008): Conversations, supervision and dissertation review.

Grand, David, (2013): Brainspotting: The Revolutionary New Therapy for Rapid and Effective Change. *Sounds True.*

Kosslyn, Stephen M. and Thompson, William L., (2003): When Is Early Visual Cortex Activated During Visual Mental Imagery? *Psychological Bulletin Vol. 129, No. 5:* Pages 723–746.

Ladany, Nicholas; Hill, Clara E.; Thompson, Barbara J.; O'Brien, Karen M., (2004): Therapist Perspectives on Using Silence in Therapy: A Qualitative Study. *Counselling and Psychotherapy Research, July, Volume 4, Number 1,* Pages:80–89.

Leitch, Laurie M., (2007): Somatic Experiencing Treatment With Tsunami Survivors in Thailand: Broadening the Scope of Early Intervention. *Traumatology, Vol. 13, No. 3;* Pages 11-20.

Lapides, Francine, (2007): Seminar: Clinical Implications and Applications of Psychoneurology: translating neuroscience to the consulting room. *PsyBroadcasting Company Jan 29 – Feb 15.*

Levine, Peter and Frederick, Ann, (1997): Waking the Tiger; Healing Trauma. *North Atlantic Books.*

Levine, Peter, (2005): Healing Trauma: A Pioneering Program for Restoring the Wisdom of Your Body. *Sounds True of Boulder, Colorado.*

Mayberg, Helen S.; Liotti, Mario; Brannan, Stephen K.; McGinnis, Scott; Mahurin, Roderick K.; Jerabek, Paul A.; Silva, J. Arturo; Tekell, Janet L.; Martin, Charles C.; Lancaster, Jack L.; and Fox, Peter T, (1999): Reciprocal Limbic-Cortical Function and Negative Mood: Converging PET Findings in Depression and Normal Sadness. *American Journal of Psychiatry May; 156:* Pages 675-682.

Moss, Richard, (1996-2008): Conversations and Presentations. *Mentor Program and Seminars.*

Ogden, Pat; Minton, Kekuni and Pain, Clare (2006): Trauma and the Body, A Sensorimotor Approach to Psychotherapy. *W.W. Norton and Company.*

Ogden, Pat; Pain, Clare; Minton, Kekuni and Fisher, Janina. Introduction by Allan Schore Ph.D., (2007): Including the Body in Mainstream Psychotherapy for *Traumatized Individuals. To be published in Psychologist Psychoanalyst.*

Ogden, Pat and Minton, Kekuni, (2000): Sensorimotor Psychotherapy: One Method for Processing Traumatic Memory. *Traumatology, October, Volume VI, Issue 3, Article 3.*

Oh, D.H. and Choi, J., (2007): Changes in the Cerebral Perfusion After EMDR. *Journal of EMDR Practice and Research,* 1 (1): Pages 24-30.

Pinco, Susan, (2008): Is It the Talking that Cures? An Exploration of the Role of Silence and Words in the Therapeutic Process.

Rauch, S.L.; Whalen, P. J.; Shin, L. M., et al., (2000): Exaggerated Amygdala Response to Masked Facial Stimuli in Post-Traumatic Stress Disorder: A Functional MRI Study. *Biological Psychiatry,* 47 (9): Pages 769-776.

Rauch, S.; van der Kolk, B.; Fisler, R.; Alpert, N.; Orr, S.; Savage, C., et al., (1996): A Symptom Provocation Study of Posttraumatic Stress Disorder Using Positron Emission Tomography and Script-Driven Imagery. *Archives of General Psychiatry, 53:* Pages 380–387.

Servan-Schreiber, David, (2003,2004): The Instinct to Heal, Curing Depression, Anxiety and Stress Without Drugs and Without Talk Therapy. *Rondale Publishers.*

Schore, Allan, (2003): Affect Regulation and the Repair of the Self. *W.W. Norton.*

Schore, Allan, (2005): A Neuropsychoanalytic Viewpoint Commentary on Paper by Steven H. Knoblauch. *Psychoanalytic Dialogues, 15(6):* Pages 829–854.

Siegel, Daniel, (1999): The Developing Mind. How Relationships and the Brain interact to Shape who we are. *Gilford Press.*

Siegel, Daniel, (2005): Presentation. *Evolution of Psychotherapy Conference.*

Siegel, Daniel, (2006): A Week of Silence. *Psychotherapy Networker, November/December 206:* Pages 34-41.

Waterworth, J.A., (2002): Consciousness, Action and Designed Virtual Space: Linking Information Technology, The Mind and Human Creativity. *Paper In Borillo and Goulette (eds), "Cognition et creation: Explorations cognitives des processus de conception".* Sprimont, Belgium:Mardaga.

Complete Bibliography available at: https://www.coherentself.com/BibliographyforChapteronSilenceinBrainspotting.en.html

Grief and Brainspotting Therapy

Deborah Antinori

Beginnings and Endings

As I contemplate the subject of grief in starting this chapter, of course, my own losses come to mind. David Grand taught my class of US Trainers to have participants tell their Brainspotting Story during their introductions at the beginning of Phase 1 trainings. So, I'll begin by saying I am keenly aware it is exactly sixteen years ago today that my mother was declared "terminal" with liver cancer by her oncologist. I felt a kind of shock and anxiety upon hearing this news that I had never felt before – it was unthinkable. Then came nineteen days in hospice watching the process of a beautiful life coming to an end. My lovely, elegant mom died two days after Christmas. We only get one mother. I'm an only child and we were very close.

A complicating factor in the loss of my mother was that it occurred in the "9/11 era". Dr. Grand speaks of "existential trauma" which people experience when an unthinkable event occurs like 9/11 - terrorist attacks and natural disasters that affect many people simultaneously. My mom went back to her regular oncologist literally on 9/11 in 2001 in her hometown in Massachusetts (MA). Her oncology specialist had moved from MA to a teaching hospital in Long Island, New York. One must navigate the many bridges and highways leading to New York City to reach Long Island from New England. With the post-9/11 events of constant bridge closings precipitated by the appearance of "suspicious vehicles" in the days, weeks and months following the terrorist attacks, my mom opted to stay with her local doctors.

There is a niggling doubt in my mind, had she been able to get to her specialist in Long Island, we might have caught this second deadly bout of cancer in time. I will never know for sure. So the loss of my mom is, for me, a 9/11-related existential loss. I wonder how many other people had some kind of connection to 9/11 with a loss – not as a direct result of the attacks, but as a possible consequence of that day and the events that unfolded because of it. I was reluctant to speak of this back in that era because others had "worse" and direct losses due to 9/11 – losing someone who was in the Trade Towers, or a First Responder – a policeman, a fireman. This is a kind of "shared existential" loss. I wonder how many other people lost someone in this indirect type of 9/11 loss similar to my mother's situation, or perhaps experienced a devastating event on that exact day in 2001 or in the "9/11 era" – deaths from an accident, a disease, suicide or murder. And how many received a serious diagnosis for themselves or a close friend or family member, lost a job, or were divorced on 9/11 or in the "9/11 era"?

An initial cancer diagnosis can give a "50 Shades of Loss" experience with the shock of finding that you or your loved one has cancer for the first time and waiting for the "other shoe to drop" ever after. And when you join the dreaded Cancer Club as a patient or family member, the new reference point in time ensues – life before and life after a cancer diagnosis. And nothing compares to the final days of hospice. You see things you have never seen before, and never want to see again. Things you wouldn't wish on your worst enemy.

I wrote a poem, "Now I'm One of Those People" as if I were in one of those "made-for-TV" movies, as we call them in the US, featuring the painful juxtaposition of the bright happy month of December holiday festivities and the unfathomable reality of a hospice facility room where Mom is dying.

So these are my first feelings and thoughts as I begin writing. This is who I am in my grief-history and how it molded me - this loss, and a myriad of other losses before and after my mom's death. This is who sits in front of bereaved clients, or those with anticipatory loss who know that death is imminent for their loved one, or themselves. An area rife for Limbic Countertransference, loss is something everyone has or will experience - no one gets away with a "loss-less life".

And what a loaded area for attachment issues – the experience of loss and grief is the natural byproduct of living a life. We find the excruciating pain of separation when the finality of death rips into our attachment experience and history to the beloved who has died. Here is fertile ground for the earliest of experiences in attachment for love, safety, and survival, all of which are evolutionarily programmed into us – to avoid death for ourselves and our loved ones at all cost. These are genetically determined circuits for love, caring, nurturance and survival of the species which Jaak Panksepp explicates beautifully in his seminal work, Affective Neuroscience: The Foundations of Human and Animal Emotions (1998) which I will return to later. Grief is the consequence for love and connection. And for those with a difficult relationship to the deceased, complicated grief can result. Neglect, physical and/or emotional abuse, alcohol and drug use by the parent, or abandonment being experienced at the hands of the now deceased can engender powerful feelings, bodily sensations and physiological symptoms for the bereaved. The yearned for connection the bereaved never received from the one they have lost is never possible in this physical world. The hope that they may have held out for some kind of "turn" or reparations made by the person who is now deceased, is gone forever.

With my mother's illness and death, I experienced what Therese Rando would term the loss of my "Assumptive World", a Secondary Loss containing our "mental schema about ourselves, life, the world and everything and everyone in it" (Rando, 2000). Basically, what we rely on day to day to get through our lives, despite the fact we know cognitively that things can change in the blink of an eye due to circumstances out of our control. A world where it was possible for my healthy, slim, happy mother to even get cancer in the first place, and to then die from liver cancer six years later was shattering to my Assumptive World. Add to this to the fact that my mom passed at the age of seventy-six whereas her grandmother lived to be ninety-six and her parents each were eighty-eight when they passed. At a time in our culture where everyone is espousing how much longer people are living these days, I was shocked, angry, and devastated that my mother died "young".

While I am a No-Assumptions Brainspotting therapist, I have had a devil of a time with my Assumptive World regarding the long-lived relatives in my ancestral family tree and my mother's relatively early demise. This Assumptive World of mine began before explicit memory was online. It began from birth, with my great-grandmother and grandparents as a part of my daily life. David Grand speaks of pre-verbal trauma, here we have pre-verbal Assumptive World, with attendant attachment and bonding experiences firing together and wiring together. These elders, from my first experiences in the world, were healthy, independent and lived a LONG time. To me, my mother at seventy-six did not live a LONG time. Turning to our clients' experiences and histories – death and loss produce a deeply nested configuration of assumptions, beliefs, and feelings with their anchors in subcortical brain regions. Our subcortical brain is where the neural precursors to thoughts, beliefs and assumptions lie. And the limbic cortex/mammalian brain is where attachment and bonding are located and experienced in the brain.

Grief and Grocery Lists

The subject of grief is the stuff of a book rather than a single chapter, so I will focus mainly on grief resulting from death in this chapter. I will also address Pet Loss as it is a specialty of mine. Rather than attempt to travel the vast landscape the wide net of grief and loss catch, I will make a small "grocery list" here of loss experiences which includes, but is not limited to:

Death – attendant attachment issues, activity of daily living disruption and reorganization, funeral and memorial arrangements, estate disbursement and on-going management, feelings, memories, the year of "firsts" without the beloved.

How the death occurred – sudden and unexpected, long trajectory of illness before death, "before one's time", i.e. children, teens, young twenties, accident, murder, suicide, ambiguous – missing persons or pets, abduction/kidnapping, MIA in wartime.

Relationships – impact on the daily life and on-going life experience without the family member:

Family Loss – mother, father, step-mother or father, in-laws, children (biological, adopted, foster, god-child), grandparents, great-grandparents, niece, nephew, cousin, sibling, aunt, uncle.

"Tribe" members – friends, doctor, therapist, coworker, pastor/priest/rabbi/imam or other religious or spiritual leader.

Type of relationship to the deceased – mostly satisfying or tumultuous and anywhere in-between.

Infertility issues – trials with fertility treatment.

Abortion, miscarriage.

Divorce, separation, estrangement.

Loss due to displacement – war; genocide; natural disaster (earthquake, fire, flood); becoming a refugee; losing one's home/becoming homeless due to financial situation, urban renewal, highway construction, or due to one's age or health status and need for supervisory care.

Miscellaneous – Loss of job; loss of social role; loss of limb or breast; hysterectomy; loss of abilities due to accident, disease or advancing age.

The above can surely have additions made to it. With grocery lists, we often come out of the store with more in our grocery bags than was on the actual list. It can make the bags heavy requiring more trips into the house to unload, and sometimes the refrigerator doesn't seem big enough to hold it all. Unpacking a loss of any kind surely finds the buried "treasure" of previous losses. This is certainly a feature of working with Brainspotting as the subcortical machinery finds relevant memories, implicit or explicit, which are lying in wait to be rescued. Loss is a "tuning fork event" and a current loss will set up a vibration in our system, an oscillation of a certain Hertz that calls out all those experiences that are resonating on the same note (Antinori, 2010).

The Longer Goodbye

We, in the Western World, live in a culture that worships the young, the physically fit, the financially successful, and are bombarded with commercial images of airbrushed models brandishing a standard of perfection that is anything but natural. With death and grief there is no airbrushing to make a pretty picture from which to aspire or to distract ourselves from the inevitable effects of time on our frail human anatomy.

In so many ways, we are not the society that we used to be, that our ancestors experienced for thousands of years as hunter/gatherers and then substance farmers. We belong to a society, since the Industrial Revolution, which has advanced in a technological manner that is so diametrically opposed to our natural biological rhythms and the rituals of our predecessors that we are in uncharted territory when it comes to grief and trauma.

The rituals of the more recent past signaled to those around us that we were bereaved and embraced many aspects of the death, dying and grief processes. Outwardly, the bereaved wore black for a year as a symbol of their altered state of consciousness. Actively, we shepherded our dead at each step of the process of death, often at home including the attentions necessary due to the illness, accident or other circumstances surrounding the death. Preparing the body of the loved one for wake/viewing, funeral and burial, and tending the gravesite were done by the family.

Today our loved one often dies in the hospital, the body is sent to a funeral home where it is embalmed or prepared naturally and buried in a cemetery, or the body is cremated and placed in an urn or scattered. We are not "hands on" with our dead, and so are removed from traditional ways the cultures we descended from dealt with many aspects of loss from death. These ministrations to the dying and care for the body post-mortem gave our brains needed motor and social activity, real-time with the changing state of the body of the beloved in the familiar context of the home. The other daily activities of living had to be simultaneously incorporated into the necessities of attending to each detail of the transition of the loved one in the process of dying, the moment of death, and the care and preparation for burial of the body. The bereaved were often not alone, extended family and community pitching in to assist the mourning family. This all took time, focus and cooperation – it was a longer goodbye to the deceased than we experience today.

Hospice and Brainspotting, Not-So-Distant Cousins

Our modern world has thankfully given us hospice care which offers us opportunities to be with our loved one during the dying process with comfort measures made through palliative care for the dying and ministrations to the family who may assist in the care and are present to the process. Hospice nurses and social workers assist the family either at home or in a facility to care for the loved one who is in the process of dying. I posit that we, as Brainspotting therapists, are an extension of this hospice philosophy and palliative care measures as we sit with our clients during the process of their feelings and expressions of grief.

Hospice attunes to the changing and sometimes moment-by-moment needs of the dying, and we as Brainspotting therapists attune to the client in their uprooted Assumptive World, where the context of their lives and their sense of time and place have become suspended and surreal. Here relationship and being attuned is of the most elegant importance. As David Grand says, "When you think you need an intervention, think relationship. I could say it a hundred times, I'll only say it thirty-six times." (2014) Being in the Tail of the Comet as we accompany the mourner on the roller-coater ride of grief through feelings of shock, sadness, anger, regret, gratitude and remembrance is likely our most helpful stance.

The Uncertainly Principle guides every step in this new world without the client-mourner's loved one – that despised "New Normal" they confront each moment. Here is where I believe we would best accompany the mourner, silently, as they sit in the unthinkable, the unbelievable – that their loved one is gone forever as they knew them. With Brainspotting, no words have to be exchanged and if we speak, it is in attunement with the client or in response to them. With a bereaved client we might indeed ask ourselves, "Why Am I Talking?" (W.A.I.T.) Our client may often hear, "He's in a better place now", "Her suffering is over", or "Your son is with God now", from those friends and associates with the best of intentions. Yet during those exchanges, the bereaved can feel very alone and misunderstood. They may even feel there is something wrong with them that they can't "get with" the fact that the suffering is over for their loved one, while their own suffering has gone far beyond a 10 on the Subjective Units of Disturbance Scale (SUDs) (Wolpe, 1969) with its numerical rating of 10 (worst) to 0 (nothing). It can be hard for friends and family members to sit with the bereaved in their sadness, or their frozen stupor and just BE with them - to endure with them without adding advise, a platitude, or their own rendition of how they have felt and coped with loss.

We, as Brainspotting therapists, can sit with "W.A.I.T." as our mantra. To accompany someone as they either talk about their beloved dead, or to sit with them in what David Grand has described as "The Million Mile Stare" (Grand, 2009) and be with them in this place, is to be in attunement. As soon as mourning clients leave our office, they are oftentimes running errands, rushing off to work, and shuttling their kids to soccer practice, or maybe visiting the widowed parent now left alone in Assisted Living. Where is the time to sit, to be quiet, or to go over the details of the loss, to remember the life of the one who has passed and feel the enormity of all it brings? And who will sit with them for as long as they need to do this, perhaps over and over again? We, as Brainspotting practitioners, will.

I contend that the Million Mile Stare is the place where we might break the "W.A.I.T." stance to suggest the client linger their gaze if they move off of such an obvious visual magnet. More than any other Brainspotting set up, the Gazespot may be the most natural and appropriate spot to harness when our client is in the "stupor" of grief. There in the longing and yearning for the loved one, wishing to turn back time, trying to absorb all that has occurred in the trajectory of "life with" - to "the death of" - and finally to "life without", our bereaved clients may evidence a pronounced Gazespot. Here we sit in a very mammalian stance just as we see elephants congregating over the body of a member of their herd. Why would they do this? What do evolution and the mammalian brain know that our neocortical minds and fast paced society don't? What signals and other non-verbal mammalian communication are we giving out when we sit quietly with one so wounded who has lost their mother, their spouse, or their child? It sounds so simple, yet is so hard for people to do. A woman told me that a month after her mother died, a coworker remarked – "Aren't you over that yet?" To which she answered, "The last I checked, my mother was still dead."

Thanatology and Grief Counseling Thoughts

As a Fellow in Thanatology from The Association for Death Education and Counseling, I am grateful for this Association and the work of the many pioneering authors in the areas of death, dying, palliative care and grief counseling. In our Western World "grief phobic" society, the bereaved can suffer from the judgments and comments of others depending on their ranking in a hierarchy ranging from culturally accepted to marginalized losses. The seminal work of Ken Doka (1989), gave us the concept of "disenfranchised grief" which is out of the realm of conventionally sanctioned mourning – miscarriages, still born babies, sibling loss, pet loss and the loss of the gravely ill or elderly have been considered disenfranchised losses among others. Though there is more understanding for these losses currently, there can still be minimization of the loss or a climate of "time to move on" because this loss was expected, or not deemed as important as other types of losses. I will discuss both sibling and pet loss, later in this chapter.

Robert Neimeyer spearheaded the "meaning-making" movement in grief counseling "...the goal is the re-establishment of a (sufficiently) coherent self-narrative and resolution of the incongruence between the reality of the loss and one's sense of meaning." (Neimeyer, et al. 2010) Within the current climate of grief counseling, clients are often encouraged to find "meaning and context" which is helpful and healing when it coincides with the client's timing. When organic, spontaneous neocortical executive and associative brain functions occur, that is the client's timing – not the timing of the therapist, friend or family member.

Meaning-making may be very helpful to the griever at the right time - when it comes from the griever themselves. Meaning making involves neocortical processing and focal attention the brain may not be capable of in the early phases of grief. In fact, in any given moment the mourner's more intense grief can be retriggered. Perhaps a song comes on the radio that they associate with the deceased or the day that the loved one died; or it could be the one, two or any-month anniversary of the death; birthdays and anniversaries of many types (first meeting, wedding, surgeries, first diagnoses) – all can trigger waves of raw feelings. Many events, sights, sounds and smells may kindle the mourner's nervous system and bring them back to the deep feelings of the early days of bereavement, and their cognitive functions can suffer at these times.

The neocortex lags behind subcortical development in evolution, in utero and in infant to adulthood brain development. The best functioning of our neocortex is in concert with the subcortical brain which lies at the foundation of our thoughts, ideas, plans, goals, beliefs and assumptions. The adage, "Don't plan a big change for a year after a significant death", is wise counsel. Our neocortical assessments are certainly colored by recent events of the loss and projections into the future that may not serve us best in the long run. This is hippocampal territory – context, time and place appropriateness and relevance. A significant loss changes us, so that the "me" we are right after a loss and the "me" we become in time can have very different needs and goals after the adjustment over time to day-to-day life without the deceased.

Grief engages the pain centers housed "in our deep limbic system" (Amen, 2016). The very pained and tortured griever may be left alone in an isolation chamber, deemed not ready for certain types of therapy yet. Add to this that a precise diagnosis may decree, "There can't be PTSD if it hasn't been three months since the death", leaving the client to be micromanaged in treatment planning that is unattuned and unhelpful.

Where there are no words, so no helpful talk therapy; where there is no impetus for movement, so no helpful gestalt, creative arts, somatic expression or other action-oriented therapies - this is where Brainspotting is an optimal fit. Sitting with someone in attunement can be the best medicine. With the relevant eye position (when that time is right/welcomed by the client) we can accompany the grieving client in not over-thinking, or perhaps not thinking at all. The more neocortically focused methods of therapy or premature meaning-making interventions may be well-intended, but can be ill-timed.

With attunement, we are also not leaving the bereaved alone in the abyss that the so-called "natural loss experience" may predispose friends and family to let the bereaved "be", assuming they need time alone. This is more akin to being in solitary confinement than having desired "alone time". And if the client is assessed as not "ready" for therapy as mentioned above, it implies that they must follow the therapist's assessment and treatment modality or protocol, not their own inner pacing and timing. Here the tail is wagging the dog or in Brainspotting terms, the Tail is Wagging the Comet. The indoctrination of therapeutic disciplines we have learned in programs of psychology, counseling and post-grad institutes is that we, as therapists, must know when and how to manage the client with diagnoses and treatment plans (Grand, 2018). If we impose these protocols and interventions on a grieving client who is already overloaded with the directives of the Western World to "get on with it", how can we claim to be an agent of healing, compassion and care? In fact, the "outcome measures" we are trying to achieve are not accomplished with the armature of many so-called therapeutic interventions, however well meaning or Evidence-Based they may be.

If we are with the bereaved client, in the Tail of the Comet, following where they go subcortically into the deep recesses of their brilliant brain that is in a "self-dialogue" (del Monte, 2016, 2017), we are, I theorize, respecting our evolutionary programs for recovery after loss. With attunement and, when appropriate, with the relevant eye position, the client and therapist together seem to locate a system in the brain that is not only innate, but genetically predetermined to assist the brain in balancing itself, with its ability to incorporate new experience, to adapt and to seek homeostasis (White, 2015). Perhaps this healing in the grief experience can have a less painful or debilitating trajectory, one that is natural, that neither pushes nor abandons the client. Perhaps that is what Brainspotting provides for grieving clients. And any meaning-making that emerges from the client is under their own steam, unprompted by the therapist.

Grief and the Brain

My work with Brainspotting Therapy has involved my intense curiosity about and study of the neurobiology of the brain – its anatomy, circuits, wiring and unique expressions in each one of us as individuals and as a human species evolutionarily. I will look at the work of a few neuroscientists, psychologists and psychiatrists with theories about brain function from which I have been fortunate to benefit. These include most importantly Dr. Damir del Monte who explicates the work of Bud Craig (2015) and Craig's mentor, Wilfrid Janig (2006), on the importance of the insula for the specificity of what and how we feel, and the "material me".

Dr. del Monte cites Antonio Damasio (2010) for his explanation of our embodied self with somatic markers in the body. Brainspotting, as David Grand reminds us, gets access to the subcortical brain most efficiently through the body. It is the felt sense of the body, experienced and represented to a large extent in the insula, deep in the limbic cortex which gives access into and information about the dysregulation clients bring into therapy. The insula has a type of homunculus which receives multiple inputs from the body including information about interoception from the internal reporting of our body including the viscera (heart, stomach, intestines, lungs, kidneys) through two pathways, Lamina 1 in the spinal cord and the Nucleus of the Solitary Tract in the brainstem (Craig, 2015). The fact that there are these two distinct pathways carrying information from the same areas of the body highlights the importance of this information as evolution has conserved two ways of doing basically the same thing - not a common anatomical occurrence (del Monte, 2016, 2017).

Information is brought to the insula about exteroception from the senses (information coming into the body from the external environment – sights, sounds, smell, touch, taste); about homeostasis from the amygdala and hypothalamus; about context, orientation in time and place from the hippocampus; and about our social rules, behavior, sensing, empathy, and our regulation from the ventral medial PreFrontal Cortex (vmPFC), Orbital Frontal Cortex (OFC), and Anterior Cingulate Cortex (ACC). Additionally, the insula receives information from the reward and motivational centers in the Nucleus Accumbens, an area of the Basal Ganglia (BG – "the heart of the limbic system") (del Monte, 2016, 2017). All of this information moves along the structure of the insula, picking up contributions from these inputs starting at the posterior insula, moving to medial and finally anterior insula. This information is synthesized and then carried to the relevant areas of the brain for further processing, regulation, and computation that influences our actions, behaviors, emotions and thoughts (Craig, 2015).

Our multitasking insula with its exacting specificity of the feel of ourselves and our body is getting a range of signals from our body and environment via these many channels. When there is a loss, the context for our life as we've known it has been ripped from us (hippocampal challenge to incorporate the new and rapidly changing context of our life without the beloved) and our internal organs are dysregulated (can't eat or over eat, rapid heart beat, shallow breathing, disrupted or no sleep). All of the systems detailed above are reporting the status of the specific feeling of ourselves to the insula. And that status has become challenged and even foreign to the bereaved in their experience of loss.

Our bond with the loved one has been broken as the Oxytocin "feel good" peptide hormone is shut down and cortisol flows. We may feel alarm, fear, uncertainty, shock, or anxiety. Oxytocin is a cortisol antagonist, having the capability of shutting down the production of cortisol (del Monte, 2016, 2017). This may be one of the reasons we see some form of a funeral across cultures. Funerals and memorial services bring together family and friends, the tribe who can feed the hungry Oxytocin receptors that are starved for something that can feel good while the mourner is facing this immediate, unwanted loss.

We have our current theories of how the Brainspotting process harnesses orienting and homeostatic functions of the brain. Included in these theories are Corrigan and Grand's (2013) identification of the Superior Colliculus (SC) in the midbrain section of the brainstem having a significant role in Brainspotting Therapy since it is a "First Responder" in orienting to threat. The SC is seen as the "bookmark to the midbrain" (Corrigan & Grand , 2013) and is theorized to begin the process of the brain's ability to initiate a satisfactory completion of the truncated orientation to the trauma in the brain. Jaak Panksepp (1998) further states the importance of midbrain engagement in therapy asserting that to have lasting helpful neuroplastic results, there must be midbrain engagement. David Grand emphasizes that Brainspotting Therapy aims to directly "drop the client subcortically" (Grand, 2018). Where other therapies may happen upon the subcortex, Brainspotting has subcortical engagement as a primary objective of the therapy.

The SC is the fast/survival-oriented track to the Primary Visual Cortex (del Monte, 2016, 2017). This is of particular significance to our work with the relevant eye position as other less urgent visual information goes to the thalamus first before being sent on to the Primary Visual Cortex. The SC is the first area for integration of visual signals. Every other sense (other than smell which goes directly to the amygdala), touch, taste, non-urgent visual, visceral and auditory signals go to the thalamus first before further relay to relevant brain areas. The urgent visual signal gets a kind of preferential treatment in four visual layers of the seven-layered SC (the other three layers being auditory, tactile and visceral). I would posit we are working with something unique in the SC by utilizing eye position and the visual field for traumatic material. Evolution has treated visual signals which require rapid and immediate attention for survival in a singular manner in the SC in our brainstem. Additionally, fifty percent of the brain is dedicated to visual processing (Amen, 2018).

Regarding relational attunement, we have theories from Damir del Monte (2016, 2017) regarding regulation through relationship/attachment and the neurochemical systems of the "feel good" chemicals produced as a result of positive social engagement – Oxytocin, Dopamine, and endogenous opioids. With repeated contact of the therapist and client in therapy, a new experience and context for the presenting distress, disturbance or trauma make for new neural connections in the brain that allow for homeostatic functions to resume and survival programs to quiet.

The therapeutic relationship can facilitate regulatory mechanisms in the limbic cortex to down-regulate the stress-axis (hypothalamus to pituitary to adrenal resulting in the release of cortisol) and the alarm-sounding amygdala. The amygdala is the original assessor of safety, danger/threat before our PreFrontal Cortex (PFC) is able to make calculated conclusions. The amygdala, and other subcortical structures, have a 50ms firing capability while the PFC has a 500-600ms rate of firing to come to consciousness (Cozolino, 2011). Another fact pointing to the inefficiency of cognitive neocortical attempts to regulate survival instincts is that the PFC has an indirect connection, one neural pathway to the amygdala and hypothalamus to try to "talk them down". The PFC with its conscious executive functions (rational, linear thinking, goal and decision making, understanding consequences) is not the most efficient, effective or rapid way to achieve down-regulation of the amygdala and the survival programs it initiates (del Monte 2016, 2017).

The dense connections to the amygdala, hypothalamus and PAG (periaqueductal grey) (assessor/alarm system, stress axis/cortisol factory mechanisms and survival programs, respectively) are those from the agranular isocortex (missing the fourth granular layer found in the granular isocortex/neocortex, hence "agranular") and allocortex (the "older" cortex housed in the limbic system). These dense regulatory connections include the OrbitalFrontal Cortex (OFC), the Anterior Cingulate Cortex (ACC), and the ventromedial PreFrontal Cortex (vmPFC) in the agranular isocortex; and the insula, and hippocampus in the allocortex (del Monte, 2016, 2017). These are the areas, Dr. del Monte (2016) states, "we are accessing when we are in a good relationship in the therapy with a client" - when we are attuned and in the Tail of the Comet. These areas are able to regulate our hyperarousal, where the granular isocortex with its functions of higher order cognitive processing and language is not – it is simply not the "job description" of that part of the neocortex.

With threat, the central amygdala will signal the hypothalamus to activate the stress axis, the HPA-Axis – Hypothalamus, to Pituitary to Adrenal - with the final result being the production of cortisol. However, if the hippocampus has given the signal to the lateral and basal parts of the amygdala to inhibit the central amygdala, the "fire alarm" is effectively shut off (del Monte 2016, 2017). This requires optimal functioning of the hippocampus regarding assessment of the current situation and its relevance to archived memories regarding safety or danger. So if you think about it – in grief, the poor hippocampus who usually encodes and retrieves memories in a reasonably optimal manner, is very challenged in trying to put a fitting context onto the "new normal" of life without the loved one. The hippocampus is struggling with time, place, memories, and any trauma connected with the death or illness of the loved one. The poor hippocampus is having one heck of a time doing its many faceted job. So the central amygdala may be running like an out-of-control child, without the parental controls of the hippocampal signals to the lateral and basal aspects of the amygdala to CALM DOWN that central amygdala – to tell it that "it's ok".

But it's not ok, it's anything but ok – the loved one is dead, forever. Here is where the attunement to the client is key as it elicits our attachment system deep in the limbic brain, in the Social Engagement system as Porges (2011) terms it. The Brainspotting Therapist sits quietly, with the bereaved client, as those newly forming neural circuits are doing their best to re-contextualize and restructure the experiences of the bereaved client and their forever-changed world. We sit with the client as their hippocampus, with its contextual and temporal contributions to memory goes through the paces this client's grief dictates.

The good news is that the hippocampus is a subcortical structure with the capacity for great neuroplasticity and even neurogenesis. It is designed to update and adapt to a changing world. Perhaps it is one of the key players in the fact that our species has been able to survive for hundreds of thousands of years despite our wobbly bipedal, thin-skinned, no fangs/no claws physical fragility. Throughout evolution our ancestors survived harsh environmental conditions, food and water scarcity, fierce animals, warring tribes, and they responded and adapted. With loss and grief, the hippocampus takes on the changed context of our Assumptive World, of our relational experience and assists us in adaptation to a world without the deceased.

Primary Emotions: The Work of Jaak Panksepp

As I mentioned earlier, Jaak Panksepp, developer of the field of Affective Neuroscience, details the primary emotions that we experience as humans and which we share with our mammalian "relatives" in his seminal work, Affective Neuroscience: The Foundations of Human and Animal Emotions (1998), and the brilliant follow-up, The Archaeology of Mind: Neuroevolutionary Origins of Human Emotions (2012). Panksepp has established seven primary emotions in humans and mammals which he describes in capital letters as SEEKING, RAGE, FEAR, PANIC/GRIEF, PLAY, LUST, and CARE. These primary emotions follow particular neural circuits that are distinct and are present in all mammals and humans.

Panksepp finds grief to be a physiological expression of the neural circuit of PANIC, the primary feature of which is the experience of separation anxiety. He delineates FEAR from PANIC/GRIEF yet both circuits can be involved in grief and anticipatory loss situations. PANIC/GRIEF follows a distinct neural circuit in the brain that is differentiated from the FEAR circuit, the latter of which is in essence an "aversive state in the nervous system" which is conserved in evolution to insure our survival – to fear that which could kill us or our progeny (Panksepp, 1998).

The FEAR circuit is found in the central amygdala and the PAG (periaqueductal gray) of the midbrain as was cited above in the section on the brain. (The PAG is discussed extensively in the Corrigan and Grand articles in Medical Hypotheses, 2013, 2015; and in Dr. del Monte's video series with Lecturio.de, 2017). Panksepp finds "multiple neural systems that can make us afraid…fear of heights, fear of pain, fear of predators, etc." (Panksepp 1998). The fear of losing our loved one in the case of anticipatory loss can produce anxiety and exhaustion in the caregiver. It is a roller coaster ride of crisis events followed by plateau periods. The caregiver's nervous system is constantly kindled in response to these predictably (expected in the course of a disease or with aging) yet unpredictable (in their timing) occurrences.

Turning to the PANIC/GRIEF system, Panksepp finds separation distress to be a key feature, and it is neurochemically distinct from the FEAR system. He found this distinction in the work of psychiatrist Donald Klein in the early 1960's when the tricyclic antidepressant imipramine was first utilized for panic attacks. In Klein's observations, patients reported fewer panic attacks but stated they were "no better". The patients' fear of having a panic attack persisted though the actual number of panic attacks was significantly less. The fear of the fear, the "anticipatory anxiety" persisted despite the actual diminishment of panic attack events (Panksepp, 1998). Therefore, FEAR and PANIC are two distinct neural systems.

Pankseep describes grief being experienced as sadness, weeping, depression and longing for the loved one as a part of the PANIC circuit. When separated from their mothers, young animals will make Distress Vocalizations (DVs) to assist the mother in finding the youngster. At some point, the DVs stop since repeated attempts to attract the mother have failed – now the young might be alerting predators to their whereabouts. A kind of torpor-like quiet sets in to conserve energy, giving time for the mother's eventual return, hopefully with food. This has been suggested as a biological precursor to the development of depression, its origins being that of survival in shutting down systems that require energy (Panksepp, 1998). The brain wants to be in homeostasis and to conserve energy (White, 2015). In this most desperate situation, the only option the young animal has is to stay alive until the mother's hopeful return. Looking to our human experience, with the death of our loved one, that return never occurs.

Studies of young birds have found that touch can quell DVs. Young birds separated from their mothers ceased their DVs when sitting in the hand of a researcher with the other hand over the bird's back. Connection, attachment and the physical reassurance of touch elicit a calming response (Panksepp, 1998). With Brainspotting, we do not physically touch the client. However, the Dual Attunement Frame provides containment, sometimes with a "tightened frame" around the client to more effectively and specifically provide the place for the brain-body to find its way to homeostasis.

We tighten the frame in a variety of ways including using the Body Resource Spot, the more resourced spot on the Z-axis, and the Resource Eye with One Eye Brainspotting (with goggles). Additionally, moving into the client's field of vision or using the Eye Contact Spot when dissociation or flashback is occurring tightens the frame. And, of course, our attunement to the client is the ultimate resource within the Dual Attunement Frame, along with the clients' own survival instincts (Grand, 2018).

Given the primary mammalian emotions born of evolutionarily programmed brain circuits Panksepp so beautifully delineates, Brainspotting offers a most natural manner with which to harness the innate regulatory systems of the brain. These regulatory functions return the brain's desired state of homeostasis and conservation of energy. While the PANIC/GRIEF and FEAR circuits are conserved in evolution to be adaptive, in the course of grief in our modern society, a type of "maladaptive homeostasis" (Grand, 2018) or overly stabilized firing (del Monte, 2017) may ensue. This overly stabilized pattern of brain firing needs instability in order to develop a new rhythm or new stability that is healthy and promotes those prime directives of brain balance and conserved energy. The introduction of a Brainspot to a grieving client, might provide the element of instability as the visual field is harnessed in concert with the client's felt sense of dysregulation (overly stabilized/synchronous firing). The processing time on the Brainspot may offer this time of "instability" as we see the SUDs decrease in numeric value and the location of the body disturbance ease.

Grief and Resource Brainspotting

I have offered the idea that Gazespotting is a natural and effective resourced way to begin the Brainspotting process with a bereaved individual. Additionally, the Body Resource can be utilized to provide a "softer" access for such raw emotions and the forever changed situation that death confronts us with. As well as being a gentler access point for the difficult feelings engendered by bereavement, the Body Resource offers a tool to find that place in the body that feels "calm, centered grounded", or "neutral", or just a bit better in contrast to what is activated or doesn't feel good. While this is, of course, used in the session to find the Brainspot, it can be utilized at home by the client to turn their attentional networks to what feels even just a bit better for them. In the midst of feeling grief, one can simultaneously tune into a part of the body that actually feels better, or even feels good. It is this repetition over time that builds the new neural network (fire together-wire together) and the beginning of feeling better naturally.

I'd like to suggest Dr. Grand's Gridwork (2009) as a way to work with the bereaved, and a tool that the client can bring home and utilize along with Biolateral Sound recordings. With Gridwork, Dr. Grand invites the client to find a Body Resource, usually with eyes closed. This Body Resource is found along a continuum of either calm, grounded, centered; or neutral; or just somewhat better than the disturbance or activation the client is experiencing. He then asks the client to let another such spot "pop" that has the same kind of calm, grounded, centered feeling or neutral feeling or better sensation than the disturbance/activation. The two Body Resource Spots are joined by an internal line "drawn" by the client in any manner they like. This process is repeated until there are four or five such Body Resource Spots connected with lines drawn internally. He suggests if they like, the client can add a soothing or healing color to that line connecting the Gridwork Body Resource Spots. He has them trace this line several times slowly. A "faucet" can be suggested for anything that doesn't feel good to find its way out - several of these faucets can be placed along the Gridwork line if the client feels so inclined. In session, Dr. Grand will then sometimes ask the client to open their eyes and locate the Brainspot spontaneously. Alternately you could use Inside or Outside Window, or Inside/Outside combo to find the Brainspot in the visual field. I have used this Gridwork often with clients with great results - decreasing of SUDs and clients reporting bodily sensations that were disturbing or painful being decreased or gone.

Recently in a Phase 2 training, two trainee-therapists related how they would never have been able to tolerate the processing of their losses without the use of the Resource Spot. (Note, permission given by both trainees to discuss their work in this chapter.) This occurred for the individual doing the demo for the Advanced Resource Model – Resource within a Resource within a Resource (Resource Eye using goggles, Resource Body Spot found with Inside Window with the pointer, and Resource Spot on the Z-axis). The practicum that followed gave the other bereaved Phase 2 trainee an opportunity to process with the Advanced Resource Model. Both of these trainees lost a sibling, which can be a disenfranchised loss as I mentioned earlier in this chapter. Several authors have recently written books about sibling loss including those with their own experiences as a bereaved sibling. There was a time when no such books could be found. Perhaps there is an unconscious assumption that sibling rivalry makes sibling loss a "lesser loss", but this is not the case.

The myriad of losses experienced when a sibling dies, including one's childhood history within the family and connection to parents (possibly deceased,) can engender the feeling that the history is somehow gone or forever changed. A sibling "gets" their experience in that family in a way that no one else quite can. Someone else who "knows from the inside" about this family and its history, without even speaking, is gone. A traumatic element can be present - losing someone from one's own generation, possibly out of the trajectory of regular life expectancy, too early, too soon. The Assumptive World is rocked – "It'll be us sibs when Mom and Dad die". No, now it won't.

These Phase 2 trainees were adamant they could never have tolerated returning to those sibling losses unless they were on a Resource Spot. It worked out well that the Advanced Resource Model provided not only a Resource Spot but the ultimate "nested" Resource Spot. One participant wrote, " It shifted my energy and felt as though I could truly let go of all the pain I was carrying around for 6 years. It was a gentle process and felt completely safe. For years I felt like there was a hole where my heart used to be and it felt like the hole was being filled back up. It is an experience like no other and felt like my sister was there the entire time. There was this sense of being rocked and soothed throughout the entire journey." The other trainee noted that the session "opened the door to new possibilities that I didn't know or remembered were there. I feel that a lot of the weight I had been carrying with me is just gone…".

Of course, not all sibling relationships are mostly positive as the two described above were. In the case of difficult and complicated sibling relationships, the chance of a wished-for relationship is gone forever. This is an area that can be fraught with very conflicting feelings. The outside world may give the message that the bereaved sibling must be sad, when in fact, they may be experiencing a host of other types of feelings. There may be relief they don't have to deal with the difficulties this sibling presented them with, or anger that the sibling was abusive in childhood and possibly into adult years. There may be guilt or anger when reparations were not initiated by the sibling or by oneself with serious quarrels, disagreements or estrangement

With Brainspotting, we can address each of these areas of concern, which can be haunting for the sibling who is left to sort it out on their own. Parts Work can be helpful with some clients, as it is surely a younger part of them that initially felt the distress with the sibling, or perhaps the relationship was better or good when they were children, but soured later in life. Utilizing Parts Work with sibling-bereaved clients can help to clarify that it is a part of them that has these feelings, and for very good reasons at that time. This leaves room for another part of themselves and more loving or connected feelings toward the deceased, if this is the case. In the situation of childhood, a very young and innocent part may have needed help with and even protection from the difficult sibling, but no one intervened. Parts Work can ease the guilt that many siblings feel that they are relieved their sibling is gone. (See p. 87, parts Work, Phase 3).

Loss, Grief and Trauma

We will all experience loss in our lives and there is no life untouched by trauma. Loss and trauma go hand-in-hand. I can think of no better way to address the trauma that is experienced in grief than with Brainspotting Therapy, a neurobiological method. Grief and mourning involve innate neurobiological processes that find their origins in the mammalian brain where we play out the evolutionary directives Jaak Panksepp (1998) defines for attachment, love, and caretaking/receiving. David Grand's Dual Attunement Frame offers both parts of the duo as neurobiological, both the relevant eye position and the relational attunement. Not only is the eye position accessing neural connections to the brain, but the mammalian brain is the seat of attachment mechanisms in the brain and is at work in our therapeutic relationship with the client as we attune to them. Clients often report the sense that the difficulty, trauma or other presenting issue is put in a better context – the "there and then" is not intruding on the "here and now" (Grand, 2018). We know that the hippocampus has done its work here in organizing the intruding feelings and images experienced as present moment events, now reorganized in memory and felt sense as something that occurred in the past. No small task.

There has been much discussed about the overlap of trauma and grief. Yet distinct specialties exist – Traumatologists on one hand and Grief Specialists/Thanatologists (death/dying) on the other. As specialists in the field of medicine have developed a high degree of specialization, the disciplines of psychology and counseling have followed the medical model with concentrations in grief counseling, trauma and PTSD, attachment disorders, OCD, thought disorders and the schizophrenias, ADD/ADHD, Autism, depression and anxiety to name a few. Any therapist with a specialty population will come across grief and loss in their clientele at some point. Whether a therapist refers to a trauma or grief counselor or has sufficient training in those areas to address the client's needs is a matter of assessment that bears scrutiny to act from attunement.

A therapist's own personal work regarding grief and loss will be as important as the grief training they have received, their keeping pace with the current grief literature, and their experience in their own clinical practice. Death and grief are areas rife with possibility for Limbic Countertransference, as the clinician surely has their own loss experiences and dreaded anticipatory losses. A clinician's similarities to and differences from the client's experiences make for fertile soil in the territory of Limbic Countertransference.

When we clinicians may have gone through a similar experience as the client, this can support a keen attunement, or it can draw us out of Uncertainty and into the Certainty that our experience gives us a unique understanding of the client. Conversly, we may hear things we have never heard before nor could we imagine. Our hippocampus is screaming, as Damir del Monte (2017, Nov) says, "I Will Not Make a Memory of This!", when we find ourselves in the midst of brainstem survival programs of fight, flight or freeze engendered by the horror story our client is detailing. In the moment, whatever we can do to ground ourselves can be helpful. I suggest reviewing Cynthia Schwartzberg's chapter on Grounding with an eye to how to practice grounding ourselves.

The awareness and wisdom to know when we are out of our Window of Tolerance regarding this client and their story brings another meaning to the term, Dual Attunement. We must be attuned to our personal disharmony in response to the client. Simultaneously we must be able to register our inability to attune to this client and either do our own supervision and personal work, or make an attuned referral to a colleague who can work with this level of exposure to the client's horrific material. We must be attuned to the client to do that referral in a manner that doesn't reinforce loss/abandonment to the client who is suffering from traumatic loss. The Brainspotting community has many resources including experienced grief and trauma therapists. Additionally, the Association for Death Education and Counseling's website and national directory of grief therapists (www.adec.org) can provide educational and referral resources.

Pet Loss, a Disenfranchised Loss

As I mentioned earlier in this chapter, Pet Loss is an area of specialty for me. I began the Pet Loss and Lifespan Transitions division of my practice and published the first edition of my audiobook, Journey Through Pet Loss (1998) twenty years ago when Pet Loss was considered a fairly new field. While there is more understanding in recent years for bereavement due to the loss of a beloved dog, cat, or other companion animal, it can still be an experience met with misunderstanding, criticism or even derision. The pet appeals to our young, precious self who needs to feel loved and safe, not criticized or judged. Our pets are perfect beings to give us unconditional love that no one person is capable of consistently giving us. Human relationships are fraught with complexity and come with each individual's history and emotional "baggage". Our pets love us unconditionally and demonstrate that love to us day after day after day. Until that difficult day comes when they die, are lost, or we need to make the decision for euthanasia.

One of the most helpful things we can do to help with the euthanasia decision with Brainspotting is to use the Brainspotting Double Spot set-up. A young and very wise veterinarian once asked my husband and me as we sat in the examination room with our failing 15-year-old Shih-tzu, Pimpernel, "Because we can't read our pet's minds and know the exact right time with certainty, where on the scale are you most comfortable being – a bit too soon , or too late?" We knew instantly for this sensitive yet stoic dog that it was "too soon" without question. For a client experiencing anticipatory loss, finding the right time for euthanasia isn't always accompanied by the feeling we are often told, "You'll know the right time", or "He'll let you know when it's time."

One day the dog is doing well, interested in eating and showing some signs of enjoyment of life, the next day he is laboring to breathe or can't use his back legs at all or comfortably. (Please know there are wheelchair options for handicapped pets, see "Wheelchairs for Handicapped Pets" at the end of References.) This up and down experience can occur hourly, greatly confusing the pet parent about that "right time". The day you decide, "This is it, it's the right time", the pet might rally and have the best day they have had in weeks. On the roller-coaster ride anticipatory loss brings, the pet owner goes back and forth agonizingly trying to find that "right time" for their pet.

Having the client find the "too soon" and "too late" Brainspots with Inside Window or Inside/Outside Window can be very helpful in finding the "rightness" of the time for this particular animal, for themselves and their family. As with Double Spotting or with Roby Abeles' Crocodile Set-Up for Addictions (2017), you can have the client spend time on each spot as they feel moved to do so. As Roby teaches, you can have one spot the client "'bookmarks" and have a post-it on the wall for that spot if they need it. Or the pet owner can hold the pointer for the first spot as the therapist holds another pointer for the second Brainspot. (Also consider using Cristiane Ramos' Pointer Stand in such situations, see References.) Being at the precipice of losing a pet can bring up so many attachment, abandonment and guilt issues for pet parents. Be prepared for other material that may come up as the pet parent Brainspots the "too soon or too late" conundrum. Be sure to be well established in your "No Assumptions" stance, as the deepest issues of attachment, love and despair can come with pet loss. Companion animals have a direct connection to our heart and our mammalian brain with its sense of "the pack, the tribe", and feelings of love, loyalty and devotion. This pet may have provided the kind of consistency in love that no person has been able to provide. Considering euthanizing the pet, even though a part of the client knows they do not want the pet to suffer, may bring a surprising amount of ambivalence.

For the neocortical portion of the euthanasia decision, you can direct pet parents to Dr. Alice Villalobos' (2018) website for a Quality of Life Scale (QoL). Clients can utilize this scale at home, work on it with their vet, and bring it into sessions with you in therapy. Some concerns and issues engendered by working with the QoL can be Brainspotted in any manner you feel intuitively would be best, just as you would do with any other issue a client would bring in as "dysregulated". Remember, the pet owner is being asked to do something we don't do for humans, to choose the date of the death.

In our modern medical world of heroic measures to extend life, we are asked to decide when a life dear to us should come to an end. While we know neocortically that our pet will die before us, the fact that we care for them as if they were another child in the family goes against any logical reasoning when it comes time for them to be euthanized. As a parent, the normal trajectory for our children is one that will go beyond our own lifespan. And our heart feels this tug as the pet's death can feel so wrong despite our mind telling us the pet is old and suffering now or has reached a disease state that will only produce pain and disability until death. We are in a crossfire of neocortical cognitive knowledge and feelings of attachment in the mammalian brain, with Panksepp's CARE circuit firing its signals.

Some information that could engage our client's neocortex in a helpful manner in conjunction with the QoL Scale, is the reality of the unnatural situation in which our domesticated animals are placed with humans in modern society. Had the pet been wild or feral when disease or old age hit, they would die from exposure to heat or cold, or become prey to a predator. We, as out pets' caretakers, are put in the position of having to do what nature would have done for them had they been in the environment of their wild ancestors. With this knowledge, any euthanasia decision is "too late" as a predator's instincts are honed through evolution to register weakness or vulnerability in prey who invariably become dinner. Of course, we do not have to say this as coldly as I do here, but as gruesome as this may seem, this is why the freeze response developed in evolution. Within the survival programs in the PAG (periaqueductal grey) in the midbrain, prey animals will experience analgesia when the predator comes in for the kill.

We humans have become very distanced from natural cycles of life and death in the "wild". This information may or may not be of assistance to a client. But as David Grand suggests, the neocortex is best engaged at the beginning and the end of the session, before we start with the Brainspotting set-up and after the Brainspotting processing or Focused Mindfulness portion of the session has ended. In the beginning of a session, certainly with a client experiencing Brainspotting for the first time, we teach about how and why we use Brainspotting, and educate them about the brain, engaging their neocortex. At the end of a session, the client may put together various insights and feelings from the session by talking about them. These are the times to introduce this information about mammal's life cycles in their natural environment, if we do it at all. As with any other psychoeducation or brain education we may impart to a client, at the end of a pet's life it may be helpful to offer these facts to a client who is struggling with the euthanasia decision - and it may not. Individual needs will guide us and only our attunement to them will tell us if we abandon the "W.A.I.T." stance "(Why Am I Talking?) and ask if they would like to hear some facts about wild and domesticated animals regarding end of life issues.

Some complicated issues can be engendered in pet owners by the loss of a pet with his or her getting out unexpectedly, or wandering. The pet parent may be distraught and feel terribly, unreasonably guilty. No matter how the pet got out, pet owners can find ways to blame themselves – even if someone else was at home when the pet escaped. "I should have known to tell Jack to leave Sparky in his crate til I came home!" The double-edged sword of not knowing if the pet is still alive if lost, and one's guilt for the animal's getting out or lost in the first place can be unbearable for people with a vivid imagination of the worst possible scenarios. Thoughts and feelings may swirl - is the beloved pet still alive? And if so, are they suffering, hungry and thirsty, or could they be prey for wild animals, or perhaps someone has taken them in?

An ambiguous loss is one that never gets resolved, where the fate of the pet is never discovered. This can bring the subject of Uncertainty front and center for this client and how they deal with "never knowing". I am thinking of working with the specific feelings that come up utilizing any Brainspotting set-up that intuitively feels right initially. For the ambiguity that may linger, the persistent wondering "Where are they?", "What happened?", I feel Rolling Brainspot could be helpful. Accessing the subcortical material that may underpin their struggles with "never knowing" by stopping whenever we see a reflex and letting the client's brain process at each spot provides the opportunity to work with multiple spots that lie outside the client's conscious awareness.

The exponential degree of Uncertainty with an ambiguous loss assures that one will never have certainty to know what happened unless the pet is found alive or dead. Rolling Brainspot may "keep up" with the haunting this kind of loss produces – "maybe he's here", "maybe he's there", "maybe he's in Heaven". The Rolling Brainspot gives an opportunity for all those "other possible Brainspots" that may be there (which we trainers get questions about in trainings) to leverage something in the unconscious survival programs of the brain. Mechanisms lying in those evolutionary programs to survive, to be in homeostasis, to conserve energy – to stop the wondering – perhaps we have a good chance at accessing them through Rolling Brainspotting.

For the client who accidently ran over their pet with their car or unintentionally killed their pet somehow – this is beyond devastating, just as those who have experienced losing a child in a similar manner suffer with the consequence of a moment in time that changes everything. A moment that seems the cruelest – that the client becomes the murderer of his or her most beloved.

We need to check on the safety of these clients referred to in the preceding paragraphs – are they a possible suicide risk? And this goes for all kinds of pet loss depending on the stability and social support available to the client. I have heard many clients say they cannot go on without their pet. And for those that had developmental trauma and abusive childhoods, who cannot trust anyone, this one "being" could be trusted. And there can never be anyone else, they tell us – they don't want anyone else. Just as you would work to assess suicidality in any client, make sure that you go through that process with pet loss. For the client who claims they want to die and who doesn't have a good support network, does the response to the loss of the pet reveal some developmental trauma that wasn't apparent when the pet was there to shield the client from the existential abyss of feeling truly alone in the world?

Be aware of the "meta-communications" (2018) David Grand speaks of with the client who will say, "I want to die", as the only way to communicate how torturously pained they are. You are dealing with a Part here, so that knowing your Parts Work or getting some supervision and further training in developmental trauma may be warranted. With cases of severe attachment breaches and early developmental traumas, particularly pre-verbal traumas before age three, consider referring to a therapist who works with that population. You may find issues of over-responsibility in the client's past going back to childhood resulting in their being The Hero or Rescuer. Or on the other end of the spectrum, they may berate themselves having been the Black Sheep of the family who could never do anything right, a "screw-up" who can't be trusted with anyone or anything, or so they were told over and over when they were young. Work as you would with Parts either implicitly in the relationship or explicitly as we learn in Phase 3. If working explicitly, you might invite the client to bring the Part into the room, with the placement of that Part becoming the Brainspot. You can certainly use a Gazespot you notice as an optimal way to work with a client who has found their own naturally resourced access spot, and this may precede any Parts Work that is more explicit.

As I've mentioned, a pet gets right into our limbic/mammalian system with a direct line to what Jaak Panksepp (1998) has termed the CARE neural circuit in his taxonomy of primary human and animal emotions. CARE, as Panksepp defines the seven primary emotion circuits, is programmed evolutionarily into the limbic system. Oxytocin and endogenous opioids are released when we are in the presence of one whom we love and care for, and who loves and cares for us. This CARE circuit has ensured the survival of our species and those of our mammalian relatives. Animals who are born precocial are up and about quickly after birth, and don't have a long trajectory of maternal care. Other animals, including humans, are born altricial, with a much longer span of time in which parental care is necessary for survival of the young. The CARE circuit developed and was conserved throughout evolution in mammals and becomes particularly piqued in us humans when we are about to lose our "baby".

Our need to care for another can be as important as our need to feel loved and be cared for. Many pet parents feel the loss of the role of caregiver to be intolerable when their pet dies. The pet has given them a purpose, a schedule, and meaning to an otherwise lonely existence, or it was "simply" more pleasurable to have this pet in their life. The change from the Social Engagement System (Porges, 2011) being "on" to being rapidly and cruelly shut "off" by the death of the pet has thrown the client's system into a kind of shock. Where there was flowing Oxytocin one day, there can be high cortisol and adrenalin levels the next – like a diver who gets the "bends" from coming up to surface too quickly.

Something no mourner gets enough of, whether they are mourning the death of a person or a pet, is the time to simply tell you all the amazing things about the beloved – their special qualities, the little jokes or games they shared, how they met, what was unique about them, what would drive them crazy, and on and on. Of course, we are not big on a lot of words in Brainspotting, but this is an area where the client's talking and our listening can be invaluable. If there is a question of our stepping in to speak, it could be to ask what else they feel or remember about their pet or the person who has died. With a very large pause on the part of the client, we might possibly begin the process of finding a Brainspot in the visual field guided by the client's eye gaze and our intuition. This kind of talking and story-telling is rich in life experience and follows Erickson's stages of development with the last stage being "Ego-Integrity versus Despair" (1959). While the client may not be at the end of their own life (or maybe they are, or close to it as a senior citizen), they are chronicling the life and the end of life of their beloved – a kind of eulogizing in real-time, not just the ten to fifteen minutes one is granted at a funeral, but a validation of the life lived.

The life of the pet and the era of the pet parent's life in which that pet companioned them is a period of time with a clear beginning and end. There was the era of all that was experienced while the pet was alive – maybe grad school, birth of a first child, a divorce, or death of a spouse. The highs and lows of life are experienced with our pets at our side as well as the daily activities of life which are mundane – getting the mail, doing the dishes – somehow these chores were not as dreary when our pets were there with us. The schedule and rituals with our pets – feeding them, walking them, taking them to the vet, and to visit friends and family, grooming them – now stopped suddenly.

And so an unwanted new era has begun – the era without the beloved – it is virgin territory and the bereaved can feel very lost. Telling the story of what was, who the deceased was, and who the client was in that era can be important. It is a kind of grounding and a natural way to mourn, grieve and heal by talking about the one who has passed by reminiscing. If we listen very closely, in that attuned place that David Grand speaks of, we will learn much about this client that may not have been evident when the beloved pet was alive and with our client in the physical world. Something deep in the attachment-world of the client has now changed and we are privy to the very depths of this person's being and soul as they search for something to grab onto in the absence of their dear one – the story of that life, and the story of their life with that particular pet. Notice their eye positions and gazes of course, their body language, the cadence of their voice as you sit in attunement with the bereaved pet parent.

Children and Pet Loss

With children, there is the opportunity to teach important life lessons as they will surely find more loss as they grow and mature. Using language appropriate to the child's developmental age is of prime importance to convey that the animal is gone now, that their body is no longer with us who are living. Finding ways to include children, in the euthanasia experience and memorialization of the pet can pave the way for how they handle future losses each step along the way. Parents can model this by sharing their own memories of and feelings for the pet. They can solicit the child's memories and feelings, or encourage the child draw a picture of the pet and their feelings about the loss. Parents can share that they, too, miss the pet very much, teaching about the range of feelings we can have when a person or a pet dies.

I highly recommend Cheri Barton-Ross's book, Pet Loss and Children: Establishing a Healthy Foundation (2005) for parents and anyone working with children. Ms. Barton-Ross describes how to speak in a manner appropriate to the child's age and developmental phase. She suggests that being aware as the months and years roll by, the child may revisit the loss from a more mature perspective and need assistance with the feelings and questions that are emerging about that loss. Brainspotting is a perfect modality for children and teens as they don't have to talk about their feelings. The Brainspot can provide the container for the feelings and experiences of the young as they work with the Brainspot in the form of a puppet on the pointer, figures in a sandtray, or a picture they may draw with its placement becoming the Brainspot.

Monica Baumann and Martha Jacobi have a helpful chapter in this book based on their Children and Teens Brainspotting Specialty Training. Various ways to work with this population, including didactic and experiential methods of teaching, will inform you about work with the younger generation in general as well as those who have lost a person or a pet

The Final Curtain

In wrapping up this chapter on grief and loss, I would like to think that the growth that comes from having endured unthinkable loss makes us better, stronger, kinder and more resilient. We have grown the muscle of perseverance in the facing of some of our worst fears in life – the end of life.

I have touched on some of the many facets of grief and loss in this chapter, a subject far to vast to cover in these few pages. The common denominator is that not only are we and our clients guaranteed more losses, but we will one day we be gone ourselves. Death crosses all boundaries of culture, language, race, religion, gender and even species. All living things die. Dying and the actual death are essentially a stage of life, albeit the Final Curtain.

In summing up I think about how Brainspotting, like loss and grief, also crosses cultures, languages, etc. I assisted in a Phase 3 training in Amsterdam in March of 2017 where twelve countries were represented in the one hundred people attending. When we broke out into dyads for practicums, the various languages spoken spanned German, Indonesian, French, English, and Japanese to name a few. Each trainee was fully engaged with their partner in the practicum and were speaking their native language in many cases. Those of us assisting spoke maybe a couple of languages – for me, only one language – English. Yet the assistants knew when to approach a struggling pair of trainees and how apparent it was when trainees were flowing along with the new method of finding the Brainspot in the practicums. And all trainees, of course, benefitted from Brainspotting. After all, this was Phase 3, which follows Phases 1 and 2 which these trainees had already taken, and here they were back for more. These representatives from twelve different countries were a testimony to the fact that Brainspotting works for clients spanning the globe from Australia to the Netherlands, Belgium, South Africa, Canada, the US and beyond.

When sitting in front of a bereaved client remember as I quoted David Grand earlier, "When you think it's in the tools, go back to relationship. I could say it a hundred times. I'll only say it thirty-six times." (Grand, 2014) With death and other losses, this client has lost a significant relationship. And they have lost relationship to themselves as the deceased was stitched into the fabric of their life. Where it is an ongoing client, they still have us. Where it is a new client, they are taking a huge leap of faith to try to connect with someone brand new. Relationship, the Dual Attunement Frame, the Uncertainty Principle and the No Assumptions Model give us, as therapists, the guidance to be with the bereaved. Regarding Uncertainty, the client may feel as though their "comet" has been relocated to another universe. Formerly streaking across the universe of their life with their loved one by their side, today they find themselves in uncharted and unwelcome territory. We, as therapists, may bump up against asteroids and fall into black holes in space as we attempt to follow in the Tail of the Comet of the client whose Assumptive World has disappeared from their sight.

Your Limbic Countertransference may be "on fire", but you work as best as you can to get back into attunement, to be in service to the bereaved individual who comes to you, puts their trust in you, and in most cases, pays you. Another "David-ism" comes to mind – during Day 3 of the Phase 1 PowerPoint with slides on the subject of Limbic Countertransference - Fight, Flight and Freeze are the unconscious responses of the therapist. David tells us to remember to be kind to ourselves, to give ourselves credit for going, as best as we can, into some of the most horrible places a person can go and not abandon them. We may experience some of don't run out of the room, *somehow* you come back, you re-attune." (Grand, 2014)

Finally, remember the brilliance of your brain and that of your client, with its' four quadrillion possible synaptic connections (Amen, 2016). The neuroplasticity that brains have been achieving through the hundreds of thousands of years of loss, grief, trauma and transition are part of our genetic inheritance. And remember the brilliance of the subcortical brain where our limbic system houses the mechanisms for attachment and bonding which have been sorely disoriented in the bereaved. Yet we have one reason for a brain, homeostasis (del Monte, 2016, 2017), and that balance is achieved by harnessing the subcortex.

To quote Hamlet with a little neuro-interpretive spin,

> *"There are more things in heaven (subcortex) and in earth (body), Horatio, than are dreamt of in your philosophy (neocortex)."*
> (Shakespeare, et al., 1883)(Antinori, 2018)

References:

Abeles, R. (2017, November 30): *Crocodile Protocol.* Lecture presented at Brainspotting and Addictions Training, Atlanta.

Amen, D. G. (2016): *Change your brain, change your life.* London: Piatus.

Antinori, D. (2010): *Journey Through Pet Loss, audiobook* (Rev. ed.). Basking Ridge, NJ: YokoSpirit Publications.

Association for Death Education and Counseling. Advanced Solutions International, Inc. (n.d.). Homepage Content. Retrieved March 30, 2018, from https://www.adec.org/

Barton-Ross, C. (2005): *Pet Loss and Children: Establishing a Healthy Foundation.* New York, NY: Routledge/Taylor & Francis.

Corrigan, F., & Grand, D. (2013): Brainspotting: Recruiting the midbrain for accessing and healing sensorimotor memories of traumatic activation. *Medical Hypotheses, 80*(6), 759–766. doi: 10.1016/j.mehy.2013.03.005

Cozolino, L. (2011, May 2): *The Neuroscience of Trauma & Effective Trauma Treatment.* Premier Education Solutions, 6 hr. webinar and PowerPoint presentation.

Craig, A. D. (2015): *How do you feel?: An interoceptive moment with your neurobiological self.* Princeton: Princeton University Press.

Damasio, A. R. (2012): *Self comes to mind: Constructing the conscious brain.* London: Vintage.

del Monte, D., (2016, 2017): *Stress, Trauma and Pain in Brain and Body Neurobiology for Trauma and Brainspotting Therapists.* 2-day seminar (and video post-seminar, at www.lecturio.de) Amsterdam, NL.

delMonte, D., (2017, Nov 3 & 4): *Brainspotting with Kids and Adolescents,* 2-day seminar with Monika Baumann, Vienna, Austria.

Erikson, E. H. (1980): *Identity and the life cycle.* New York: W.W. Norton.

Grand, D., (2018): *Brainspotting Training Phase 1 Manual.* New York, BTI.

Grand, D., (2014): *New York Brainspotting Trainer Training,* New York, BTI.

Jänig, W. (2008): *Integrative action of the autonomic nervous system: Neurobiology of homeostasis.* Cambridge: Cambridge University Press.

Neimeyer, R.A., Burke, L.A., Mackay, M.M., van Dyke Stringer, J.G., (2010, June): *Grief Therapy and the Reconstruction of Meaning: From Principles to Practice,* Journal of Contemporary Psychotherapy, 40(2), 73–83. DOI 10.1007/s10879-009-9135-3

Panksepp, J. (1998): *Affective neuroscience: The foundations of human and animal emotions.* New York: Oxford University Press.

Panksepp, J., Biven, L., & Siegel, D. J. (2012): *The archaeology of mind: Neuroevolutionary origins of human emotions.* New York: W.W Norton.

Porges, S. W. (2011): *The polyvagal theory: Neurophysiological foundations of emotions, attachment, communication, and self-regulation.* New York: W.W. Norton.

Ramos, Cristiane: *Brainspotting Pointer Stand, Brazil,* cristianeramospsicologa@email.com, +55 61 99969-9512.

Rando, T. A. (2000): *Clinical dimensions of anticipatory mourning: Theory and practice in working with the dying, their loved ones, and their caregivers.* Champaign, IL: Research Press.

Villalobos, A.: *Quality of Life Scale.* Welcome to Pawspice and Animal Oncology Consultation Service. (n.d.). Retrieved March 30, 2018, from https://pawspice.com/

Wheelchairs for handicapped pets: https://www.handicappedpets.com/blog/

White, L., (2015): *Medical Neuroscience* online course, www.coursera.org, Duke University Medical School.

Wolpe, J. (1969): *The practice of behavior therapy.* New York: Pergamon Press.

Finding, Holding and Adjusting the Frame; Utilizing the Core Elements of Brainspotting to Facilitate Healing in Individuals with Complex Trauma

Susan Pinco

Now that you have had the opportunity to read about how Brainspotting helps people heal at warp speed and have seen how it can be a powerful resource for individuals struggling with a wide variety of issues, I would like to take you on an exploration of how the frame of Brainspotting can be adjusted to accommodate the needs of people with Complex Trauma.

Before we start this journey, I would like to remind you of a few of the core elements of Brainspotting -- dual attunement, frame and focus, no assumptions and following the head of the comet – as they will form the scaffolding for our exploration of this topic. Each of these elements of Brainspotting will first be reviewed in a general way followed by a brief description of how they relate to complex trauma. We will then explore the concept of complex trauma and its impact on individuals, and then take a deeper look at how Brainspotting can be adapted to facilitate healing for these wounded individuals.

As I hope that you have already learned, dual attunement has more than one meaning it refers to the therapist attuning to the physiological and psychological experience of the client and, it relates to the way that seasoned Brainspotting therapists attune to what they are experiencing inside themselves as well as to what they are experiencing in the space between themselves and their client/patient. When thinking of attunement in this manner, we can see that it has many facets. And, just like a well-cut diamond, the more facets we hold in our awareness the more brilliant and illuminating the experience. When working with complex trauma, this type of attunement is one of the cornerstones of effective treatment. The present, grounded and connected therapist acts like an anchor, tethering the flooded client, helping them to begin modulating sensory stimuli, orient in the present moment, and emerge from the storm of looping flashbacks into the relative calm of the consulting room.

To illustrate: I will introduce you to "B", an individual who had some of the worse exposure to horrific sensorial assaults related to 9/11 (The attack on the World Trade Center in New York City in 2001). Initially, "B" was so activated that the early part of our sessions were spent helping her come into her body and recognize that she was in my consulting room, not in her childhood home or at "Ground Zero" which is what we called the World Trade Center site. We did that by my noticing, out loud, her breathing patterns, body tension, posture, movement, 1000 mile stares and so much more. I would invite her to just notice what was happening inside as her breath become more shallow, as her body tensed, or as she took a nice, deep breath. Often I would also ask her to notice what it felt like for me to be aware of these subtle changes. Occasionally I would also share what I was noticing in my body and ask what she noticed when I shared my experience. This explicit use of dual attunement is quite different from the more subtle forms that are found in a typical Brainspotting session with someone who does not struggle with complex trauma. In those sessions, the therapist's active tracking, moment to moment, is conveyed in a non-verbal manner with mirroring of posture, breath, and the occasional nod.

Shifting to an exploration of frame and focus, you might pause for a moment and imagine traveling with me to an art store with a picture that I have mixed feelings about. I'm not sure that it is something that I really love, the colors are a bit off and it lacks the lyrical beauty of some of the other Japanese wood block prints that are in my collection. None-the-less, it is a print that I have had stored in my portfolio, waiting for a time when I felt called to take it out and give it a place on one of my walls. As I chat with the framer, I begin by trying a number of different colored mats, noticing how the print transforms, becoming either more or less appealing with each one. One in particular makes it "pop" and we begin to play with the size of the mat, and then the frame itself. As we approach the conclusion of this exercise, I am struck by how "right" the selected mat and frame feel and how much I like the print. This sense of "rightness" is what often accompanies the framing of a Brainspotting session. Framing in a session entails identifying something that is activating, irritating, unsetting or distressing to a client/patient. Often we just use the term "activating' as it is neutral, but as a client recently pointed out to me, this implies that activation is bad, which it is not. With this in mind, I encourage you to find just the right word to refer to this specific part of the frame for each client. One final thought before we move on to the other scaffolding elements. Timing is critical. Just as it wasn't the right time to have the print I had mentioned framed when I first acquired it; needing to develop other aspects of my collection before bringing this particular print out, framing it and hanging it on my wall. You will find, when working with clients, particularly those with complex trauma, that it often isn't the time to focus on certain pictures, memories, experiences, traumas, until it is. Often foundational work must be done before a particular focus and frame will be beneficial, rather than destabilizing and re-traumatizing.

To illustrate: I have been working for three years with a client/patient, "M" who is highly dissociated and has survived long-term, repeated trauma which began around age 2 and continues to this day. Up until recently even simple conversations about self-care and family lead "M" to switch into an "alter" or fragmented part of himself. These fragmented part(s) are only dimly aware of other "alters" and of the ANP (Apparently Normal Part(s)), and act and feel as if they are separate people. In those moments when "alters" are active the frame and focus is on safety, detoxifying shame, listening to what the alter wants to share, and increasing connection in the present moment. This frame and focus has helped "M's" ANP to increase its capacity to be with the "alters" and to now engage in a conversation about Brainspotting and how it might be utilized to help the "alters" to heal. If I had tried to introduce this concept earlier, there would likely have been a revolt. The system would have flooded more than it already was and it is likely that "M" would have become incapable of work and self-care.

"No assumptions" and "following in the head of the comet" are the final two elements of Brainspotting that I will focus on here. With both, there is an implicit injunction to slow down, to follow the client's lead, permitting their process to unfold with minimal interaction, interpretation and reflection. Since each utterance by the clinician will alter the trajectory of what is unfolding moment to moment, we are trained to be attuned observers rather than interactive fellow travelers. This is an incredibly powerful and effective approach for most people. It is, however, devastating early on in treatment for individuals who have experienced complex trauma and the accompanying unbearable aloneness, shame and dislocation that accompanies it (Fosha, 2011) For these individuals, the initial imperative is for the clinician to be a fellow traveler, someone who actively sees the client/patient, who in the seeing and accepting begins to detoxify the shame and engender a sense of safety moment to moment so that the "alters" engage with the therapist and where possible the ANP, allowing themselves to be seen and heard.

A typical Brainspotting session where

- an issue is identified;
- SUDs (Subjective Unit of Distress; 0-10 with zero being not at all and 10 being off the charts) calibrated;
- body sensation(s) located;
- a visual focal point that correlates to the body sensation(s) identified and held; and
- mindful processing occurs with the clinician mostly silent

will not be effective with individuals who have complex trauma. They will dissociate at some point in the process, often sooner rather than later.

At this juncture you may be asking yourself: How do I know if someone is struggling with complex trauma? What follows are some basic signs. As always, if you have not worked with complex trauma or have not had a lot of experience working with it, please request supervision from someone who has and consider taking some courses related to working dissociative disorder, particularly the course in Brainspotting Advanced Resource Model which is under development by Pie Frey, a senior Brainspotting Trainer.

There is no template for identifying individuals struggling with complex trauma. They could be an accomplished emergency room doctor, a construction worker, a teacher, an artist, as struggling student or an unemployed adult. They could be anyone. The persona they put forth to the world can seem incredibly competent, but there will be cracks in their façade. Their family and close friends may be aware of the cracks. You will become aware of them as well as you being to work with individuals on the trauma spectrum. For others there will be a sense of fragmentation, an as if presentation that is both brittle and fragmented.

Everyone has trauma; it's part of being human. What distinguishes simple trauma, PTSD and Complex PTSD or Complex Trauma is the severity of trauma, the number and severity of prior traumas, and the impact that the event(s) have on the individual. You might consider someone who had a reasonably safe and supportive childhood, who at the age of 10 had a blood test during which the technician stuck her repeatedly over the course of what felt like hours as her mother sat close by. Since that time this girl cannot have a blood test without lying down as her pressure will drop so much that the test will be impossible. This is a relatively simple issue and falls well within the "standard" frame of Brainspotting. This individual is well grounded and her personality is intact.

In another case, which illustrates the way that trauma can impact individuals in different ways, there are two individuals who worked at Ground Zero. One of the individuals had numerous losses, but came from an intact home. She also had a meditation practice and a strong support system. This individual, when not working at the site found herself to be very reactive, easily frustrated, highly sensitive to perceived injustice, sad and highly self-protective. Despite this, she was able to sleep well, and over the following month as she shifted from working the site to working in other areas of the city, she began to return to her "normal" level of functioning. The other individual grew up in a home where, from a very early age, he witnessed his mother and older sister being beaten regularly by his father; where mom was trying so hard to keep herself together that she couldn't validate her child's experiences. In his early teens, this individual was raped and experienced serial sexual abuse from the one person in his life whom he had come to trust. 9/11 was a destabilizing force for this individual who became unable to sleep through the night and was unable to maintain connection with his support system. His body and emotions became so destabilized that he was no longer able to work and spent most of his days in flashbacks, where he felt as if he were still at Ground Zero or in dangerous childhood experiences. When not in flashback, he was stuck in a highly reactive emotional state where he felt under attack, rejected and terrified of abandonment.

What underpins the startling difference in these two individuals' reactions? It is the foundation that was laid in their childhoods. The first individual had an intact home for much of her childhood. While the community was not idyllic and there were numerous issues at school, she had loving and present parents and extended family. The second individual came from a home where violence was the norm, where there wasn't always enough food to eat, and there was little safety. In addition, there was confusion as the primary abuser was also a protector, when the child faced danger from outside the family. Secondly, while no one escapes childhood without some trauma, the first individual had what we often refer to as small "t"s; the loss of a pet, the death of someone important to her, bullying on the playground. For the second individual, there are many big "T"s; moments when he felt that he might not survive.

Herein lie the seeds of complex trauma, trauma that is the result of repeated intolerable experiences that feel life-threatening and are inescapable. In most cases, the earlier the trauma begins the greater fragmentation of the self.

Complex trauma can be found in individuals from all walks of life, all socio-economic status, all regions of the world. The trauma can range from loss of primary care givers, medical procedures, war, incest, neglect, and ritual torture. In complex trauma, there is not only the traumatic event but also a lack of even one caring, nurturing individual who is capable of recognizing the pain, terror, and confusion engendered by the traumatic event. Imagine that a three-year-old child, who is living with her mother and her mother's angry and aggressive boyfriend. Mom is focused on keeping her boyfriend calm and happy. The child is often ignored and when she is given attention, it is negative. She is told to be quiet, to go to her room and to leave mommy alone. When she cries, she is punished severely and told to stop being so bad. When mommy goes out to work, the boyfriend drinks and backhands (slaps her with the back of his hand) her if she gets too close. At night, she hears screaming and the terrible sound of mommy being beaten. There are no caring adults to see her pain, to help her make sense of this very frightening world. As this cycle continues it is likely that this little girl, who has little capacity to metabolize and make sense of these traumas, will become more and more skilled at dissociating. It is also possible that parts of herself will fragment and alters will develop.

Taking a step back, we can examine these cases through a slightly different frame: the frame of ego-state psychology, first articulated by Watkins and Watkins. In this school of thought, we are all seen as having numerous ego-states or self-parts. These parts develop as a normal outcome of our experiences. Our biology, genetics, "personality" and life experiences coalesce to generate perceptions of ourselves and the world which then seed the formation of self-states. These self-or ego-states can be called forth by an array of unconscious and conscious stimuli. You might be acquainted with a grumpy ego state that shows up when you are late, when there is a lot of traffic, when you are hungry. You might also be aware of a joyful ego state that emerges when you hear the first few bars of a particular song, when the sun is shining, when you gaze at someone or something that touches your heart. For the vast majority of people, when we pause and think about our reactions in a situation, we can recognize these self-parts and their role. There is something called co-consciousness, an awareness of an "observer self", an awareness of the various parts of ourselves and an awareness of how the parts contribute to our lives. Even when we are highly reactive to a situation, once we are away from the stimuli we can, with or without help, recognize our reactivity and are able to hold the polarities that might exist when two or more states are activated. Often the work of therapy is to help various ego-states to heal so that there is more freedom to respond rather than react.

Individuals with complex trauma often have barriers between many of the different self-states, making it difficult for them to be aware of and co-exist with the others. This fragmentation will vary from moderate to severe. Regardless of where an individual falls on the dissociative continuum, you will find symptoms of flashbacks, nightmares, and difficulty sleeping. There may also be an inability to recall aspects of the trauma, negative thoughts about themselves and or the world, irritability, risky or destructive behavior, self-harm, hypervigilance, heightened startle reaction, feelings of isolation, difficulty feeling and accepting positive affect, exaggerated blame of self or others, and difficulty concentrating.

To illustrate the borderline between dissociation and DID: a young man was referred to me due to seizures with no clear medical basis. He appeared congenial, smiling and making good eye contact. And yet, his smiles rarely reached his eyes and there was a certain vacantness that settled in as he told his story. We worked for many months utilizing Ego-State approaches and slow movement Eye Movement Desentization Reprocessing (EMDR), as I had begun seeing him before the development of Brainspotting, There were some parts that didn't want to participate in the sessions, and others who were happy to have center stage. All appeared to be co-conscious, i.e., aware of one another despite the fact that there was some amnesia around early trauma which he felt had occurred but had happened. Nearing the end of a non-remarkable session I told him that we had five more minutes and asked him to check inside to see if there was anything that was needed before we finished. In the blink of his eye he had transitioned into a fugue state. His posture became limp and he was non-responsive. Having worked with DID, I knew that this was an "alter" and I continued to talk, orienting him to the sound of my voice, to the room, to the year, to safety in the moment. After about 45 minutes he became responsive; however, he appeared as a 6-year-old who had no idea who I was but felt safe being with me. At that time I called his wife and asked that she come to the office. While we waited the 6-year-old and I interacted with my following his lead while interjecting orienting comments: 'what are you seeing as you look around the room', 'what do you notice when you run your hand over the couch', 'what year it was'. When his wife arrived he had no idea who she was but felt safe with her and willingly left my office. I later found out that his ANP returned when they had walked halfway through the parking lot outside my office. The ANP had no memory of what had transpired. This client and I continued to work with his "parts" who were willing to participate in session and acknowledged those who were not. Some were willing to work with EMDR and later Brainspotting, and others were not. The hallmark of our sessions was my modeling respect and compassion for all his parts, and a cautions engagement with his protector parts. More often than not, this entailed being in the moment, recognizing the parts presence, and being curious. Since the protector parts didn't want to engage and weren't so willing for the others to engage, we did Brainspotting less and less. Sadly, he is currently taking a break from treatment.

This contrasts with another young woman who was referred to me for dissociation, changes in her visual and auditory input. She would see kaleidoscopes of color, feel as if she was distant from others; that they were shrinking or expanding and their voices appeared to be drifting in from far away. This young lady and I also worked with ego states but did not do any fixed eye position Brainspotting, as it would have been too destabilizing in that it would have required her to anchor her attention on a fixed visual point rather than my presence. While no "alters" appeared in our sessions she clearly met many of the criteria for complex trauma.

As I hope I have illustrated with the vignettes noted above, people who experience complex trauma are easily flooded or emotionally and physiologically overwhelmed. This happens when isolated parts of themselves are triggered and take over the executive functioning. I sometimes describe this as different parts driving the car and not sharing the access to the accelerator, the steering wheel, the break or the navigational system. In fact, there are some parts that have no awareness of the time spent in the car, where they have gone or what they have done. For these individuals, there can be confusion about what happened in the last 15 minutes, last hour or perhaps the last few days. Objects appear in their lives that they have no memory of acquiring and they find themselves in places they have no memory of going to.

In addition to intermittent loss of time and orientation there may also be a polarization of self-states similar to what is seen in Borderline Personality Disorder, and perhaps even a switching where one moment the person sitting with you is an adult and the next a young child or a teenager, as seen in the vignettes I presented above. In some occurrences, people's eye color may change. And, even more radically, they may also have certain diseases in one state and not in another. In fact, Dr. Bergman reports that there are individuals who have diabetes in one alter and not in another.

So, how do you work with someone who lives with frequent disturbances in their relationship to time (flashbacks and dissociative amnesia), body (depersonalization and derealization), thought (shame, distorted and over generalized sense of self and the world) and emotions (numbing and hyperarousal) (Lanius 2017) ?

You begin by expanding your capacity to trust. Trust that the client will move toward healing, that the 'alters' and symptoms are a form of communication, that if you listen with all of your senses as you accompany these incredibly complex and courageous individuals you and your client/patient can and will be safe. This deep trust is often something that must be developed through experience. Just as you don't have the strength to lift 20 kilogram weights the first day you walk into the gym, you may not have the capacity to sit comfortably the first time an alter appears in your consulting room. This trust will grow; perhaps the seeds for it have been planted today as you read my words.

What does treatment for individuals with complex trauma look like?

As with any client/patient, the initial sessions will often be spent creating connection, navigating distance and closeness, and determining the frame. To illustrate: "Q" came in for her first session a few weeks ago. She had indicated that her psychiatrist had suggested that she call me and that she was struggling with fear and anxiety. When she arrived she had difficulty maintaining eye contact and looked much smaller than her actual height. I also noted to myself that her voice sounded quite young. As I ushered her into the room I asked where she wanted to sit, gesturing to the couch and the 2 chairs that flanked it. After initially shrugging her shoulders and my telling her it was ok, that I wanted her to choose what felt best, she selected the couch. I then asked where she wanted me to sit and she chose the couch as well. We then navigated the distance between us with her telling me what felt right.

Settling in, I said hello again and "Q" looked at me and smiled tentatively. I invited her to take a few minutes and notice what it is like to be in the room: what does she see, what it was like to sit with me. She did this for a while then proceeded to share some of her trauma history with me. As a portion of her story was told a young alter emerged, shifting the frame and focus, transporting us back in time to the world of that young child. In that moment the therapeutic frame shifted from holding the narrative to being with the alter, whom I shall call "R". Initially, "R" is calm and curious, but then she is seized by a flashback and is terrified. The frame shifts again, tightening so that the focus is on anchoring "R" in the safety and connection of the moment. In order to do this I speak in a clear, calm manner, asking her to notice the tone of my voice, to look at my face, to notice the way I am holding my body. I ask her to see if I am afraid, if I am frightening, if I am calm or angry. I invite her to look around the room with me and see if it is familiar or new and, looking outside the window, if she can tell me what she sees. My intent is to differentiate "then" from "now" i.e., this is 2018. As I work I realize that "R" is not able to take in my words, although she nods when I ask if I should sit closer as she keens and curls up in a ball. I then begin to speak to her in the language of her childhood and she is more responsive. I ask her again, in that language, if she knows what year it is and while she doesn't respond overtly there is a slight lessening of her rocking. We sit like this, with my accompanying her with my words, my tone and my proximity until near the end of the session when I am able to help her age-progress so that she becomes 12,16,18,20 and so on until she reaches her ANP's (Apparent normal Personality) current age. The last portion of our session is framed by my encouraging her to take in my response to her and her insistence that she is disgusting.

As you can see, rather than following in the tail of the comet, giving "Q" the space to notice what was appearing at the physiological, emotional and cognitive levels, I was highly interventive. While I attuned myself to "Q" on multiple levels, I was rarely silent, using my voice to tether her to the current moment and our connection. My relationship to her Gazespotting was also quite different that it would be with a client who wasn't struggling with complex trauma. When I saw her fixed gaze I realized that she was shifting into an alter, and that she was losing connection to me and to the present. I moved myself to be in her line of sight, which occasionally facilitates connection and grounding. I quickly discovered that she wasn't seeing me in that moment, and returned to sit next to her on the couch as I continued my monologue.

While our initial session occurred many years ago, there are still times when one or more alters appear during a session. At times there is co-consciousness between them and at others, particularly in the midst of a flashback, there is none. With other clients/patients the 'alters' are much more situationally specific. For example, "B" never switched in session but his wife reported that he frequently switched around bedtime. In my initial session with "B", like the one with "Q", we also focused on connecting, navigating the distance, and determining the frame. "B"'s ANP was present for the entire first session where we spoke about symptoms; his difficulty sleeping, his hyperarousal, flashbacks, shame, guilt, and rage. We also identified historical antecedents as well as areas of traumatic amnesia. Given "B"'s hyperarousal I asked him to pause intermittently and just be aware of his breath, the rise and fall of his chest, the surroundings and what his words were engendering. For this individual, and many others with complex trauma, "slow is fast" (Grand 2002-2018). Meaning, that if you move too quickly the therapeutic process will stall and the client/patient is likely to become flooded. As a result, going slowly will enable people to reach their therapeutic goals much more quickly.

In the months that followed and as our therapeutic alliance became more established, we were able to utilize the Brainspotting frame and focus of finding an issue and the associated ego-state or part. After that we would identify a resource memory or body resource and its associated brainspot and notice what came up. In addition to the fixed eye position, "B" found the biolateral sound soothing and helpful. At times we also integrated Ericksonian Hypnosis to deepen the connection to resources and facilitate processing. This was particularly important when the traumatic events were threatening to swamp him or when the processing seemed to loop, in the way that a phonographic needle gets stuck in a scratch on a record. Those moments were often related to sensorial triggers which, while disturbing in their own right, were also linked to dangerous and traumatic events in "B's" early childhood. Many of these events were reported to have occurred after age 4, but given the family system, it is likely that there were many traumas prior to that age.

"B" participated in treatment for over 3 years and found that the work was helpful but ultimately, when we got too close to one of his alters, decided that he was fine and that it was "too much work" to continue.

As with all clients, there is the opportunity to co-create clinical goals. That being said, it is often advisable to develop goals with as many alters or ego states as possible and to choose who you will be working with on a session-to-session basis. Ideally, it is best to work with protector or aggressive parts first as they will fear loss of control and will frequently side-track or obstruct the work. While engaging them is not always possible, it is worth the effort to try, because even in the trying you are beginning to build a therapeutic alliance with them. That alliance came come about in unforeseen ways. With one individual, it was my watching a movie with her that transformed my relationship with her more aggressive parts.

Using the Brainspotting frame, I am curious about how our eyes, fixed on the screen, permitted a transformation inside of this individual: one where here-to-fore hostile and hidden alters were willing to speak with me directly and begin to engage in healing the system of which they are a part.

It is also worth noting that while working with protector parts is a priority, it is often the younger parts that show up, craving connection and support. Occasionally, simply focusing on them is effective; however, it has been my experience that at some point, the protector parts will show up either obliquely as an increase in flashbacks and self-harm, or more directly in session. When they do, it is good practice to make every effort to engage them.

Clinical Goals

The primary goal when working with someone with complex trauma is to help them stay within their window of tolerance, to enable them to limit flooding and flashbacks so that they can begin to address the underlying trauma in what Sandra Paulson calls a "fractionated manner". While this window may vary moment to moment, once it is experienced it can be a reference point, something to anchor the individual as they move through their terrain, traveling from survival to healing. As they move closer this goal, individuals are better able to titrate or fractionate (Paulson 2009) the traumatic material, regulate affect and utilize what April Steele calls "imaginal nurturing". This can lead to reduced switching, anxiety, hyperarousal, and hypoarousal, as well as increased co-consciousness of parts and improved sleep and cognition.

The road map for doing this varies from individual to individual. For those whose ANP is able act as a spokesperson for the various ego-states and alters, facilitating an internal dialogue between the parts and the ANP, it is possible to collaborate on goals and direction. Thus Brainspotting may be utilized to vivify resource states and increase a sense of connection to them before working with small pieces of the trauma. As noted earlier, it is important to be aware of protector parts and engage them whenever possible. Early on, these parts may not come forward and you may only intuit their existence as you encounter what feels like resistance to letting go of old patterns or fear of change.

When working with individuals with complex trauma, even those whose ANP participates in all sessions, it is important to explicitly recognize that some parts may want to participate in what is happening in session and others may not. Further, some may be able to work while others may need to be sheltered. Sandra Paulson uses an imaginary conference room with one-way mirrors and a sound system that can be turned on or off. Alternatively, you can work with the client/patient to identify a safe, comfortable, fun place for those alters who would be overwhelmed to "hang out in". One of my clients chose the beach, another "I dream of Jeanie's" bottle, from an American TV show, and a third, a well-appointed play room. Some parts prefer to be alone, others to share the space with other parts and a nurturing figure. Before starting to work, I often remind the client/patient that anyone who elects to participate and later decides it is too much can leave and go to the designated place. At the end of each session it is important to check in with the parts and see where they would like to spend the time between sessions. For one client/patient it was under a big tree by the beach, for another it might be tucked in to a big, fluffy cloud.

Where the ANP is frequently replaced by various alters, the therapist must both follow *and* lead the alters as they appear. For example, when "R" appears, I might say 'hello "R" what happened to "Q"?' In some instances she might shrug, in others she might say she (Q) got scared, and in others she might simply change the subject or descend into a flashback. My reaction will depend on what "R" brings forth. If "Q" was scared I would ask if "R" was scared too and work with her response. If "R" shrugs and demonstrates that she has arrived so that she can have my attention and feel our connection then I will draw or read with her. As you can see, regardless of where the alter is leading, I become highly interactive.

Attuned Presence and Trust

Just as working with silence requires the therapist's comfort with and trust in the process, so does working with fragmented parts: parts that dissociate, are angry, vulnerable, inflict self-harm, and dispense self-hate. This comfort is often the result of good supervision and experience. It can also be found in therapists who work with children, as they are skilled in the rapid shifting of focus, ego-states and metaphoric communication that is part of all play. They are also well versed in the utilization of "imaginal realms".

These highly sensitive and attuned clients/patients, with extrasensory antenna, are constantly scanning the environment for danger and will pick up on any discomfort and concern which they will then amplify and distort. This means that the therapist should be as transparent as they can allow themselves to be. If you have an upset stomach and are unable to set this aside in session, tell the client that if you seem a bit "off" it is because of a belly ache and that your lack of smiles has nothing to do with them. This admonition also applies to changes in the therapist's responses to the client. If you smile broadly, check with them and see what they are noticing in response to your smile. This metacommunication, communicating about the communication, will help build trust and a sense of safety. It will also help to unravel the knots that form in relation to miss attribution and hypersensitivity/hyperarousal.

Some final thoughts regarding frame and focus

Our work with individuals with complex trauma is never linear. The frame and focus will constantly change as trust is built, and their systems reveal themselves. Often it will feel like one step forward and three back as the clients/patients recoil from sharing another aspect of their internal "Pandora's box". In the best of all possible worlds we will model Rumi's poem, "The Guest House" where all visitors are welcome, even those sorrows that violently sweep out our homes. Within that frame, the Brainspotting therapist will utilize dual attunement and curiosity in an explicit and active manner: I am here, I see you, we are here together. In this manner the therapist sometimes follows in the head of the comet rather than in the tail, enabling them to employ techniques that slow the process down and enhance the connection to and utilization of resources.

While Brainspotting talks about "no assumptions" there is one that underpins all Brainspotting work; it is the assumption that an individual's internal system is more complex, unique, intelligent, and solution-oriented than the therapist can ever conceive. Furthermore, that if we help create the conditions of curiosity and mindful attention, then add in the neuro-physiological "starter" e.g., a Brainspot, and get out of the way, healing will occur. This assumption has validity for many clients/patients. However, some individuals need more active and explicit connection to the therapist in the moment. This is particularly true for individuals with complex trauma as their internal system is so chaotic and sensitive to triggers that there is little possibility that the conditions of mindful attention and curiosity can occur for more than a brief moment before a significant state change will occur. In some cases this will be dissociation and numbing, in others redirection or switching. For those whose trauma is a little less complex, and who have developed significant co-consciousness of parts, resourcing and Brainspotting with specific parts can be highly effective, although it is likely that you will encounter looping and SUDs that do not go down to zero. When this occurs it is usually an indication that the internal system has parts that believe that the symptoms are necessary. Identifying and engaging these parts will be a necessary but often allusive part of the work.

I want my mommy

Working with individuals with complex trauma requires focus and framing for the therapist as well as the client/patient. As Cheri Lindberg and Cynthia Schwartzberg teach in their Brainspotting Advanced Clinical Seminar, it is important to be aware of our own limbic countertransference: the ways that we unconsciously respond our clients.

As trauma upon trauma is shared with us we may feel anger at the perpetrators, a desire to shield and protect the young parts, deep sadness, the desire to flee, to stop hearing. This can be framed as the impulse toward fight, flight or freeze. Within this potentially toxic stew we may also feel frustration, as many of these individuals may be in situations where the trauma and abuse are on-going and/or they are caught in a trauma bond with their perpetrators who did unimaginable things to them but were also one of the few individuals who also paid attention to them, and who, from time to time, acted in a loving manner. We may also struggle with explicit requests from young alters that we be their mommy or daddy and protect them. Bringing our reactions into consciousness will help us differentiate between our experience and that of our clients/patients, between then and now. It will also help us to hold the space for them as they work toward healing. When our reactions inhibit our ability to respond in a manner that doesn't implicitly invite compliance on the part of the client/patient, it's important to seek supervision and/or therapy. Regardless, it is always helpful to have a support system that includes colleagues who can undo the aloneness of the consulting room for you, the therapist, so that you can fully appreciate the honor and grace that is possible in your work with these incredible individuals.

Bibliography

Bergmann, Uri: Treating Dissociation in the Spectrum of Personality Disorders. *Unpublished Paper.*

Bergmann, Uri, (2001–2010): Numerous lectures and conversations.

Fosha, Diana, Siegel, Daniel J. and Solomon, Marion, (2009): The Healing Power of Emotion: Affective Neuroscience, Development & Clinical Practice. *Norton Series on Interpersonal Neurobiology.*

Fosha, Diana, (2011): Lecture on Neurophysiology of Healing NYC

Gendlin, E.T., (2000): When you feel the body from inside, there is a door. In Jeffrey K. Zeig (Ed.), *The evolution of psychotherapy: A meeting of the minds.* Phoenix, AZ: The Milton H. Erickson Foundation Press. From http://www.focusing.org/gendlin/docs/gol_2232.html

Grand, David, (2013): Brainspotting: The Revolutionary New Therapy for Rapid and Effective Change. *Sounds True.*

Grand, David, (2003–2018): Personal conversations, numerous trainings and supervision.

Lanius, Ruth A., (2015): Trauma-related dissociation and altered states of consciousness: a call for clinical, treatment, and neuroscience research. European Journal of Psychotraumatology. 2015; 6:10.3402/ejpt.v6.27905.

Mosquera, Dolores, (2017): Challenging Issues with Complex PTSD & Dissociative Disorders. Online/live class.

Paulsen, Sandra, (2009): Looking Through the eyes of Trauma and Dissociation. Booksurge Publishing.

Pollani, Eva, (2010-2018): Lectures and personal conversations related to Ego State theory and treatment.

Rumi (13th Century): The Guest House.

Schore, Allan, (2003): Affect Regulation and the Repair of the Self. W.W. Norton.

Schwartz, Richard, (1997): Internal Family Systems Therapy. Guilford Family Therapy Series, Guilford Press.

Steele, April, (2006): Developing a Secure Self. *Seminar June 2006.*

van der Kolk, B. A. (2002). Beyond the Talking Cure: Somatic Experience and Subcortical Imprints in the Treatment of Trauma. In: Shapiro, F., (Ed.): EMDR as an Integrative Psychotherapy Approach: Experts of Diverse Orientations Explore the Paradigm Prism. Washington, DC: *American Psychological Association Books.*

Watkins, Helen H. and Watkins, John G., (1997): Ego States: Theory and Therapy 1st Edition. Norton.

Multifocal Brainspotting and Dissociation: Moving the Internal System from Entropy to Synergy

André Maurício Monteiro

> *"Everything around me is evaporating. My whole life, my memories, my imagination and its contents, my personality – it's all evaporating. I continuously feel that I was someone else, that I felt something else, that I thought something else. What I'm attending here is a show with another set. And the show I'm attending is myself."*
>
> Fernando Pessoa, The Book of Disquiet (2002)

In this chapter I'll outline the way I usually work with dissociative clients, and how Brainspotting can be used as an appropriate psychotherapeutic approach to deal with the challenging clinical situations these complex clients present in therapy. I'll start with a brief overview of dissociation and the different levels of complexity of more dissociative clients. This introduction is followed by theoretical and clinical examples on how Brainspotting can encompass this complexity, and how it may provide clinicians with the support they need in order to cope with this therapeutic endeavor. This is followed by a session segment, which exemplifies what multifocal Brainspotting is, and how Brainspotting may have its unique way of dealing with dissociative clients. Data from the clinical excerpts were disguised in order to protect clients' identity.

Are you talking to me?

Dissociation is not a unified concept. It can be viewed as a spectrum phenomenon, meaning that some clients may dissociate more than others, but all of them do dissociate to a certain extent, just like we all do! This means that dissociating is not pathological in itself. All of us switch off from the surroundings on a daily basis, from time to time. This distancing strategy helps us think creatively, make plans for the future, contemplate our lives in a mindfully based way, or simply divert boredom.

This innocent detachment from reality, and its corresponding dissociated emotional states that may vary along a continuum, ranges from crying at the movies (though we all know they are just make-believe stories, and no one really gets hurt or dies in the end), all the way up to more severe expressions of dissociation, such as feeling a constant sense of strangeness, of doubting whether existing is a confirmation of reality, of perceiving reality as a figment of one`s imagination, to which one does not belong, of being under the impression of living in a dream, or cognitively attempting to deal with self-derogatory voices inside one's head. The symptomatic plasticity dissociative clients may bring to therapy gives rise to multiple inaccurate diagnoses, followed by improper treatments. The elusiveness of dissociation may be a comorbid state that mingles itself with other disorders, such as anxiety and depression, thus confounding clinicians, and frustrating clients.

Dissociative clients may be compelled to pursue defensive actions of fleeing into fantasy, usually for the purpose of avoiding stressful contexts, such as transferential issues that come up in therapy, fighting the eclosion of traumatic memories into awareness, adapting to sudden changes in behavioral patterns for coping with daily life issues, such as compulsive behaviors, and many other strategies.

At a clinical level, some of these defensive dissociative expressions may be identified in therapy sessions, such as clients losing their train of thought, crying for no apparent reason, berating the therapist, changing the tone of voice, suddenly acting in a childish way etc. All of the previous instances and many more reasons to disconnect from reality help clients maintain a tight grip on a very fragile balance they manage to attain in life.

The practice of switching off, for example, rather than staring at a ghost from the past straight into its eyes, may be carried out through the development of ingenious maneuvers for emotional distancing from the here and now, such as pretending to pay attention, but not really connecting to what is being said. A client who was a journalist would talk to people and pretend to pay them her utmost exclusive attention, when in fact she was thoroughly counting how many letters the person would utter while speaking. In another instance, whenever I offered a possible explanation for a confusing issue, a very dissociative client used to say: "What you`ve just said is interesting, but I was actually thinking about..." – something totally off- topic.

To these clients, being in the present may be deemed as uncomfortable or totally unbearable. Dissociative schemes become a great fire escape to them, whenever unwanted emotional interactions begin to trigger defensive reactions. Therapists should bear in mind that most of these reactions, though pathological in their display, may be both persistent attempts to preserve adaptation and profound personal investment to look normal. But there is more to dissociation than appearances.

In general, dissociative symptoms may manifest themselves either through intrusions or withdrawals in relation to the clients' level of awareness. Inspired by the acronym proposed by the BASK model (Braun, B. G., 1988), dimensions pertaining to behavior, affect, sensation, and knowledge may evoke full awareness of clients, partial denial, or complete repression.

For instance, the manifestation of intrusions, which refer to the "knowledge" category, may influence the emotional state of the individual by means of invasive repetitive thoughts, by intense feelings and emotions irrespective of whatever the person is living at the moment (affect), by physical sensations, such as pain, that may strike without warning (somatic), by involuntary recollection coming from traumatic memories of the distant past that push their way into consciousness, by impending catastrophic fantasies related to the future which destroy recently attained peace, or by impulsive actions that wreak havoc on the relational lives of these clients, who cannot figure out why they exhibit such maladaptive "behaviors".

Instead of intrusions, there may be complaints of withdrawal symptoms related to the same BASK components. In these cases, a pervasive sense of physical numbness (somatic), for example, may be accompanied by an elevated threshold to painful stimuli or by a total lack of initiative and constant procrastination (behavior) or by boredom denouncing the ongoing absence of emotions (affect) or by concentration problems that result from a sense of heads filled with an undefined void (knowledge). These emotional, cognitive, and physical states of inappropriate intrusiveness or of persistent withdrawal from the client's field of attention may be accrued by comorbid psychiatric conditions, such as borderline personality disorder, eating disorders, fibromyalgia, anxiety disorders, depressive episodes, or compulsive behaviors.

These dysregulated ways of perceiving the outer and inner reality, of feeling either too much or too little, push clients into oscillations, hopping between excessive sympathetic, or pervasive parasympathetic activation. Dissociative clients have a hard time remaining in the present and may polarize their emotions rapidly, overwhelmed with emotions, or by fleeing from emotions, and shutting down.

Ogden, P. and Fisher, J. (2015) understood these oscillations not as distinct categories, but as a fluid process they termed a window of tolerance. This concept describes an emotional flow, with a variety of intensities of emotions, ranging from excessive activation of the sympathetic autonomic nervous system and its corresponding intrusive symptoms, to the physical and emotional shutdown, promoted by excessive activation of the parasympathetic autonomic nervous system.

When these polarized manifestations of emotions become long-lasting states, rather than isolated moments, clients remain outside an ideal integrative processing zone. During these extreme states, primitive defensive action systems are activated and set in motion either flight or fight responses, coupled with sympathetic activation. Conversely, clients may react with freeze and collapse responses when parasympathetic activation becomes more radical.

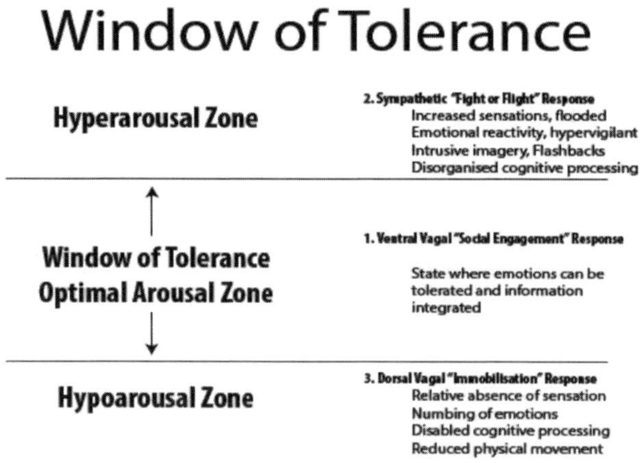

Fig. 1: The Window of Tolerance (based on Ogden, P. & Fisher, J. (2015, p. 48)

The ideal processing zone in between these two poles of autonomic activation is equated to what Stephen Porges (2011) termed the ventral vagal response, represented by social engagement. Derived from his polyvagal theory, social engagement implies the activation of the X cranial nerve, along with cranial nerves V, VII, IX, and XI. When activity from these cranial nerves prevails, especially when the person feels safe, an individual may rise above the primitive emotional reflexes by activating the attachment system and exchange with others in a way that brings about an interactional containment, a socially-based emotional regulation. Speech and facial expressions strengthen bonds and facilitate a sense of belonging to the community.

Social engagement promotes social interchange, and a diffusion of core anxiety among peers, who manage collectively to calm down, ascertaining the power of the group and the absence of danger in the surroundings. The group offers containment, just as the therapeutic relationship does. Polyvagal theory proposes that we may reframe the opposite of autonomic activation as social engagement, instead of relaxation (Rosenbery and Shield, 2017). When we manage to overcome animal defenses, we encounter attachment and social safety. The emotional regulation may also be obtained through self-soothing activities we may psychoeducate clients in, such as the practice of mindfulness exercises and breathing and relaxation techniques.

Instead of flowing within the window of tolerance, dissociative clients tend to switch between emotional extremes. It is as if the source of emotional regulation that social engagement can provide, is beyond their limits. Since closer interaction in the past once was coded as dangerous, filled with betrayal, and treachery, social proximity can trigger entropic defenses that harness dispersion and avoidance instead of synergic interaction.

Still according to Rosenbery et Shield (2017), ventral vagal social engagement enables dissociative clients to develop a kind of Goldilocks relationship with their surroundings. According to the tale, the girl with the golden locks first tries the extremes outside the window of tolerance in the house of the three bears, before settling for the middle term. The best option is not too cold, nor too hot, nor too hard, nor too soft, but just "window of tolerance" right. The same principle is valid for the quest for association and connection with others. Therefore, social engagement is the opposite of dissociation, of polarized emotional experiences.

By having difficulty in maintaining themselves inside a window of tolerance, dissociative clients suffer from reflex responses with respect to the twisted perception of excessive or deficient stimuli. They seldom ever find the "just right" amount of stimuli! A plethora of dissociative responses may take place in contexts where clients detect the slightest emotional or physical alteration, which they interpret as a sign of a threat. Clients may become paranoid with everyone because they detect threat in every relationship. No matter how well guarded they are, they still fear the dangers of a harmful close relationship that misleads them into a false sense of safety. They miss attachment opportunities, and do not spot destructive bonds.

Overreactions to harmless stimulus suggest that dissociative clients find it hard to regulate and keep their emotions within the boundaries of emotional tolerance, both in and out of sessions. Dissociation may be their ultimate security blanket, something that provides them with a refuge from any kind of risk. Defective risk assessment leads these clients to episodes of revictimization. The failure to protect and seek protection is a common theme among dissociative clients, regardless of their excessive futile defenses.

This contradiction between enhanced alertness and faulty protective measures can been seen in other expressions of dissociation. Though dissociation provides an emergency escape from impending doom, at the same time it becomes not an exception, but a constant way of being in the world. The initial path to salvation from emotional annihilation becomes the client's ultimate trap. Dissociation apparently shelters clients from mundane perils, but there is no easy way out of its cushioned claws. The safe haven of disconnecting from immediate reality becomes an automatic condition that denounces a deficiency of risk management and perpetuates the mistaken perception of the environment. The client may prefer to space out rather than deal with relational conflicts, resulting in perpetuation of vulnerability.

Apart from the perceived looming threat of imminent danger, these clients may also be triggered by recollections from the past and current reminders stemming from their polytraumatized childhoods. This temporal confusion caused by the invasion from the past disrupts the accurate distinction between past and present. The dysfunctional nostalgia blends signals between current triggers and recollections from the traumatic past.

The lowered ability to stay in the present ensnares these dissociative clients in a repetitive, never-ending nightmare. Due to this temporal blending, therapeutic initiatives to help these clients may also be encoded as some sort of grooming attempts from dissimulated perpetrators from the past who plan to become abusive, if given the chance. This is one of the bases for the phenomenon that in the clinical setting psychodynamic therapists called transference. The abusive relationships with significant others from the past are replayed in the present in the therapeutic relationship. Therapists offer themselves as blank screens upon which clients project internalized relationships form the past. To dissociative clients this means a repetition today of what once were inappropriate relationships in childhood and adolescence. With respect to the capacity of dissociative clients to assess risks, protectors from the present and perpetrators from the past become one and the same.

Consequently, it may be a daunting task for these clients to engage in a therapeutic relationship that is viewed as helpful, yet at the same time potentially harmful. Similar to what happened in the past, therapy may update parental noxious relationships in the therapeutic dyad. Dysregulated caregivers once were the simultaneous source of help and protection, combined with abuse and neglect. With all of this at stake, dissociation is one of the best fire escapes there is: dissociative clients may resist and put up a fight or flee the office, disconnect, pretend this is not happening at all, resign, and wait to be attacked.

It is up to the therapist to help clients orient themselves to the present, and process these abusive records they drag around with them. Psychoeducational strategies, such as relaxation and mindfulness exercises, may provide the support that is lacking. Clients may gradually learn to keep themselves regulated enough to stay in session.

What`s Brainspotting got to do with it?

So what happens if we attempt to use Brainspotting with these clients? First of all, with respect to the principle of uncertainty and its relationship to theory, Einstein once stated that: "whether you can observe a thing or not depends on the theory you use. It is the theory that decides what can be observed" (in Rosenberg et Shield, 2017, p. 29). The evolution of theoretical guidelines related to Brainspotting seems to have taken up uncertainty also via dialectical principles, which means the search for syntheses with hypotheses on the one hand and facts on the other. Whenever a fact discredits the hypothesis, or the client reacts in a way that was not previously predicted by what theory expected, if anything at all was expected, therapists should be ready to throw away hypotheses, and keep their minds open for new ones. Whenever working with uncertainty and its unpredictabilities, therapists need to not have a theoretical attachment, other than the pursuit of the unpredictable trajectory of the comet that clients provide.

The concept of dual attunement is another example of simultaneous foci (potentially multiple) of the therapeutic interaction that addresses the need to widen the scope of observation from the perspective of the therapist. Dual attunement provides emotional support that helps clients reorient themselves to the present. When we put the Brainspotting theory into practice, we may understand all of Brainspotting as being grounded in the present through the therapeutic relationship, as well as inherently multifocal, both from the perspective of the therapist and the client.

While working with Brainspotting, therapists maintain different foci of attention. Based on the principle of uncertainty, at the one level the therapist is invited to maintain a constant state of curiosity about what happens, and to wait for the process to unfold. At the same time, the uncertainty principle at a cognitive level does not prevent therapists from being subcortically present and attuned with the client. As implied by Schore (2012), subcortical reprocessing corresponds to a connection between the right hemisphere of the therapists with the right hemisphere of the clients.

In the meantime, clients may be encouraged to maintain the awareness of what is happening at different BASK levels, varying from evident traumatic recollections, all the way down to impalpable speechless subcortical processing. In the case of dissociative clients, the multiple foci of awareness may have to do with the recognition of the internal isolated parts of the self, each one filled with specific needs and demands, and different levels of consciousness. They also live in different time zones, some stuck in childhood, others in adolescence.

Multifocal Brainspotting and dissociative clients

Clients with a dissociative disorder may find it harder to maintain themselves the present, in a state of dual attunement with the therapist. Instead of feeling safe and understood, distinct parts of the self in the respective closeness of the therapeutic relationship may easily trigger well-organized emotional and behavioral sequences that Panksepp (1988) defined as emotional operational systems (defensive action systems) of fear and rage, which mediate the three Fs: flight, fight, or freeze responses. When these feelings are activated, the reaction will push client out of the window of tolerance.

Close relationships are viewed as overwhelming, and survival instincts may cause these clients to disengage from the ventral vagal therapeutic alliance and slide back into more primitive reptilian responses of fight, flight, or freeze. When this happens, reprocessing stops its flow. The comet becomes a floating asteroid.

Due to a damaged sense of a fragmented identity, it is not clear to these dissociative clients who they actually are, let alone what their relationships are with other people. Consequently, establishing and maintaining an intense close encounter with a caring therapist may be viewed as an unattainable task. The contrast between therapists who seem to know who they are and clients who do not, can make these insecure clients in a close interaction look even more damaged, and they clients are aware of that.

The interaction with a therapist may be too complex for clients who consider themselves as suffering from chronic disconnection at several levels, in relation to themselves, in relation to others, and to the world at large. The disconnection may be worsened by an uncertainty of what reality actually is, coupled with a fragile sense of self, on the constant verge of collapse. All of these contrasts may sustain obstacles to the continuous, meaning-making therapeutic process clients should be benefitting from in the Brainspotting context.

So, should we give up? Paraphrasing David Grand, whatever the client expresses does not have to be regarded as a problem in itself, unless we conceptualize it that way. Dissociative behavior may be considered as a form of adaptation to imagined threatening situations that are involuntarily updated from a traumatic past. Therefore, this challenge may be an opportunity for the brainspotter to reevaluate the psychotherapeutic relationship with a positive regard and confidence in the process. We can look at dissociative phenomena as attempts of a wounded hero to survive early childhood adversities.

The dual attunement frame may help these clients foster exploratory ways to promote constructive manifestations in the therapeutic alliance, should they manage to keep within their windows of tolerance. The relational aspect of dual attunement can help clients explore the subjective relationship with the brainspotter in the outside world, in the context of the therapeutic relationship, and with other internal parts of the self that may not be readily available for external contact.

One client or multiple clients?

> *"My soul is a hidden orchestra; I know not what instruments, what fiddlestrings and harps, drums and tamboura I sound and clash inside myself. All I hear is the symphony."*
>
> (Fernando Pessoa, The Book of Disquiet)

Despite the external apparent lack of existence, dissociative clients may identify voices in themselves, or inner parts of the self. These parts can be decisive in allowing therapists to understand the psychodynamics of the client. During a more focused clinical interview, a few of these parts may come forth into the awareness of the client, and spill over the therapeutic relationship in the shape of the children, usually the client once was. They may attempt to contact the therapist and forge alternative non-therapeutic relationships, in order to fit their needs of protection or autonomy, depending on the circumstances.

They may also present themselves as parts the clients do not recognize as belonging to them, such as wandering orphans or refugees. Moving beyond the fragility category assigned to certain frail parts, other ones may also turn out to be more abstract, such as abusive monsters or shapeless aggressive voices that trigger panic and avoidance defenses, in both clients and therapists. Oftentimes, clients in panic may be an indication that a scary part is pushing into the client`s awareness. The multiplicity provided by these emotional representations introduces us to a whole universe of interactions that were previously invisible to the unwitting eye.

Though usually perceived through internal voices, some dissociative clients may have more self-like parts, with higher degrees of autonomy. They have a somewhat defined personality structure that is more organized than others. Some may hold opinions and values that are distinct from those defended by the self, yet preserve this covert nature from the outside world, making them intriguing to apprehend. Though hidden, they maintain a close relationship with the client, sometimes a torturing one, through vociferations or prolonged crying. For a more comprehensive understanding of the composition of parts and the various possible interactions with the self, please refer to Steele, K. et al. (2016).

In order to reduce the effect of the entropic tendencies of dispersion and more dissociation promoted by internal conflict among parts, brainspotters should remind themselves that the bottom line is that the client is always one. Entropy is characterized in general as a tendency for systems to move into more disorganized, randomized arrangements. The opposite of that would be the principle of synergy.

From a systemic perspective, we understand that these inner characters assemble in the form of an interactional system, an uncovered domain filled with internal conflicts. Power struggle and unmet needs promote entropy of the internal system, or the tendency of this internal system to produce and maintain a form of unbalance, one that tends to be stuck, pulled apart by opposing dispersive forces, accompanied by a reluctance of its components to associate. The individual has a hard time coalescing these inner parts into a more harmonic state of internal synergy of conjoining efforts towards integration. Our overall goal in Brainspotting would be then, with the help of the relational frame, to reduce entropy and to foster synergy among the parts of the system, so as to make it more syntonic to adaptive emphasis.

Brainspottingwise, despite efforts from the client to avert internal interaction, therefore preserving entropic principle of dissociation, the dual attunement frame provides a safe area where clients can attempt connections with their inner parts, thus bolstering some synergic convergence. The presence of the therapist may be labeled a concrete link back to reality, a safe base which enables clients to explore their relationship with inner parts. These inner parts may try to destabilize the therapeutic relationship if they suspect there is a chance the client will try to gain control over them with the help of the therapist. Parts may try to weigh in, by means of imperative voices, on how the self should behave, or by repeating self-defeating phrases into the mind's ear of the client, to sabotage the constant presence of the therapist. The surrounding frame around the client may provide containment that promotes the establishment of a collaborative interaction, and mutual growth between self and its internal parts.

The internal system is governed by rules pertaining to the preservation of the individual, just like the parts that compose the system. Inner structural features of the system, such as one part not being fully aware of another one, may express internal dissension, with power struggles among parts who want control the self, and to rule over other parts. Actions resulting from this entropic interaction among parts, issuing commands for self-destruction, impulsive behavior (self-cutting, binge eating/drinking, suicidal ideation, unsafe promiscuous sex, dramatic mood swings) may seem chaotic to an outside observer. If appropriately contained by the dual attunement frame, the commands of the destructive parts, and the impulsivity that tries to sequester the self from agency of the individual, may be underscored as extreme attempts by parts to prevent the person from facing inner dilemmas in the present and from becoming whole. The reduction of systemic entropy can enable parts to engage in a more ventral vagal form of verbal negotiations pertaining to social engagement and a synergic disposition to more integration.

Theoretically, the principle of uncertainty and entropic forces within the system of parts lures the therapist into preserving a state of relative ambiguity with what the client allows to surface. The result of the uncertain interaction proposed by the therapist that observes the entropic movement of the internal system of the client opens up the activation of meaning-making synergic tendencies, which resonate in both client and therapist. One example is by trusting the client`s subcortical wisdom to move wherever it drifts during processing.

One of the issues related to dissociation is to what extent we are dealing with one client or partial aspects of a client. Brainspottingwise: are we following the head of a comet or a meteor shower? If the latter would be a way of conceptualizing dissociative clients, then setting up a looser frame would probably make more sense, in order to encompass all of the complexity involved. On the other hand, we could dance back and forth between a larger scope of the frame, so as not to lose sight of the whole, but eventually to intervene with temporary focal frames for each meteor.

Focal frames would provide transient support to parts with specific needs that are reluctant to integrate into the wholeness of the self. This would imply the observation of at least a dual perspective of the client, as being individual and being multiple, composed of a non-integrated system of parts, thus adding more uncertainty regarding the client, the specific needs of some of her parts, and her integrative capacity as a whole.

Since we are attempting to establish and maintain a therapeutic relationship in approaching this ever-unknown person before us, so is the person dealing with the same enigma with respect to our presence. We may, therefore, ask ourselves how hard it is for someone who realizes s/he is not in full command of reality, does not hold a clear sense of self, and yet attempts to obtain support from an unknown person called a therapist.

The use of primitive avoidance defenses hinders the internal system from going into a state of more synergy. Avoidance defenses of entropic nature are set in motion whenever vulnerable parts of the system get a sense there is danger of imminent realization of their existence. The realization of such existence by the adult self may destroy the current status of homeostasis. The pressure to integrate the parts means the extinction of their entropic autonomy, their growing disconnection from other parts. The risk of integration may threaten realization of a situation once evaluated as unbearable, thus throwing the system into a state of disarray.

First example of a multifocal Brainspotting session

A client, for instance, who was very poor in childhood, struggled to make it to the university, and was about to finish a MSc in biology. She had a panic attack the day before defending her thesis. While setting up the frame during the investigation of what might have been threatening her, it dawned on her how much a child inside of her felt that an impending professional success would mean a kind of betrayal of her family values of humility, of the unsuccessful alcoholic father and of the enabling, compassionate mother who stayed home to take care of the client's various siblings. There was also a part of her that wanted do overcome all of this and eventually become a university professor. Both this inner child and the professor-to-be were in a meteoric collision course that caused a reaction of comet paralysis, much aligned with the forces of entropy and synergy at play.

During the Brainspotting session, the client told her internalized mother that the daughter was entitled to more in life, as homage to all of the sacrifices mom had made in the past with the goal of taking care of the children. She also told her internalized father how sorry she was for the bad choices he had made in life, but her professional success should not be a source of shame for his failure in life. On the contrary, it should be a source of pride that his daughter had made it into the world of the grown-ups.

The little girl inside of her realized she could break the eggshell to reach a new state in life without having to destroy the nest. As the fears of her instinct towards growth subsided, and were viewed positively by the parts of the system, a shy teenager appeared for the first time. This synergic synthesis realized she would have to explore the limelight if she were to overcome the family financial and social shortcomings. The panic attacks did not occur again. She got her MSc title and moved to another city for a PhD program.

This example shows that the system provides the client with a contradiction between these synergistic and entropic vectors. Initially, there is overt motivation to change, but a substantial part of the system considers change as a move towards entropy, towards dispersion, annihilation, and ultimate demise. On the other hand, as therapy progresses, it becomes gradually evident that some of the defensive reactions are the ones that actually maintain inner dispersion. The entropic gradient is high, with parts maintaining their attempts to avoid engagement, to avoid interaction, to surrender to the unknown of the self, or to the perceived expectations of the therapist.

The concepts of entropy and synergy offer the clinician an indication of the status of the system, so that therapists may evaluate the availability of parts of the self to participate in the reorganization, and their ultimate conversion into a more cohesive whole.

The client is always one to whom we may return

Many therapists feel drawn to the multiplicity used by the client to represent the internal reality. This allure tempts the therapist into taking up a position of believing that multiplicity corresponds to various personalities trapped inside a single body. Though this attitude may sound coherent with the empathic therapist, it can hamper the progress of clients who feel trapped inside an imaginary room of mirrors that distort their personal image. Therapists should be careful not to add another mirror to the already fragile system, even if at times there may be some direct interaction with a single distressed part. When an inner child manifests itself, the adult does not vanish from consciousness. It may recede into a quieter background, and observe the interaction with the therapist.

Where to start and how to proceed

Since the internal negotiations involve parts that vary in levels of developmental stages, of distinct degrees of consciousness, with differing steps towards integration with the self, it would make sense to intuitively address the most fragile parts first, so as to grant them synergy and empower the system. However, though counterintuitive, it is safer to first address the "gatekeepers", the most reluctant and powerful parts of the system, and ask them for permission to continue. If we overstep their territory without a free pass, they will raise infinite barriers of resistance, wasting energy and creating power struggles within the client and against the therapist.

But how can this permission to move on be granted from such reluctant parts? Some psychoeducation and actual sharing of the therapist's point of view may help these reluctant parts to review their strategies for protecting the inner system from synergy.

1. No parts are to be destroyed or disempowered from the outside;
2. Every part is relevant for the maintenance of the system, and every part has the right to exist;
3. No matter how a part may act, it is a sign that it is doing its best to preserve the integrity of the system;
4. The therapist is willing to help by promoting more communication between the parts, and to reduce the suffering that results from internal alienation;
5. No one in the system has to trust the therapist, and any therapeutic activity may be subjected to thorough surveillance from internal parts; and
6. Should there be any form of infringement of rules the therapist may not be aware of, the system must inform him/her, so as to maintain a spirit of collaboration;

With this kind of basic information out in the open, components of the system usually acquiesce to the presence of the therapist, if the intervention is more collaborative in nature.

Once the therapist has the authorization to continue, and the parts have engaged in the therapeutic relationship, we may move a step further and set up the frame.

Multifocal Brainspotting as a promoter of systemic synergy

What follows are basic guidelines to set up a frame that encompasses multifocal intervention. The steps will vary, according to the client's inclination to participate and the degree of internal entropy of the system.

1. Invite the client to go inside, to access his/her self and to be in contact with the self for a while; then find a spot that goes with the self. This self-spot should be a resource spot that offers anchoring in the here and now and to which the client may return any time during the session;
2. After focusing on the self-spot, and realizing the state of being on this spot for a while, the client is instructed to go back inside, or to become aware of the presence of another part that may want to participate in this activity. Unwilling parts do not have to participate; they may go to sleep or play somewhere else, so that only those who are engaged in the process should be involved. The client usually finds the spot via an inside window, but may be helped with fine tuning the spot through the outside window;
3. The client returns to the self-spot for a while, to reorient to the here and now;
4. The client is invited to look inside and see if there is an additional part that is activated, and that would like to participate. The client feels the part and finds a spot that goes with that feeling;
5. The procedure is repeated until all parts have a corresponding spot, and the self-spot is well established.

Clients are free to choose on which part to focus, how long to stay on each brainspot, what to comment on, and what sequence to follow.

The observation and processing of unmet needs of parts tends to gain momentum with changes in the configuration of the system. What happens next varies from uncertainty to the occurrence of the unexpected. A few examples:

There tends to be a decrease in an initial sense of isolation;

There is usually visual rearrangement of spots, changes in proximity and distancing, which suggest rearrangement of entropic and synergistic vectors;

The self tends to take the initiative to change patterns, and to listen to an estranged part, reducing what Fisher (2017) in her wonderful book termed inner alienation;

There is more curiosity and the will to negotiate the needs of certain disowned parts;

In more defensive clients, with more entropic systems, the client may recognize the impossibility of offering the system the help it needs for the time being – it is vital for the client to forgive him/herself for not being able to correspond to internal demands;

In less entropic systems, with less ambiguity, requests for help from fragile younger parts may be received with parental capacity from the adult self to shelter them;

Self and parts may decide to become more integrated, or to keep their communication channels open, but in a state of relative dissociation.

Example of a multifocal Brainspotting session – welcoming the damaged internal system

The client is a successful professional in the area of physical health. She initially comes to therapy due to thoughts of suicide. She believes her hostile daughters learned to bully her from the estranged former husband. She divorced him on the grounds of domestic violence. She has had previous experiences with talk therapy, but complains they were not sufficient to give her the answers she is looking for. She now lives with the younger of two daughters. The younger daughter was diagnosed with borderline personality disorder and an autoimmune disease. The elder followed in Mom's professional steps. She is an accomplished student who does not know what career to pursue. She is quitting her studies altogether, and beginning a course in computer science. The client is currently married to a second husband. Together with the younger daughter, all three maintain a tempestuous interaction under the same roof. The elder daughter lives in the neighborhood, in an apartment that is rented by Mom. She resents what she believes Mom's having neglected her in favor of her "manipulative sister". Being a good girl did not guarantee the attention she always wanted from Mom.

According to the client, "no one respects Mom". The younger threatens to commit suicide every time Mom attempts to exercise some autonomy, such as asking her to find a place of her own to live. The client suffers from chronic pain and was diagnosed with fibromyalgia. The presentation of the complaints is confused, painful, and catharsis brings little relief, suggesting an ambivalent style of early attachment to her caregivers.

After a few introductory sessions, we decide to focus on the client's feeling of impotence with respect to her daughters as well as her personal neglect with respect to her physical health. As soon as we start to set up the frame, she is suddenly seized by an uncontrollable feeling of drowsiness, shuts her eyes, and reclines prostrate back into the armchair. With her eyes closed, she asks me if I am attempting to hypnotize her. She feels all of her thoughts have vanished from her head, and she can no longer think straight. Despite the inability to keep her eyes open, she maintains a fairly normal tone of voice.

I tell her I am not trying to hypnotize her, but add that if I were, what she thinks might happen. She shares a fear of being controlled, as her father had done to her in the past. I encourage her to simply observe what happens to her, and where this fear comes from. I reduce the scope of the frame by interacting more and keep her going, instead of attempting to pull her out of the apparently spontaneous trance, which does not have to be seen as a problem. I also ask her how she would feel less in danger of being controlled. She says that if I speak too much, then I would be hypnotizing her. I reassure her I am not moving from my chair, and will not speak too much, so she may feel in more control.

She moves on, and shares the fear of not doing what she is supposed to be doing in therapy. This is a voice that comes to her. I reply that I do not have expectations of what she is supposed to be doing. We may entertain the idea of finding out what happens if she keeps on observing herself, and if we pay more attention to the apprehensive voice. She says it` s from a little girl who tries to be nice. This is a girl inside, to whom she sometimes talks in her head. I realize she may be more familiar with dissociative parts and not get too scared to notice them.

She says "something" holds her eyelids down, so she was cannot open her eyes for the Brainspotting to take place. I clarify there is no such prerequisite to Brainspotting, and that all she has to do is to observe what happens, and wonder who keeps her eyes shut. She says it is another part, a teenager who is afraid I may abuse her, like an uncle of hers did in the past. If the abuse happens again, and her eyes are closed, she will not have to see it, so the little girl will still be nice. She feels a choking sensation, like her throat being strangled. When encouraged to observe the feeling, she realizes it is caused by a male voice who says she's a prostitute, and orders us to stop.

I concentrate on tranquilizing the abused parts by saying the uncle and I are different from one another. I tell the client to check with the male voice to determine what his concerns are, were we to continue. He says he is not in the mood for talking today. I reassure the voice that I am keeping the promise that was made that we would only work under previous authorization from the system. We negotiate to continue our conversation in another session, when these parts may have their chance to been seen and to be heard. Everyone agrees with the plan, and the teenager lets the client open her eyes. The client is still a bit stunned with everything that has happened, and so we try to orient her to the present and close the session in the here and now. It is usually safer to interrupt the procedure and to preserve the deal, than to trespass the protective borders and lose the client.

During the following session, we check inside to see if everyone is ok to continue, as was agreed upon last time. A child that was not present last time reports she prefers to stay away. She is afraid to see what may come up. The strangler will monitor the session, which is great, since it is a gatekeeper, and has to evaluate what is happening. Upon request, we are good to go.

She finds a self-spot at the center of the visual field, a little to her left side. The teenager prefers to find a spot inside, with her eyes closed, whereas the nice little girl looks up to the right, and an additional ashamed abused part looks down to the left. The strangler does not want a fixed spot. His job is to oversee the others.

The ashamed part suffers from self-recriminatory remarks that we later on in the process recognize as coming from a male part who does not accept the abuse. I try to reframe the inner criticism by saying that instead of being stubborn and critical, perhaps he is just being cautious, trying to be protective of something the client has not yet fully grasped. It is the reluctance to realize what happened in the past, and integrate it with the present.

She explores the inner space a bit further and finds a three year old who does not understand what is happening. She was left in an empty attic in the past. She is scared, and not really sure if the self is her mommy or something else. I try to utilize the intensity of the strangler and the scared one, and somewhat connect them. I ask the adult to explain to the 3-year-old how many strong protectors she has inside. The little child cannot cope with all of that, but the client returns to the protective teenager, now rebellious with blue hair, to take care of her. The self does not have the capacity to hold the 3-year-old, for she had to cleanse some of the inner dirt, before helping her other parts. The teenager finds and lends the 3-year-old a protective brainspot. The child could not do it on her own.

I join in by saying it is always prudent to respect the wisdom and rhythm of the inner system, and that things have to move according to the limits set by the parts. The adult complains she is drained and wants to finish. I asked her to thank the new parts for presenting themselves, as well as those who are not ready to show up.

Before we finish, I ask the self to make a summary to all of the parts of what had happened, and then to concentrate on the part of the body that feels most tranquil. We gradually return to the outside and debrief quickly. The client still thinks it is all too crazy, but her intentions of suicide have subsided a little. She feels we have performed major surgery, and she needs some time to recover. Her initial apprehension is replaced by relief, and some hesitant hope. Before leaving, she asks what to do with these parts, and I tell her to observe them and to check how they react in her daily life.

In the following session we do more grounding exercises and go over what happened, so as to fully reorient the self to the present. It is a long-term process. In other equivalent situations, clients have to undergo some more integration of parts, and the employment of synergic forces of the inner system before they feel strong enough to confront the traumatic contents from their past history.

Concluding Remarks

The theme of dissociation is complex by its very nature, with different foci of divergent schools of thought, and various books on the subject. Brainspotting is an encompassing, psychotherapeutic approach that provides a theoretical and technical substrate that helps brainspotters support these clients, though dissociative clients may bring a complex mixture of simultaneous attachment seeking demands with flight/fight/ freeze avoidance defenses. The dual attunement frame therapists set up provides a breathing space for exploration, negotiation, and eventual integration of disowned parts of the self.

This chapter offers Brainspotting clinicians an introductory step in this direction, but far from an exhaustive one. Different contemporary renowned authors use innovative ways of conceptualizing and treating dissociation [Richard Schwartz, 2013 (Internal Family System); and Kathy Steele, Ellert Njenhuis, and Onno van der Hart 2006 (Structural Dissociation)]. Brainspotting may also be regarded as a therapeutic approach that offers specific technical alternatives to grant clinicians access to inner parts of dissociative clients, even those parts that make up an entropic inner system. Brainspotting intervention promotes the establishment of communication channels and provides opportunities for integration between parts and self, whenever that is a possible outcome of internal negotiations.

The interaction between parts and self points to a characteristic indeterminacy of the self. From the vagueness of its composition and the uncertainty principle that guides brainspotters come the support for clients to plunge into the unknown inside of them and come out of it with a sense of integration and peace. Based on the dual attunement frame, we encounter the indeterminacy of the client and the relativism of a therapeutic relationship, a fluid connection that provides both clients and therapists with the opportunity to interact in a meaningful way, making meaning where once entropy prevailed.

Based both on options ranging from the resource up to the activation model, different intervention Brainspotting strategies help dissociative clients find their stabilization within a flexible window of tolerance. Multifocal Brainspotting is just one of these tools. It can offer support to our clients so that they learn to acquire trust in external relationships with therapists and in internal relationships with their own conflicting parts. Based on this relational paradigm, clients are encouraged to face their ghosts and to gradually transform them into helpers. Processing traumatic content and integrating dissociative material may bring peace to their troubled pasts. The entropic nature of these inner systems can be changed into synergic forces that help clients find untapped resources.

The Brainspotting way of moving the system`s entropy to internal synergy may be achieved both at a clinical and at an affective neurobiological level. Clinically, brainspotters set up a relational bond that establishes a collaborative relationship. At a neurological level, ventral vagal activation enables clients to engage in self-contemplation in a non-threatening environment provided by the therapeutic support. Dissociative clients benefit from these processes of affective neurobiological interactions in order to foster synergic integration of disassembled parts of the internal system and to enjoy the freedom of self-regulatory activities.

The internal system acquires the confidence to let some light shine through the cracks of dissociation, so that isolated parts gradually feel they may belong and become players in this game of interactions with other people. The avoidance defenses of chaotic maintenance of inner struggles may gradually subside, and be replaced by the possibility of internal commitments between parts and the self.

Brainspottingwise, a preferred way of applying multifocal Brainspotting works by means of gazespots because it is hard for therapists to memorize the exact multiple angles chosen by the client to correspond to each dissociated part. As the client is invited to follow what happens on the spots, multifocal Brainspotting may be considered as a combination of gazespotting and rolling Brainspotting, but with the spots scattered throughout the visual field instead of placed along a straight line. I also refer to the self-spot as a resource spot, to which the client may return at any time, with the main purpose being grounding. Should the client not find the self as a grounding place, due to its fragmentary composition, other Brainspotting interventions may be used in order to adjust themselves to the unmet needs of the client. Multiple Brainspotting is a comprehensive strategy encompassing the complexity of dissociative clients and bringing them to a state of integration and grounded peace.

The literature on dissociation is expanding rapidly, and brainspotters who identify themselves with the dissociative clientele have plenty of sources to support their interest. These sources will boost the necessary knowledge required to improve the quality of lives of these clients. For the additional information and training these complex clients require, please check International Society for the Study of Trauma and Dissociation (www.isst-d.org), the European Society for Trauma and Dissociation (www.estd.org), and the International Society for Trauma and Dissociation Studies (www.istss.org).

References

Braun, B. G. (1988). The BASK (behavior, affect, sensation, knowledge) model of dissociation. *Dissociation,* 1, 4-23.

Corrigan, F. M, Fisher, J. J., & Nutt, D. J. (2011). *Autonomic dysregulation and the Window of Tolerance model of the effects of complex emotional trauma.* Journal of Psychopharmacology, 25 (1): 17-25.

Fisher, J. (2017). *Healing the fragmented selves of trauma survivors: Overcoming internal self-alienation.* New York: Routledge Taylor and Francis Group.

Grand, D. (2013). *Brainspotting: The revolutionary new therapy for rapid and effective change.* Boulder: Sounds True.

Ogden, P., & Fisher, J. (2015). *Sensorimotor psychotherapy: Interventions for trauma and attachment.* (Norton Series on Interpersonal Neurobiology). New York: W. W. Norton & Company.

Panksepp, J. (1998). *Affective neuroscience: The foundations of human animal emotions.* New York, NY: Oxford University Press.

Pessoa, F. (2002). *The book of disquiet.* Penguin Modern Classics. London: Penguin.

Porges, S. (2011). *The polyvagal theory: Neurophysiological foundations of emotions, attachment, communication, and self-regulation.* New York: W. W. Norton & Company.

Rosenbery, S. & Shield, B. (2017). *Accessing the healing power of the vagus nerve: Self-help exercises for anxiety, depression, trauma, and autism. Berkeley:* North Atlantic Books.

Ross, C. A. (2017). *Structural dissociation: A proposed modification of the theory.* Texas: Manitou Communications, Inc.

Schore, A. N. (2012). *The science of the art of psychotherapy.* (Norton Series on Interpersonal Neurobiology). New York: W. W. Norton & Company.

Steele, K, Boon, S. & van der Hart, O. (2016). *Treating trauma-related dissociation: A practical, integrative approach* (Norton Series on Interpersonal Neurobiology) 1st Ed. New York: W. W. Norton & Company.

Schwartz, R. (2013). *Internal family systems therapy* (The Guilford Family Therapy Series). NY: The Guilford Press.

Van der Hart, O., Nijenhuis, E. R. S., & Steele, K. (2006). *The haunted self: Chronic traumatization and the theory of structural dissociation of the personality.* New York: W. W. Norton & Company.

BSP, Dissociation and Ego States

Mario C. Salvador

"The 'descent into the underworld' is the journey towards our parts that are separated, repudiated, that are unknown, undesired, banned and exiled in the different underground worlds of consciousness ... The goal of this journey is to meet with ourselves. This return home can be surprisingly painful, even brutal. To undertake it, we first have to accept not exiling anything"

(Stephen Cope, mentioned in van der Kolk, 2015, pg. 139).

The soul empties itself of all its own contents in order to receive into itself the being it is looking at, just as he is, in all his truth.

Simone Weil

Brainspotting and highly complex Post-Traumatic Stress Disorder

Brainspotting is a very efficient technique for reprocessing the traumatic memories and the painful experiences that still limit the performance of the individual in his current life (as well as for expanding the optimal performance based on peak experiences). As we teach in the basic Brainspotting training, the standard model is very efficient in the treatment of PTSD and complex PTSD and even highly complex PTSD, owing to the fact that BSP is highly focused and inclusive, and the therapist's active use of presence and attunement helps with focused mindfulness and with self-regulation (see chapter about Attunement and BSP in this book). But with patients who easily come out of the "Window of Tolerance", which David Grand calls "highly complex PTSD", "extremely complex PTSD" and "DID" (Dissociative Identity Disorder) the standard model becomes insufficient due to the self-regulation issues of these patients, the difficulty of developing and staying in a dual awareness in mindfulness, the strong dissociative barriers and the issues of trust and staying in a relationship even if it is therapeutic.

Brainspotting is a powerful therapeutic technique to access the non-processed experience registered in the subcortical brain and to promote their adaptive processing in a fast and efficient way. But when treating severely traumatised individuals with highly complex PTSD diagnoses, processing in its turn will awake the rigid and extreme defences that the individual developed to survive: denial, neglect, disconnection, and affective lethargy, all of these expressions of an extreme dissociation. These dissociative mechanisms helped the victims to survive but now they also maintain the trauma. Therefore, in therapy when we wish to approach the original trauma, the dissociative mechanisms will be aroused and they will awake in a way similarly to how they acted to protect the client's brain from feeling overwhelmed or overpowered with terror and pain. Therefore, therapy with these patients becomes more complex and technical and the therapist will have to apply knowledge and specific therapeutic capacities to work with a highly deregulated and only slightly resilient brain. This will require, among other things, the therapist to help the patient to work on more focused and defined frames as a way to promote the healing and the processing by parts or pieces of the experience. One way to do so is to consider and identify the inner complexity of the divided system: the Partsi of the personality that have been fragmented and that cohabit the intrapsychic world of the client, turning it into a complex or a very complex inner system, which normally is in conflict.

All the processing with Brainspotting naturally comprises an implicit process of the experience contained in the different survival subsystems involved in coping with the traumatic threat (they match the biological survival systems: attachment crying, fight, flight, faked death, freeze, total submission and collapse. See figure 1). In the processing we can observe how the different survival subsystems reveal the information associated with the experienced story. However, patients with very complex PTSD present important issues concerning:

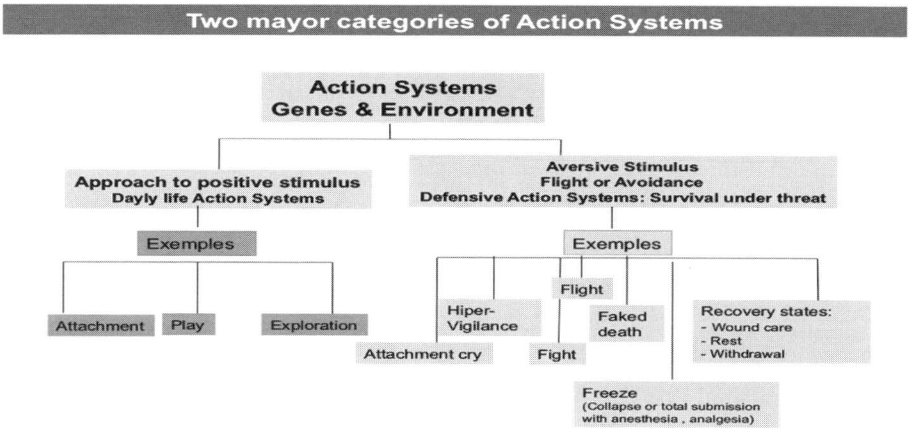

fig. 1

Two Major Categories of Action Systems
Action Systems
Genes & Environment
Approach to Positive Stimulus
Daily Life Action Systems
Examples
Attachment
Play
Exploration

Aversive Stimulus
Flight or Avoidance
Defensive Action Systems: Survival under Threat
Examples
Attachment Cry
Hyper-Vigilance
Fight
Flight
Faked Death
Freeze
(Collapse or Total Submission
With Anesthesia, Analgesia)

- Emotional deregulation and its capacity to support the needed mindfulness, which is essential for reprocessing and containment and pacification of the overwhelming emotional responses or management of dissociative defences that have turned off the emotional experience.
- The capacity to trust and to stay in a trusting human relationship can help support emotional regulation of very intense emotions. These people have learnt to distrust human beings due to the fact that they generally have been betrayed by their closest caretakers. With them, a special emphasis should be put on restoring their social engagement system response (Porges's ventral vagal system), by helping them differentiate their transference response of the past context from a new relationship that now is present, safe and supportive (see chapter on BSP and attunement). One way to help this is to use their mechanisms of attention to collect data proceeding from the current context, what their eyes and ears let them know about having a therapist present, interested, involved and safe. It requires paying attention to the signals they perceive emerging from the facial expression and the voice intonation of

the therapist. Once this is established, the therapist can invite them to observe how they feel in their bodies, the experience of being in a new relationship in which they are with someone present. This can be used as a somatic-relational resource for re-processing.

- Their motivation is to accept some inner aspects that retain memories of horror, terror, shame, desolation, and desperation. In this sense, they also do not trust themselves, nor their capacities to tolerate the pain that they have kept denied, set aside, and dissociated for so long. The therapist must express the hope that they can go through the experience together and that something healing will take place, but must also teach self-regulation mechanisms that will help develop a sense that they have a self-regulatory control and that the way to promote healing is to listen and to embrace what for so long was disowned. Here psycho-education is important, being able to see that the way they judge, despise, and ignore their own experience is a replica of how others treated them in the past and how this contributes now to re-traumatisation.
- The consciousness of their inner system is divided into different survival subsystems that have been established as ego states or Parts that are in internal conflict, that live in a chaos that fights to take control, and that search for attention in the client's system. In extreme cases they may be unknown to each other. An important task in the therapy process with these clients is to help them recognize their inner map of the different Parts in competition with each other, and to know their inner constellation of Parts. The next step will be to create with them an inner self-relationship culture with each of the Parts of this constellation, by showing interest in knowing its functions and fears, the relationship among them, and their contribution to survival. This will increase co-consciousness and communication among the Parts.

With these patients it will be necessary to adapt our way to treat them, to be more careful and patient, and to proceed slowly. Generally, we will not be able to use Brainspotting in the standard way, just to promote and expand the resilience states and the positive resources of the individual. The work with the therapeutic relationship and also with helping them treat their traumas in a more focused way becomes especially important. One way to do so is to identify the involved subsystems: the Parts of the personality that carry traumatic memories or act as intrapsychic defence systems or interpersonal defences that prevent access the pain. Each of these Parts hosts its own vision of the sense of the ego, of the others, and of the world.

Structural Dissociation and Actions Systems for Life.

Mammals are equipped for life with the background of neurobiological systems that help us to handle our lives since our birth. These systems are the result of selection through thousands of years of phylogenetic evolution of what is adaptive for life and survival. Jaak Panksepp (1998) in his book *Affective Neuroscience,* named some of these systems *"primary emotional systems"* for life, and he stated that they are embedded in specific psychobiological systems that monitor the activation of particular emotions. These basic emotional systems – or primary as termed by Panksepp – are very "sensitive" as they offer a neuronal substrate to arouse several kinds of coherence or organised patterns in the body's function. They also allow animals – and human beings – to be "active agents" in the world, as contrasted with simply "information processors"; that is to say, they enable active interaction with the environment. "Without conditions" (that is to say, in a programmed and automatic way) they identify specific primary threats for survival, and they initiate actions that help us deal with the environment without participation of will or of thought (tertiary processes).

In general, we have two large branches in the "primary emotional systems": systems organised for defence or survival and systems that function in everyday life; other authors call them 'action systems' (Ogden et al., 2006; van der Hart et al., 2006). One branch inhibits the other, that is to say, either we are arousal-oriented towards defence and survival or we are arousal-oriented towards dealing with normal life (care, learning, procreation, play ...)

Among the action systems for defence (figure 1) we include:

- Attachment crying (call the care-giving figure)
- Hyper-vigilance and exploration of the environment
- Fight
- Flight
- Faked death
- Freezing or total submission with anaesthesia
- Recovery states:
  - Wound care ("lick the wounds")
  - Rest
  - Isolation from the group

Among the action systems for daily life, we have:

- Attachment (approach and get closer to others, separation stress disorder, longing)

- Exploration (interest and curiosity)
- Play (characterised by joy and laughter)
- Energy regulation (eat, rest, consume, etc.)
- Sociability (motivated by affection and cohabitation)
- Care of others and oneself (boosted by tenderness and compassion)
- Reproduction/sexuality (handled by sexual desire)

We know that in individuals subject to chronic and cumulative threats to their lives (those who have experienced and grown up under chronic mistreatment, neglect, or abuse), the action systems with which we are equipped for survival and life may not integrate in an organised, coordinated, and sequenced survival response. They can become fragmented, resulting in the individual living alternatively with different senses of himself (fig. 2). These senses of one's self result in the subjective experience of the different Parts of the individual's ego. Many times, we can literally listen to the client talking about different Parts of himself thinking, desiring, or perceiving in ways that are in conflict, the ones with the others. In figure 2 we can see the relationship between the survival subsystems and the emotional and psychological experiences associated with them.

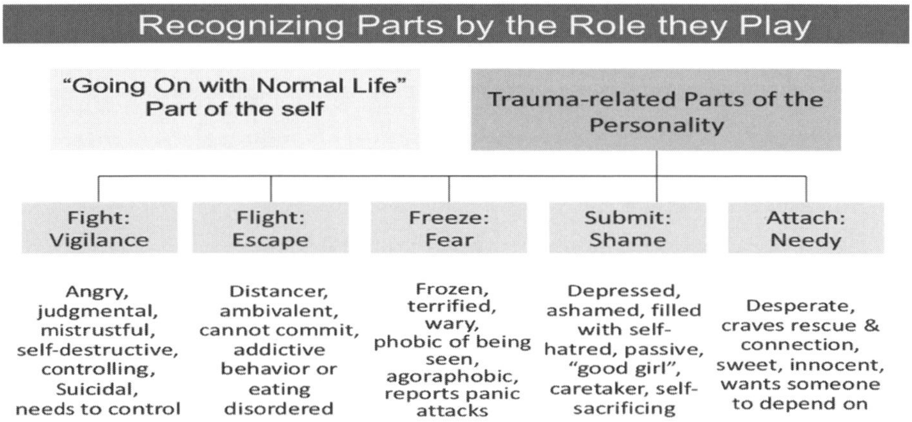

Fig. 2, adapted from Janina Fisher (2017)

The therapist will have to listen with attention to the language of this fragmented inner world. With this language, he starts not only identifying, but also understanding the conflict and inner complexity of his client. More importantly, the therapist helps the client to recognize what activates and inspires his behaviours, to differentiate what drives his actions, to create an internal relationship environment with his different Parts, the co-consciousness among them and interest in the survival function they have had and how they all helped in their own way. All of them have acted in the most intelligent way possible at the time of the trauma in order to help him to survive.

The personality contains a series of characteristic and enduring ways of thinking, feeling, acting, and perceiving; these can be situational and can depend on the context; that is to say, they are triggered after a specific stimulus that reminds them of other similar moments. This happens when we have experiences that have not been processed and updated. We have a biographical story (mediated by the hippocampus and the dorsolateral prefrontal cortex). Here we feel like authors and we can distinguish the past from the present, keeping ourselves in the present. And we have an implicit somatic story, that contains the procedural learning and the emotional scars of our personalhistory. Dissociation is a survival mechanism that involves appropriation and disowning the experience alternatively: while a Part of us retains the experience, the other one denies it and avoids it by all means, codifying it as an implicit, somatosensory and procedural memory, leaving it as a living story in our corporeality. Individuals with dissociative disorders and complex post-traumatic stress disorder survive by splitting their memories and feeling fragmented and divided; they have memories, thoughts, feelings, behaviours, ... that live alienated to them, as if they did not belong to them. This way, they experience more than one sense of 'ego' and they do not feel that some of these "egos" belong to them. Our thoughts, emotions, and behaviours, apart from their resulting pleasant or unpleasant feelings, belong to us; in some way they tell our story. Even if we try to disavow our experiences and our history, it is impossible to do so. The integration work will consist of reclaiming of our experience and accepting with it our different Parts, listening to the story they could not tell in order to extract an adaptive life lesson and be able to inhabit our body bountifully and lovingly. This is honouring our survival story and our intelligence.

A first goal in therapy is to be able to relate to the experiential stuff which is avoided or rejected by the defensive Parts better in order to create a sense of co-consciousness, cooperation and inner harmony, and a new way of relating to oneself, a new internal attachment system. This will contribute to starting the path to carry out a friendly and more efficient and self-regulating neuroprocessing.

The Parts' Language

Parts, or ego states, are bundles of neural connections that hold consistent patterns of information, affect, attention, behaviour, and sometimes identity, which belong to specific developmental ages or situations. Human beings, like other mammals, are wired for all kinds of states. We are wired for waking, sleeping, eating, connecting, playing, aggression, curiosity, and, when needed, inhibiting those states (Shapiro, 2016, p. 27). When we are in an ego state that involves behavioural patterns, thoughts, feelings, and physical sensations, we usually refer to them commonly as "a part of me". We can say that each of these Parts has a different way of behaving under some circumstances; they, sometimes, have their own 'minds'. Thus, in a similar situation sometimes we can feel offended – for example – while other times we feel calm and reasonable. The Parts, ego states, or subpersonalities are alive (they contain experience) and they are personal; they have relationship with "oneself" and among each other. As the Parts are like individuals in the inner system, we can establish contact with them, help them communicate with each other, and provide what they need to heal.

Each Part has a role to carry out in its own life; they all open the door to an attribute in our psyche and in our actions in the world. Many Parts are specialised systems that perform a positive role, healthy and functional when we are in times of serenity and calmness. In this case our life works better; they help us have contact with other people, perform our work efficiently, take care of others, etc. But frequently when we are under stress, some Parts adopt an excessive and extreme role in a desperate attempt to protect ourselves from pain, vulnerability, and being damaged (protective Parts). These can behave in a way that self-depreciates or criticises or creates problems with other people; they can involve distorted perceptions of reality, inaccurate and prejudiced beliefs, or obsessive thinking patterns. Some others (repudiated Parts) can overwhelm us with pain or body tension by subtracting capacity to live our life with flexibility and creativity. When a protective Part becomes intense because it tries to protect, it also creates an inner imbalance in the system itself.

In general terms, we can talk about two main categories of Parts with respect to how the trauma was managed and to the "window of tolerance" (Siegel, 1999; Ogden, 2000). That is to say, if the experience exceeds the upper threshold of the "window of tolerance" and organises its response in hyperarousal or if its way to survive was more related to dissociation and freezing (Porges's dorso-vagal immobilisation defence), which involves hypoarousal, we will then have:

a) *Hypoaroused Parts,* which corresponds to what Lanius et al. (2010) call "dissociative blackout". Their features are:
   - They do not feel many emotions, and physical sensations; they live with emotional numbness and physical anaesthesia. Disconnection from emotions can produce an experience which to the individual feels like living only in 'his head', as if he were dead inside, as if he were wrapped in a cloud, or he feels 'stiff' or one-dimensional, or has the sensation of living on autopilot or as a robot. These people can be insensitive towards pain or feel numb in some parts of their bodies.
   - They have amnesia or memory loss, lost moments (more frequent in DID)
   - Time distortions, they have an altered consciousness of time.
   - Alienation or detachment from the self. The individual feels strange within himself, numbed in his emotions, feeling blank or clouded. Or he feels like he is observing himself from outside of the body. They can feel as if their environment or the people that surround them were unreal; people's voices can seem distant even when coming from nearby, or they can visually appear distant.

All these symptoms refer to Parts of the individual that live as if they were frozen during the trauma time.

Activation of these Parts produces changes in consciousness: feeling like one's the head is in the cloud, being forgetful, losing consciousness of time, and having issues with concentration, having day dreams, having fantasies, being in a trance, and experiencing a low level of mental energy.

They refer to immobilized states (Porges, 2011) such as: hopeless/helpless, inert/depressed, shame-filled.

b) *Hyperaroused Parts.* They correspond to when the experience interrupts or interferes abruptly with the life of the individual. They can be memory intrusions, thoughts or beliefs, feelings, perceptions, ideas, desires, needs, movements or behaviours, or physical symptoms. Their features are:
   - It is as if they suddenly appear out of nowhere and the individual feels physically controlled, possessed, or abducted by an experience that he cannot manage and that he feels overwhelmed by. He can feel how the other person controls him; he can hear voices that comment or discuss, criticise, cry, or talk in the background; or he senses other shocking inner experiences that do not feel like theirs.

These symptoms may manifest more easily when the individual is tired, suffers from a disease, because of high stress, drugs, or alcohol.

These kinds of Parts generally refer to mobilized, protective states (Porges, 2011) such as: hyper-alert, terrified and ready to run, angry and ready to fight; they could become extreme and inappropriate for current circumstances.

The usual situation for a person with complex PTSD and worst conditions is to alternate between hypo-aroused and hyper-aroused states. This shows the lack of emotional regulation capacity (something that is learnt during the first years of life in the bond with "a good enough mother", in terms of Winnicot, 1953). The level of severity of dissociation is marked by the degree of inner fragmentation and segregation (the experienced aspects that are repudiated and disowned). This involves some degree of lack of knowledge and lack of coordination among the different systems, to the extreme that in the most acute DID patients some Parts may not know others completely and establish in themselves a system that works separately from the rest. The post-traumatic spectrum disorders follow a continuous degree of severity from the simplest to the most complex and severe.

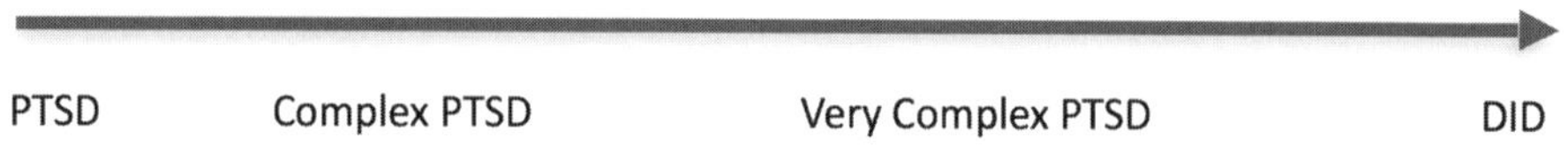

About Dissociation and Parts

Some parts may be dysfunctional, but they are not necessarily dissociative. Dissociation arises from a person's reflexive attempt to deal with attachment ruptures or trauma by shifting into a separate neural network, feeling disconnected from the sense of the core self. Dissociative Parts are more strongly wired, because survival was at risk when they arose. All dissociative Parts are ego states, but not all ego states are dissociative Parts. Ego states have permeable boundaries, unlike many dissociative Parts. They do not involve amnesia; that means this Part doesn't operate in the world without the awareness of other Parts. Dissociative Parts create a jarring intrusion into the person's experience and can cause the person to experience first-ranked Schneiderian symptoms: hearing voices commenting or arguing, feeling that the body can be controlled by someone else; that it can made to have thoughts, feelings, or impulses. Dissociative Parts can have a separate sense of self while ego states experience themselves as the person, albeit perhaps in a different state, age or time.

When a dissociative Part is active, the person can experience spacing out; the reaction could be a reflexive opiod response to a distressing emotion or situation. This is particularly the case when early trauma or attachment disruption (Schore, 2001). These may also be affective states such as anger, deep shame, fear, ... tied to another time.

In conclusion, dissociative Parts are more complex and can involve: their own identity, can have a characteristic self-representation sometimes not consistent with the self-representation of the individual, can have their own autobiographical memories, and may have a sense of ownership of their own experience.

Goals of Therapy in a First Stage:

1. *Training to be grounded to the present.* The sensations associated with the trauma are normally interoceptive sensations, sensed in the guts. As is explained well by Stephen Porges in his polyvagal theory, these sensations are informed very quickly by the efferent pathways to the stem and subcortical brain involved in the survival responses. The subcortical brain responds in a conditioned way as a dangerous life experience associated with the context in which the trauma happened, and it is now disconnected from an assessment of the context of the present reality. In this sense, they send the interoceptive perceptions that awake the warning in the brain stem and the reaction without mediation of consciousness. In these cases, it is important to help the client direct his attention towards the sensorial senses (sight, hearing, smell, touch) in order to be able to assess the perceptions related to the objects or stimuli that belong to the present context. This is one way to restrain the sensory flashbacks. It is about training the brain to direct the attention towards the present; it's about describing the nuances of sight, hearing, smell, touch, or even the inner stimuli that inform about physical sensations of the striated muscle not associated with the trauma, such as the strength sensed in the peripheral muscle, the feeling of balance, muscular contention, etc. Also the client can describe pictures or objects that remind him of the individuals in the social environment that support and love him. All of this is a way to put more energy into the perceptions of the current context to contradict the perception of the dissociated Parts held prisoner in the trauma context.
2. *To become conscious of the dissociated Parts of the personality.* Individuals with extreme traumatic dissociation can perceive their inner world or inner landscape with some degree of conflict; this way they can perceive aspects of themselves as hidden in caves, dark wells, children huddled in bedrooms. These scenes or inner landscapes are useful in therapy to help the client create a distance between the current sense of self (and even better the observer self, hereinafter called the Essential Self) and the ego that belongs to the past.

The chronic and intensely traumatised person generally organises his personality in types of specialised Parts.

Types of Parts according to the experience and functions that they involve:

a) *Parts in charge of managing everyday life and avoiding any connection with the traumatic experiences.* We may call them 'proactive protective Parts'. These Parts are in charge of managing the challenges of life proactively, that is to say, doing things or mobilising behaviours that help avoid contact with the pain. Even if they are trying to avoid contact with the Parts that remember the trauma, they are always influenced by them. As an example, some of these Parts are demanding or perfectionist as a way to protect themselves from a deep pain of another Part that feels 'unsuccessful', 'useless' or 'worthless'. Other Parts can be over-solicitous of others to also pseudo-satisfy a need to 'feel important or necessary for the others' and to mask the pain of having 'felt ignored'. Even other Parts can be strong and hard with oneself or others as a way to protect them from 'feeling that they needed others that were not there, the abandonment and the neglect'. Some of these protective Parts emerge or act internally, for example 'the inner judge or the internal criticism'; this inner judge can be very hard and hostile with the person saying things like "you're a piece of shit, you don't deserve love", or "you're a slut and no one is going to love you". Even though the attack itself is harmful, the ultimate goal is still to convince the more vulnerable Parts (disowned), those that need love and attachment, not to emerge and ask things, as there will be nothing for them and they will suffer more. We can still find fighter Parts that try to keep the others far away in order to frighten them and make them want to avoid the pain or the proximity and the fear of being betrayed or abandoned again.

In conclusion, these defensive Parts are the method by which the survival system made decisions, sometimes very radical and rigid, about how to cope with pain and avoid suffering. However, even though these decisions once were an intelligent adaptation to the environment given the resources available, in the current life of the person, they keep the system in a survival state, and they hold the intrapsychic environment in the same relational context as the one that happened in the past, contributing to a re-traumatisation.

I say that every trauma was once interpersonal, but now it is kept intrapersonal, replicating an inner relationship, among Parts one with the others, that makes the person relive the past traumatic relationships. I also affirm that every interpersonal trauma is at the same time a transgenerational trauma; our caretakers do not do anything other than to reenact according to the ways they were treated and express the unresolved traumas of their ancestors. There are also Parts that support our ancestors' story, and they carry stories provided by the others. It is well-known that the transgenerational transmission pathway goes both through the relationship with the parents as well as through the epigenetic pathway. Many times, part of the healing work requires helping to understand that the experience does not belong to the patient and helping also to unload from these Parts the pain passed on by the ancestors.

b) *Parts tied to trauma* and which keep patients in intense pain, terror, shame, extreme sadness, freezing, collapse, ... I call these Parts: *disowned or repudiated*. These are those Parts that remember the trauma and what was experienced. They can be Parts that long for bonding and love – they cry unceasingly for an attachment figure – some others that feel terror about trusting and being betrayed again, Parts with shame, etc. These are frozen in time and distant both from the interpersonal bonds and from feeling accepted by the client himself. They tend to burst abruptly into the system overwhelming the patient with too many intense emotions, that in their turn can arouse dissociative protective Parts related to hypoarousal: not feeling, blank dullness, floating outside the physical body, ...
c) *Functional Parts*. In nearly everybody, even if not in all of them, we can also find Parts with resources that can help the system. Very commonly they are Parts that have lived and registered experiences with people that have provided good care in the past (sometimes a grandmother, a teacher, ...). These are Parts that can hold empathy, acceptance, and feelings of affection towards the Parts tied to trauma and have a self-comforting capacity. They are commonly Parts with empathy, caring capacities, or Parts that contain resources of strength, peacefulness, joy, love, spiritual feelings, or specific skills or knowledge useful for dealing with a situation .... In Brainspotting, they are important Parts for use in the first stages of therapy with the most acute patients or when resourcing is needed; we can find the "brainspot" of some of these Parts and expand their experience; it is a way to promote the resilience of a deregulated brain.

Beyond Parts

Beyond the Parts of our personality that by definition are associated with life experiences, there is a dimension of the individual's self that we all have before any experience and beyond all experience. It is the non-conceptual and compassionate observer that we all have, without exception; it is what we usually call a state of mindfulness, which corresponds to the arousal of one of the prefrontal cortex functions: metareflection. It is the specifically human capacity in which the possibility of the mind to observe one's self resides. We are not talking about another Part of the personality, but about a state of consciousness and a state of the self that can observe, embrace with compassion, and hold onto our experience with the attention and intention of accepting it as it is and 'listen to' the story which is still alive and needs to be revealed, completed, and finally unloaded and transformed. From this state of consciousness, which I call the 'Essential Self', the individual relates with the different Parts that are activated at a given time and now constructs a loving and friendly inner bond with his experiences (an internal attachment). This welcoming and compassionate attention is the most powerful resource that contains the self-healing capacity of the system.

As he reprocesses the experience, we must help the individual to place himself in this self-observing and compassionate self-study dimension so that he may enter into contact with his different "egos", help him feel that he can be having a painful experience but 'he is not' the experience. Any non-processed and non-metabolised experience comes from another time and another context, and "has a story to tell"; to be transformed, it needs for both the therapist – in his own Essential Self – and the patient, also in his compassionate Essential Self, to be present and interested in knowing and accepting the story.

Eastern philosophy teaches that when the mind becomes silent, a direct experience of spirit emerges. That signal, like the stars which appear when the sun goes down, is really always present. But it is concealed by the noise we make. And the biggest noise is the clamouring of the ego-absorbed mind, the reaction that comes from our different inner parts. In distancing ourselves from all that creates our everyday habitual ego (our reactive parts), we begin to recognize the dimension of the self that does not change, the powerful and universal self that permeates all (the Essential Self). There is a basic freedom that comes from relaxing our attachments to who we think we are and how we think things should be. There is a lightness of being, a new peacefulness and a feeling of spaciousness that makes room for humour and compassion. This spacious mind is about celebrating mystery and humour and an Essential Self beyond the boundaries of the ordinary ego. The first part of emotional healing is being limbically known – having someone with a keen ear catch our melodic essence (Lewis, Amini and Lannon 2001).

Dealing with the Parts

First stage: Identify the Parts and differentiate among them

The goal during the first stage is:

- Identify the Inner Constellation. This would mean creating the system's map or the inner constellation of Parts. We can perform it either in written charts by pointing out the Parts we identify in the verbal and body narrative of the client. During the time when the client expresses his understanding of the problem we point out and differentiate the various aspects of the inner constellation. We can help the client identify the manifestations of each of the Parts. The Parts can be expressed both as sensations, a belief, an emotion, a thought, a behaviour, a physical symptom, a memory, or an image. The therapist who acts here as detector and detective, helps to clarifyg the arguments or inner conflicts and the sub-systems involved in the client's difficulties. In this process the patient is helped to identify, name, place the age of each Part and how every one of them relates with other Parts or which place it has in relation to the other Parts of the internal system. Diagramming the Parts is less threatening than talking about their emotions. In some way it helps to get distance and to start relating to them from a curious and observing self that begins to have a relationship with the different elements of his inner system interested in knowing them and in what they do for the system: how did they help to survive. A variant of the Parts' map is to ask the client to draw his inner system (see figure 3) on which an inquiry could be developed.

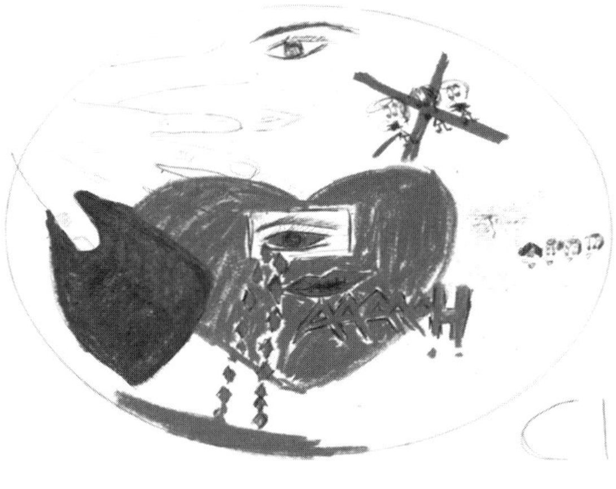

Fig. 3

- *Create a Sense of Differentiation and Distance between the Essential Self and the Experiential Ego.* In the former step, representing the Parts would have already created a sense of differentiation between the dimension of the individual who knows and starts to relate with his Parts and the Parts themselves. Now we want to continue promoting the construction of an "internal healing environment" At this point, some people will need to learn how to regulate the arousal of their autonomous nervous system (ANS) and to lower the arousal of the amygdala in order to be able to "plug in" and activate their prefrontal cortex (called "the watchtower" by van der

Kolk), the seat of the capacity for metareflection, in order to be able to regulate and support the intensity of their experience while maintaining their natural curiosity and capacities for self-compassion. The activation of the prefrontal cortex is the entrance gateway to awaken the brain's capacity for integration and healing: the brain that observes itself with "curiosity, acceptance and self-compassion". The Essential Self is the dimension of the self that is already present in each of us before having experiences, before having a name, and before any idea of the ego (it is our human spiritual condition, innately curious and kind).

Second stage: unloading and integration

As our parts are usually in a state of inner conflict and struggle to see who controls the sense of the self and the life of the individual, it will be essential to ask the inner system to which Part we should pay attention first and foremost. It is a way to create order and to establish priorities, making sure to express to the system the attitude that all Parts are important and that they will have the attention at another time. Generally there is a primary Part (in terms of Hal and Sidra Stone) which controls the performance. They are usually controlling perfectionists or pleasing protective Parts; sometimes they can also be Parts addicted to substances (reactive protective Parts) or in more extreme cases depressed or terrified Parts (disowned Parts).

Therapy and Unloading of the Protective Parts

Generally, some protective Parts are very closely identified with one of the primary caretakers or have developed ways to adapt to their requirements and desires. These dominant protective Parts try to be proactive in protecting the system of the self from entering into contact with and experiencing the Parts that contain more pain; thus, they try to avoid the suffering. In therapy, protective Parts should be treated first. They, on the other hand, are more superficial and more visible, as they are the ones more often dealing with everyday life and the relationships with others. Thus, they will be the ones more often emerging in the relationship with the therapist and with the world or they will appear in reprocessing when trying to reach the pain of the trauma. Some of these Parts have the energy of one of the caretakers (introjects) that were important in life (parents, grandparents, older siblings, etc.), but they could also contain energy and issues of other important educators in the life of the individual. It is this way because they have been in charge of trying to adapt to the relational environment's requirements and demands in order to be accepted. In other cases, they can also carry traumatic burdens of unknown ancestors who have passed on their experienced legacy through epigenetic and trans-generational pathways. The function in this case has to do with assuming roles or demands to promote the "belonging to the family clan", "carry family secrets" that they are forbidden to talk about, "remember unresolved or shameful matters", etc.

Concerning these Parts we must try to enter the closest time possible in which the Part was loaded with the energy of the introjected parental figure. By doing this, we work with the Part at the time when the features of the character, the habits, and the defences were still malleable. To work with the Part identified with the abuser in the earliest age state not only eases the alliance and the access (Calof, 1992), but also leads to a deeper generalisation of the resolution (Paulsen and Golston, 2014; mentioned in Lanius, Corrigan, and Paulsen, 2014). Working with the introjected Parts and with the patient's loyalty towards the abuser is a central issue in the treatment of the ego-system and child abuse (Paulsen, 2007, 2009, Putman, 1986; mentioned in Lanius, Corrigan, and Paulsen, 2014). The process of changing the alliance with the Part identified with the introject of the abuser towards the compassionate Essential Self of the patient is crucial. Due to the fact that the introjects of abusers are allies in the way of seeing things by the abuser and that they are heavyweights and leaders in the inner system in relation to the vulnerable and helpless child Parts, working with them directly and relatively soon in the treatment is very important in order to deactivate resistance to work. The cure for these introjected protective Parts will not be reached without the therapist's honouring, acknowledging, and appreciating them. However cruel its internal action seems, it was the little child's best way to cope in that situation in order to protect himself. At the time of that trauma, the child's own view of himself is truncated due to the shame that his needs and feelings are never seen, valued, nor satisfied. For reasons of survival, the child adopts the point of view of his abuser as the only possible one, and identifies with a sense of himself congruent with that of his abuser. These Parts identified with abusers can be understood better if we accept them as dissociative post-traumatic defences. On the other hand, it is often necessary and very healing to invite the Part with the introjected burden to reveal his own traumatic story and how it helped the client survive while it is in the presence of the compassionate Essential Self of the client. This will help with the healing of the system and the trans-generational healing.

Many times, the Parts of the client that have a trans-generational legacy have it as the function of someone bringing to light the ancestors' secrets or griefs that were encrypted as at that time, when the caretaker or ancestor lived his trauma and the circumstances did not allow its resolution.

Other protective Parts have learnt to avoid pain through adopting requirements demanded by the individual's caretaker environment. This is how they have become demanding, perfectionist, compliant, ... in order not to experience the most unbearable pain of rejection, devaluation, or judgement. There are two basic inquiry directions with these Parts:

a) *The protective function* they have been performing in favour of the client up until now. Generally they have been helping the person not to suffer more from looking for something that is not there in others, or to avoid facing rejection or criticism; or even the neglect of the caretakers. Even the very self aggressive Parts try to convince the individual of things such as "you are not worthy of love" or "you are defective" in order to discourage him from looking for something he will not be given. An important question is "what benefit does he get from what you are doing?.
b) *Fears* of what could happen if they stop doing what they were doing up until now. Some of these Parts may fear 'can not bear the pain', 'never stop crying', 'stay trapped in depression', etc. This is due to the fact that they have never been in contact with any other person who knew how to accompany and understand them in their pain, nor with their own Essential Self. Generally they have always met with their own denying protective Parts, the fierce internal criticism or other dissociative defences of not wanting to feel or trying to forget. Thus, an important role in treating them is to convince them that the way they did it up until now was good for surviving, but now they maintain the trauma as they continue treating the vulnerable Parts in a similar way as they were treated in the past by other people. Another important issue is to convince the protective Part that this time the client is interacting from a new place that never existed before (the Essential Self).

In any case, we always have to first treat the protective Parts that interfere with access to the most traumatised Parts that hold the most intense pain and the traumatic memories. Protectors have to feel that they are seen and validated before 'giving their permission and trust' to allow the access to the disowned Parts.

Therapy and Unloading ofthe Vulnerable Parts, the Disowned Ones

Once the protective Parts feel appreciated, seen, and acknowledged – and sometimes after they have unloaded their own story – they can allow access to the vulnerable Parts that they had been protecting, but at the same time had "repudiated" or "exiled" from the system. These are the Parts that retain the traumatic story and memories, or the encapsulated family secrets. The work to be done in processing is to support the compassionate gaze of the Essential Self and maintain the inner bond so that they can deliver the story they had been withholding for years.

When they are available, they become the target of processing under the accepting and compassionate gaze of the Essential Self. They are invited to speak in their language of sensations, emotions, images, beliefs ... the long time ignored and repressed story. The therapist must help the patient support the presence of the Essential Self to encourage the disowned Part to tell his story. Sometimes, it is advisable to ask the disowned Part to tell its story little by little so as not to overwhelm the system. These Parts, since they have been repressed for so long, may have the impulse to show their emotional burden abruptly. Therefore, inviting them to express themselves in small, measured amounts and little by little or helping them with the cyclic rhythmic breathing is a way to maintain them within the "window of tolerance".

The role of the therapist is to support the healing space and support the internal relationship between the Essential Self of the client and his disowned Part (see the healing bubble in the chapter on attunement). The therapist will do so by maintaining the state of presence and inviting the disowned Part to express as much as needed and the Essential Self to accept and embrace the experience as it comes, without judgement or expectations. Generally, the processing follows a "transformation arc", in such a way that every story has a beginning, a development or expression of the painful plot, and an outcome to reach completion and transformation. We must encourage the entire story to be expressed until the bodily sensations associated with the psychological distress are released and processed.

If the processing has reached its conclusion, we will focus the consciousness on the current pleasant sensations, a product of transformation, to give them time and space for the positive psychological qualities associated with them to surface (joy, freedom, love, spontaneity, strength, ...). Finally, we will invite the healed Part with its positive sensations and qualities to project its transformation in the individual's current life situations: "ask the child who now feels freed and loved to show you how he can help you in your current life with these sensations he has now", "can you see yourself handling your current life with these new sensations?".

Finally, it is advisable to acknowledge all the Parts that have been involved in processing for the trust they placed and their effort to help to survive.

Brainspotting and the Work done with the Parts

A patient, Susana, was expressing her relational issues and her frustration with her husband. She reported that he was never able to understand her completely and that there was a part of her that felt angry and frustrated with him. She explicitly stated "there is a part of me that he doesn't see and that he cannot reach". We continued exploring what she was experiencing in that place of herselfwhere she felt a tightness in her chest, this Part becoming thus more glaring and explicit. She felt alone and misunderstood, and she felt small and helpless. At some point I asked her "how old does that Part feel, which you feel in the tightness in your chest? She stated that she felt it as 6 years old. I explored what Susana felt from the current woman she was toward the 6-year-old part and she stated "wanting to help and take care of her". Grasping that Susana had enough energy in her Essential Self, I suggested letting that Part know that she now was there and that she would help her, and that we would give her the 'space and time' she needed to receive attention and care. I suggested helping her find a "brainspot" where she could feel that little and misunderstood Part more and we proceeded to look for the eye position in which she felt her Part more when exploring the line at the height of her eyes, the X axis. She pointed to a spot at her right and then we explored whether she felt more if the pointer went up, at the eye level or under the eye level, at the Y axis. She chose a high spot and there we located the "brainspot" to access the experience. From that point, I invited her to welcome with kindness and interest the information and the story that the Part retained in the feeling of tightness in her chest, in its language of sensations, images, emotions, or any other kind of it. The Part soon started showing an image the kitchen in her house when she was a child. There she learnt mathematics when she was 6-7 years old; she was also with a friend and her father was helping both of them. Because her friend was more skilled at mathematics, her father paid more attention to and gave more acknowledgment to her friend. The child Part of Susana started expressing feelings of pain and anger because her father expressed preference for her friend. And then she described other scenes in which she felt that her father had not supported her. He would not go to her sports competitions or he would not play with her. This child Part concluded "I am not important for Dad", "I cannot rely on him". Additionally, her father was not sensitive towards her complaints and crying; he would tell her she had to be strong and not cry. Thus she finally decided that "I have to be strong and independent; maybe then Dad will see me as worthy." Susana was embracing and witnessing the story of her child part embracing her pain and loneliness and helplessness while she was absorbed in the "brainspot" of her child part. During the process she awoke more love and compassion towards her child Part, and at some point she felt that the child was sitting on her lap and was crying. At the end of the session, the tight feeling in her chest reached SUD 0 and what surfaced and was replaced was a feeling and a sense of "I deserve love and I am worthy". When we again applied this transformation to the relationship with her husband she could see and felt that she could express to her husband her need for him to provide more physical contact and could also assume that she could ask him because he was willing to respond.

Procedure for Working with Parts in Brainspotting

1. Identify with the patient, as he relates his experience, describing which Part or Parts are involved in the problem he expresses. It is possible that more than one aspect or involved Part may appear. If this is the case, we can reflect on it by saying "what I've heard is that it seems there is a Part of you that feels sad and tired and I also hear how another Part of you calls it 'weak' and compares it to other people who suffer more. If the patient accepts the feedback, we can ask him "do you feel that we have to treat that sad and tired Part today?"
2. Confirm the therapy contract with respect to the process. If the patient accepts the former step proposal, this is taken as a therapy contract for the session. Before entering and treating the 'target' part (the part on which the "brainspot" will be looked for), the therapist must consider the involved 'protective' Part (in this example, the Part that criticises: "you are weak and others suffer more!") to see if this one is having some resistance or impairs access and to treat the Part that is suffering. If the involved Part has a problem with that, we have to negotiate with it in the sense that we are going to treat the Part with pain to help it and heal it. Usually, this is enough for the protective Part to be willing to leave the place and allow us to go to the painful Part (disowned). If this is not the case, we should continue treating it or, in a more resistant case, we have to move the protective Part into the therapy and processing 'target' in order for the protective Part to express its story too. In any case, either in the same session or in another one, the goal is to reach the Part that holds the pain (the disowned Part).
3. We explore where the client feels the target Part in his body, and we help this part to show itself as explicitly as possible. For example, we can ask the client to observe the Part's feeling in his body and to observe if there is any image or any scene associated with it, or if there is any emotion or belief connected to the physical sensation. I usually ask the patient "what do you feel towards that Part now?" as a way to check if he is in his Essential Self or in another protective Part. If the individual shows that

he feels "interest, curiosity, love, acceptance" or a non-judgemental, non-anxious, positive attitude, we realize that he has enough active energy in his Essential Self in order to start processing an 'internal relationship' between the Essential Self and the target Part. Thus, we are able to start looking for the "brainspot". It is advisable to measure the SUDS from 0 to 10 at the beginning as a way to measure the processing that will happen and/or to evaluate at the end of the process how much has been processed or how much there still is to process. We ask the patient to focus his attention on the physical sensation of the Part and we look for the eye position where he feels it more or where he feels it is the best position.

4. We invite processing in focused mindfulness. "Give space to that Part (or use the words that the client has been using to refer to it) and to the sensation (or the image, belief…) in which it is expressed and allow it to express itself in sensations, images, emotions or in any kind of way that she needs you to know about it, and simply embrace with kindness and curiosity, whatever it delivers".
5. During processing from time to time we will probe what is happening or what the Part or the body sensation wants to express. We should not over-use this inquiry in order to leave sufficient space and silence for the Essential Self to be able to listen and observe whatever comes without feeling interrupted or invaded. And from time to time the therapist will also check how the patient feels in his body, what he is expressing, to keep the focus on the body. Alternatively, we may ask "how is the child now?"; when he answers, we help check how the client feels that child state in his body and we invite him to continue observing and embracing whatever it still has to express.
6. Towards the end, we will check what the SUDS level is to assess how much has been reprocessed. If the SUDS has reached 0, we will tell the patient to invite the Part if it still needs to express some more ('squeeze the lemon"). If there is nothing more, and the sensations are pleasant and positive, and there is still time left in the session, we invite him to continue staying in the pleasant sensation and to see what happens from there on (always without expectations, or impatience). Here, we enter the 'expansion' mode of the experience. Normally, new functional behaviours will become associated with being used in current life. It is always appropriate to suggest that the patient focus on the starting scene where the target Part was suffering and to see how the situation is now with the new sensations. And finally, we suggest that the patient visualize himself in his current daily life with what he is experiencing right now (action planning function of the prefrontal cortex)
7. If the SUDS doesn't reach 0 during the session, a partial closure may be offered, giving to the Part the opportunity to suggest what else should be expressed in the

SUDS that still remains active. We assure the Part that we will not forget about it and that we will treat it again during the next session.

In particularly difficult patients (those with more difficulty maintaining their intense emotions modulation or calming their most injured Parts) it is advisable to promote the inner connection between the Essential Self and the Part during the week. We may ask "what do you feel now towards the child?", or "ask the girl now sitting on your lap how she would like you to interact with her during the week". Generally, these more dissociated Parts need the stable contact of someone who sees them, takes care of them, and gives them some attention. So we promote a commitment to meet each day – should it be possible, but we respect what the individual accepts or says -, to the Part that we are working with. This is about promoting 'the internal attachment' between the Essential Self and the Part we were treating, and developing a new neurological network between the traumatised part and a loving and caring dimension in the patient.

If during processing other defensive Parts, or rage, or fear, had risen in the client, we suggest checking how these Parts are after the work that has been done and the connection established between the Essential Self and the target Part. Usually if the processing has not been completed, these Parts involved in the problem will manifest that they will remain cautious or that "they will need to see what happens" before being able to transform the function they were carrying out. In some way, the system must consider whether the transformation is stable and helps in everyday life.

In other events, it is possible that a protective Part will be particularly resistant during processing. Should that be the case, we must leave space for this protective Part, and maybe transform it into a target Part, so that it can express how what it does helped and also its painful story. In this case, we must be cautious abaout expressing and assuring the disowned Part with which we started that we will get back to it later, and that if not possible during this session, we will do it in the following one.

A version of the processing expressed above is to use more than one "brainspot" for each of the different Parts involved in the problem. For example, in case of Parts that are very angry with each other, what is traditionally known as polarised Parts, the "brainspot" may be located for each of them and then the process of going from one to another is boosted. An elegant way to do so is to ask the internal system "which one do you feel needs to receive the attention first?" And once it has expressed and discharged enough, invite the patient to ask it if it is all right to go to the other "brainspot" for a while to see what happens in the other one. Usually, we may start suggesting that the patient ask the other Part if it heard what the former one was expressing and if it can also reveal what its sensed feeling retains. We tell the patient that when it has had enough in one, it may go to the other "brainspot" and observe what is happening there now, or simply just remain curious as to what will come now from that "brainspot". This way, reprocessing in two "brainspots" is promoted, which generally takes us to harmonization or integration of the system.

Additionally, we may work with "multiple brainspots", which is the technique I call "The Meeting Room". There we may invite the Parts involved in the client's problem to 'emerge or jump anywhere' in the room the client is in and suggest that he feel in which place and eye position he finds each of them. Thus, we will have several 'brainspots', one for each Part that has emerged. Then, we will ask if the client can feel curiosity and interest in knowing and interacting with each of the active Parts and will ask the inner system which is Part needs to express itself first (always expressing that all the other ones will have their space and time). We will invite the client to process the first one in mindfulness. When a great part of the story including functions and/or fears of this Part are expressed, we will suggest that the client ask the system which Part should continue expressing. We will invite the client to go to the "brainspot" of the Part whose turn it is and once again we will invite the client to the process (with the indication "invite this Part now to express in its own language of sensations, emotions, images, or thoughts what it needs you and the other Parts to know"). And, in that way, we will continue with each of the Parts that will have emerged at the beginning. Once all of them have expressed themselves, we will continue asking the system which one still needs to express itself. At the end of the session, we will check how each of the Parts is and how it is in relation to the others. If the processing has reached an integration, we will invite the system to express how it will help the client in daily life from now on.

In conclusion, the work with Parts is a more sophisticated and contained way of treating the problems of the clients with complex or very complex post-traumatic stress disorder, with those with whom it is necessary to tighten the frame for processing in order for it to be more contained and focused and for it to help the brain work on more concrete aspects of the trauma experience. Additionally the explicit work with Parts helps to establish peace and stability in the intrapsychic system and to establish a cooperative environment in the internal constellation. At the same time, it also develops an internal communication system with the survival roles that promotes a friendly relationship with their own experience and the different ego states.

Bibliography

Calof, D.L. (1992). Adult children of incest and child abuse: *Holograms of the trace generational family. American Family Therapy Academy Newsletter, 50,* 34–40.

Fisher, J. (2017). *Healing the fragmented selves of trauma survivors. Overcoming Internal Self-Alienation.* Routledge, NY.

Genpo Merzel, D. (2007). *Big Mind, Big Heart, Finding your way. Big Mind Publishing.*

Lanius, U. F., Paulsen, S. L. & Corrigan, F. M. (2014). *Neurology and Treatment of Traumatic Dissociation. Toward an Embodied Self.* Springer Publishing Company, NY.

Lewis, T., Amini, F. and Lannon, R. (2001). A General Theory of Love. Vintage Books, New York.

Ogden, P. & Minton, K. (2000). Sensorimotor Psychotherapy: One Method for Processing Traumatic Memory. *Traumatology,* Volume VI, # 3, art 3.

Ogden, P; Minton, K. & Pain, C. (2006). *Trauma and the body: A sensorimotor approach to psychotherapy.* New York: Norton.

Porges, S. W. (1995). Orienting in a defensive World: Mammalian modifications of our evolutionary Heritage –a polyvagal theory. *Psychophysiology, 32,* 301–318.

Porges, S. W. (2001). The polyvagal theory: Phylogenetic substrates of a social nervous system. *International Journal of Psychophysiology, 42,* 123–146.

Porges, S. W. (2011). T*he polyvagal theory: neurophysiological foundations of emotions, attachment, Communications, and self-regulation.* New York, NY: Norton.

Panksepp, J. (1998a). Affective neuroscience: *The foundations of human and animal emotions.* New York: Oxford University Press.

Schore, A. N. (2001). Effects of a Secure Attachment Relationship on Right Brain Development, Affect Regulation and Infant Mental Health. *Infant Mental Health Journal, 22,* 7–66.

Schwartz, R. (1995). *Internal Family System Therapy.* New York: Guilford Press

Siegel, D (1999). *The Developing Mind. How relationships and the brain interact to shape who we are.* Guilford Press, New York.

Stone, H. & S. (1989). *Embracing Our Selves: The Voice Dialog Manual.* New York: The New York Library.

Van der Hart, O; Nijenhuis, E. & Steele, K. (2006). *The haunted self: Structural dissociation and the treatment of chronic traumatization.* New York: Norton

Van der Kolk (2014). *The body keeps the score: brain, mind and body in the healing of trauma.* Viking Penguin.

Winnicott DW. Transitional objects and transitional phenomena; a study of the first not-me possession. *Int J Psychoanal.* 1953; 34 (2): 89–97.

[i] We write Parts with the first letter in capital letters to show that these are specific subsystems of the ego.

Brainspotting with Children and Adolescents

Monika Baumann & Martha S. Jacobi

Preface

The use of Brainspotting with children and adolescents poses further challenges to therapists and their young clients beside the normal Brainspotting process. What are these and how to deal with different age groups and regressive behaviour as well how to allow a creative approach in the Brainspotting therapy are explained and illustrated by many case studies.

Introduction

Research in recent years confirms that childhood trauma, seen as developmental and emotional injury, has a significant negative influence on psychological and physical well-being and illness, throughout the entire lifespan. A recent article in Spectrum, "Frühe Brandmale," sums up these newest alarming research results, which are consistent with an extensive body of pre-existing research (See, for example, the various works of Allan Schore, Robert Scaer, Louis Cozolino, Linda Chapman, and Daniel Siegel, among others).

More and more correlations are found answering the question "Why are we emotionally and physiologically affected by our emotional development during childhood?" Initial results indicate that mindfulness, presence, and psychotherapy can help to stimulate emotional self-healing. Daniel Siegel's work is exemplary in this regard.

As co-authors, we are contributing to this research in a practical way based on our daily experiences using Brainspotting with children and adolescents in different clinical settings including private practice, post-disaster community response (such as that provided after terror attacks and school shootings), and times of crisis in children's lives (such as placement into foster care, orphanages, and children's homes).

At the time of this writing, research about the use of Brainspotting with children is limited to one community study (from Sandy Hook, Connecticut, where there was a school shooting in 2012) and an anecdotally based report of the common experiences of Brainspotting therapists from four continents in their work with children and teens. The latter is available online in English, German, and Spanish on the authors' personal homepage: www.solucionbaumann.com. However, we and our colleagues consistently observe and feel the effectiveness of Brainspotting in our work with children. During treatment we observe body changes, as well as changes in children's art, play, perspective, cognition, emotion, verbalizations. As treatment progresses we observe children's behaviour that is age or developmentally inappropriate, regressed, or pseudo-mature, transform to become age and developmentally appropriate, without having explicitly addressed the behaviours and relational interactions. We watch somatic "tension" move to dissipate, emotionally "frozen" children become "warm" and start to move, aggressive behaviour turn into appropriate interpersonal relationships, with children letting themselves ask for help, and, and, and ....

This chapter, therefore, offers an additional description of practical therapy to supplement the existing research and reports. To stay within the limited scope of this chapter, the authors decided to restrict themselves to the following topics:
1. Basics of Brainspotting with children and adolescents
2. Developmental issues (different ages – different access)
3. Creativity using Brainspotting

Practice experience in using Brainspotting with children, of course, ranges far beyond these three areas. Thus, this chapter is presented as a glimpse into our work and our approaches to using Brainspotting with children and teens. In describing case studies which should help the reader to understand the theoretical contents in a practical way, for all cases names and identifying information in the case presentations of the chapter have been changed/modified to protect the privacy of the children and their families.

Basics of using Brainspotting with children and adolescents

In order to use Brainspotting with children and teens a therapist needs to be trained and skilled both in treating young people and in Brainspotting. We assume that the reader of this chapter is at least somewhat familiar with the principles, practice, and vocabulary of Brainspotting.

Even though Brainspotting was discovered during a session with a 16 year old girl, it was originally developed for adult clients. Brainspotting therapists who work with children quickly realized that how Brainspotting happens with children is different from what happens in adult sessions.

Brainspotting's pairing of a client's physiological activation with a relevant eye position, is the same for children as for adults. What's different is how a child's developmental stage affects his or her ability to identify and verbalize physical states and to locate and sustain the relevant eye position. What is also different is the rapid growth and change in children's brains from the time of a trauma to the time of treatment and during the course of treatment, as well.

Case Example 1 (mj)

Harry was 9 years old when he started therapy, but he was 41/2 when his parents' divorced and his mother moved to another town. He had lived with his father since then. Harry's teachers said his behaviour at school was normal for a child of his age, but Harry's dad said that after Harry turned 9, he began to cry every night, play aggressively, and refuse to follow the rules at home. At the beginning of treatment, Harry used "feeling words" easily, but his facial expressions didn't match his words. In his play, Harry chose toys designed for 3-5 year olds, and handled them the way a 4 year old would. He created buildings with blocks, covering them, hiding them, putting small objects in them ... and then stared intently into them. His body looked tense and stiff. "Where are you looking?" I asked. "Over there, in that corner," Harry said. I was sitting on the floor next to Harry. "Hmmm ... let's just look there for a while, and see what happens ..." After about 30 seconds, Harry turned his attention to other toys, and created competitive, aggressive games with them. Harry repeated this sequence, with some variations, for 5 sessions. During the 6th session, he ignored the blocks and other toys for younger children and created a game from some old poster-board in the office, inviting his dad into the session for a game. In the meantime, Harry's father reported that the night-time crying had stopped, and that Harry was behaving well at home and excelling in school. Harry came to a few more sessions in which his play was relaxed and age-appropriate before his treatment ended.

As in all therapy, children might or might not know what is bothering them, or be able to express it in words. Children may not have the vocabulary for the abstract language of emotions or bodily awareness. Very young children might know how to count, but can't yet use a number scale, like Wolpe's "SUDS" (subjective units of disturbance) scale, as adults would do in Brainspotting. And many young people have difficulty sustaining quiet attention on the relevant eye position for any length of time – but we have observed that often they do not need to do so in order to heal.

What children *can* do, however, is play – and draw, dance, create stories, make music – and imagine whole worlds and fantasies within their play. Their worlds and fantasies serve as openings for healing. We observe that activation, body sensation and awareness of its intensity, and relevant eye positions (brainspots), often emerge spontaneously in children's play, and/or in the co-creative process of the child-therapist dyad in session. It is the task of the child therapist to notice these things when they happen, and/or to intentionally elicit them, if necessary.

This chapter, therefore, discusses the integration of Brainspotting theory and technique with some of the long-established ways of helping children heal, such as play therapy and the creative arts therapies.

The informal motto of Brainspotting, "Where you look affects how you feel," is an easy way to begin introducing Brainspotting to children and teens, as well as adults. It is simple to hear and understand, and children have fun experimenting with eye position around positive feelings.

For example, a child might be asked: "*Imagine something that you like or something that makes you happy – maybe something you like to do, somewhere you like to go, or something you like to eat. Where do you feel that 'happy' that good feeling, in your body?*" The child can then be prompted to look right, center, and left, to find the relevant eye-position that matches the newly identified, positive body awareness. In working this way with children, a body resource and a resource brainspot will be identified even as the child is learning, experientially, what Brainspotting is, and the dual attunement frame is beginning to take shape.

In this process, also, the core Brainspotting principle of "uncertainty" comes into lively focus, because entering into children's "worlds," into the "theatre" of their minds, within the therapeutic space, necessarily calls upon the therapist to embrace the tentative and developmentally fluid nature of the child's brain-body system.

Perhaps nowhere is this more true than in working with children with reactive attachments and/or highly oppositional behaviour. There is no question that these children are like little "comets" hurtling through the room, often "faster than the speed of light." There is no predictability of what they will do next, no way to "direct" their action, without eliciting a non-productive power-struggle with them. What is a Brainspotting therapist to do? Attune and follow, setting limits for safety and respect of boundaries... waiting patiently for a moment of wonder and surprise when the child's gaze locks into some spot ... And then attune and follow some more.

Case Example 2 (mj)

At 5-year-old Nancy's first session she ran into the office ahead of me and locked herself in. Opening the door was the last cooperative thing she did that day; so the usual ways of engaging with a young child clearly were not going to be effective. I let Nancy move freely in the office, placing some things out of her reach for her safety and mine, gently but firmly telling her what was "off-limits" (e.g., my desk drawers), and moving quietly behind or beside her. I played biolateral sound recordings through some speakers in the room. When Nancy stopped to look intently at something, I stopped and looked at it too. When she noticed me doing so, she moved on to something else ... I became her shadow, close but not too close; attuned to her gaze, wherever it went. One day, Nancy brought her favourite stuffed animal with her, and said was it always tired and needed to sleep. I encouraged Nancy to let the stuffed animal take a nap; she said I didn't have the right bed and blanket. I bought supplies for a toy-bed and small blanket, and had it in the office at Nancy's next session. To my surprise, Nancy gave me the stuffed animal to hold, then had it look at the "bed" while she looked at the stuffed animal, and then she put it down for a nap. After several sessions, Nancy's mom decided she wanted to "try" another type of therapy. At Nancy's last session, she took my shoes and put them on, took a pen and drew on some "sticky-notes" that she made into jewellery for me. Then she drew something else – a large head with limbs sticking out from it, as a younger child would do. "This is you," she said, and gave it to me to keep. Nancy's mom began to cry softly. "She's never done that before," her mom said.

Because children's brains are still "under construction," they lack the vertical (subcortical with the neocortical) and the horizontal (cross-hemispheric) integrative processes of the adult brain. Moreover, the younger the child, the less language the child will have to adequately articulate the large and confusing feelings that rise up and result in "symptoms" and problematic behaviours.

These realities are foundational to all therapy with children, but according to Brainspotting theory, they are not limitations requiring special interventions. Instead, they invite therapists into the "uncertain" mystery of the unknown, the subcortical "land of no words" (the limbic system and the brain-stem) – the places where the impact of trauma resides and where healing begins. As therapists attune to their young clients, relationally and neurobiologicaly, each session can become a profound experience of therapeutic co-creativity, neuro-developmental reconfiguration, relational healing, and brain-body integration.

In the remainder of this chapter, the reader will have the opportunity to consider several more cases through the window of Brainspotting theory applied integratively and creatively in practice with children and adolescents. The cases have been chosen to illustrate the developmental impact of trauma and the potential of Brainspotting to restore young people to healthy, non-trauma driven, developmental trajectories. The cases have also been chosen to illustrate various technical issues about which we often receive questions, including:

- specific ways in which the uncertainty principle and dual attunement frame guide all clinical choices;
- when and how to interact verbally with children in a Brainspotting session; how we understand the important therapist question, "*W*hy *A*m *I* *T*alking?" (W.A.I.T.) in the context of the developmentally necessary role of verbal, visual, and behavioural interaction with children;
- the variety of ways that a Brainspotting therapist moves and behaves in the therapy room with children; we note that a therapist may be active and interactive, standing, sitting, or working on the floor;
- the congruence of Brainspotting theory with client-centered, non-directive but co-creative play, art, and exploration;
- the high degree of quick, spontaneous creativity that may serve as a Brainspotting "set up" when working with young people, as therapists "attune, follow, and wait …" for the moment in which where a child looks affects how the child feels;
- the amazingly creative, survival-oriented, and mysterious process of neurodevelopment as each child interacts, for good and/or ill, with caregivers, teachers, healthcare providers, social service workers, other non-related adults, as well as schoolmates, friends, and the physical environment around them.

As noted above, we offer here a glimpse of our work, necessarily limited by the size and scope of a book chapter. We invite you to learn more as our larger "work-in-progress" moves to publication as a book, and/or by attending specialty training in Brainspotting with Children and Adolescents.

Developmental issues (different ages – different access)

Although this might be a general topic of children's therapy, questions often arise about 1—whether there are different ways to access brainspots in children of different ages; and 2—whether there are any special ways of treating a 4-year-old, a 9-year, or an adolescent with Brainspotting. Responding to these two questions includes awareness of the basics of Brainspotting theory and practice, such as: "staying in the tale of the comet," "uncertainty," and the "dual attunement frame." Discussing the topic of "different ages – different access," however, includes much more general information about treating children with Brainspotting, and therefore was chosen as the primary emphasis of this section of the chapter.

The age of a child is less important than the stage of development

It is part of every therapeutic act with children to meet the children where they are in their development. Treating with Brainspotting means accessing traumatic events through the dual attunement frame of neurobiology and therapeutic relationship. The following two examples explain in a practical way how important it is to use the developmentally (and not the age) appropriate dual attunement frame and techniques with children.

Case Examples 3 (mb)

Sue, an 8 year old girl, came in the office with her mom, father, and two sisters. The family had suffered a life-threatening situation during an assault (attack). When they entered, Sue appeared like an "iceberg", physically extremely stiff, mentally delayed, and hardly spoke. The family's history informed me that Sue is a bright girl, part of a dancing and singing group with excellent school performance and good social skills. As this girl expressed her trauma consequences drastically with her body as well as with her emotional expressions, it was decided to start treatment with her.

Although Sue's appearance during the first moments of treatment was that she was "delayed," the therapist decided to trust the information from the family and tried to address the girl in an age-appropriate manner. The Brainspotting process was explained to her with the help of a brain model. During the brain explanation the therapist realized that Sue was understanding even better than most 8 year olds would do, and started conversing with her like she was an adolescent. Sue started to emotionally defreeze. Being treated like this, she could express her feelings of fear, insecurity, sadness, and overall, talk about her question, "why this must have happened?" As it was observed already at that point, Sue was not at all delayed. So I offered to have her to work with the pointer, telling Sue, that I had the feeling she is as bright as an adolescent. Sue was willing to do so and was able to "process" the presenting traumatic situation as well as earlier events in her life when she felt completely helpless. Although she was very young, the actual processing took at least 30 minutes. For Sue, the access point turned into a resource point. Feeling strong again, she imagined a sunflower to be her "inner picture" of help.

Sofia is a 14 year old girl with special needs, due to a slight mental delay caused by seizures. Her classmates are her age and she has been with them since she started school. Although Sofia was 14, she was not interested in boys nor in popular adolescent things, as all her friends were. She had no words to express that she felt out of place compared to her friends, but she felt that something was strange and shared her confused and anxious thoughts about it. Sofia was obviously in a critical emotional situation, as she felt deeply neglected by her friends, but had no idea why. Sofia knew and loved her Brainspotting sessions. Seeking for an appropriate way of access to work with her on her actual situation, she chose to paint an acrylic picture and used an eye as her motif. Her style of painting, talking, and asking was like that of an 8- to 10-year-old girl. After she was finished, her art piece was used as a pointer and a place (a brainspot) was found where she felt a strange feeling in her body. The actual processing of Brainspotting then began. Sofia started talking about her school situation and bullying friends. Talking concretely about her daily hassles helped her to calm down. After processing all her feelings, she discovered it was possible to change the activation access point into a resource point. Her art piece turned into a "secret adviser". She decided to look directly into her friends' eyes and talk to them about her misunderstanding instead of running away due to shame. To close the session, the therapist did some role play exercises with Sofia experiencing different difficult situations in school and trying to react in a better way than shyness and shame ("squeezing the lemon."). For that task, the same place where the painting was, was chosen to "squeeze the lemon" and strengthen the Brainspotting process.

This session brought about a new period in the therapy. Sofia became open to behaving differently, and "just like that," could confront her daily situation.

What we want to express to the reader with these examples, is:

>*To stay in the tale of the comet:*
As demonstrated in the two examples above, Brainspotting allowed the therapist to choose completely age inappropriate accesses compared to chronological, age-related developmental scales. The 14 year old girl was treated more like a nine year old, and the eight year old, more like a teenager. In both cases the therapist used the principle of being – and staying – in the tail of each girl's "comet."

It is assumed (and again this is nothing new) that trauma processing for children is only possible if they feel safe, accepted, and free to talk or express their feelings. Being with them where they are in their state of development eases the opening of a Brainspotting process. The therapist's observations, feelings toward the young client, and openness are the main tools to be with them, wherever they are in the moment so that they have the possibility for a Brainspotting process.

As it was shown in the first example, the therapist observed that the eight year old girl seemed mentally delayed and strange in her movements. A first feeling of: "How could they not have told me in advance, that this girl was physically and mentally delayed?" appeared. Talking with the whole family and hearing that everybody was proud of the smart and socially competent girl, and observing her for more time, allowed the therapist to "give it a try" and treat the girl as having normal, or maybe even advanced development. The therapist's feelings were right and it was worth giving it a try.

>Fulfilling the Dual Attunement Frame:

In Brainspotting we use development and awareness of a "dual attunement frame" during the treatment. Specifying this, Brainspotting therapists are not only mindful and emotionally attuned, but also observant of the neurobiological processes that may be going on within their clients. Body reactions, changes in facial expressions, etc., are a main focus of observation during treatment.

Not only being with the children emotionally, but also being aware of their neurobiological state of development and capacity to process is part of the art of practicing Brainspotting and using the dual attunement frame with children. At each point of a Brainspotting process you can adapt your therapeutic presence in response to the client's reaction. This means the therapist can either act more childish or more "grown up" at any point of the process. In this way, by trusting the child's capacities and being curious about which therapeutic strategies to use, the therapist and child can co-create the dual attunement frame.

Reading the second example, above (Sofia), shows that the girl could process with the help of her self-made painting. This was an important part of her Brainspotting process. After that, role-playing and reinforcing her newly gained resources (possible ways of reacting in difficult situations) was extremely important due to her lower learning capacities.

In the first example (Sue), the girl was shown the brain model. It could have happened that she would not have liked or understood it. The therapist has the possibility to adapt his/her way of acting in every step of the way: before, during, and after the Brainspotting process. So – suppose that the eight year old girl would not have understood the brain model. The therapist could have named it "the boss of our feelings" like "a king or queen of the realm" and that this "king" or "queen" would be able to help with managing the feelings the child has about the assault. Therapeutically, this would be a "step back" to attune with the neurobiological development, and at the same time it would be a "step forward" in developing the emotional part of the dual attunement frame.

>*During processing children, adolescents, and also adults, sometimes "step back" in their behaviour to the state of their development where they were when the traumatizing event happened.*

Thinking of children role-playing, it is impressive how they can "be" a grandmother in one moment and in the next second they "become" the happy grandchild. Applying Brainspotting sometimes seems exactly the same. Going through the Brainspotting process can change in-session behaviour. The clients suddenly "become" the age that they were during the traumatic event. The following example demonstrates clearly the way children can step back in their development.

Case Example 4 (mb)

A 17-year old once spoke about an abusive event during his childhood. During this difficult situation not only he was abused, the abuser also integrated the boy's much-loved stuffed bear in the action of cruelty. The boy had to watch this before being abused himself.

During the Brainspotting session, he could pick up one of the therapist's stuffed animals and the therapist worked with both – the boy as well as the stuffed bear. The client's feelings for himself, and for his bear, were expressed. The adolescent "became" very young for some minutes, caressing the little bear as 6 year olds do when they are role-playing. As the therapist was invited, she stepped into this Brainspotting process. Both the boy and the therapist helped the little abused bear to overcome this trauma. After this, the boy could process the abuse done to him in the language and with the feelings of a 17-year-old.

Concerning these observations, we often wonder how the process of neuroplasticity is involved in children's processing. "Critical periods" during brain development are described as times in which some capacity (physical as well as emotional) is gained. We do not yet know, but speculate, that these "critical periods" in which, for example, relational behaviour is learned, can be reactivated during a Brainspotting process. If so, then children might use their natural capacity to step back into their behaviour of the time trauma happened. Maybe this is a way of activating some self-healing or reactivating and reopening apparently closed brain processes. As Cozolino (2013) writes, "Those of us who study interpersonal neurobiology believe (and research supports) that ...psychotherapy...can reactivate neuroplastic processes and actually alter the structures and biochemistry of the brain."

Again, there is no formula for how the therapist should engage with this "step back behaviour.". "Uncertainty," in Brainspotting, uses the philosophy "we know that we know nothing,", and therefore observing and waiting to see what is happening is the helpful therapeutic act. Having a child processing and stepping back into the helpless situation is often a challenge for us as therapists, because we want to protect them. Still it is recommended that we observe what is happening in such moments, and let the child be the one who decides if s/he wants to invite the therapist to be part of the process or if the child feels better being observed.

In the case above, and in the earlier case of "Nancy," the children needed the therapist's help to cure the trauma of the stuffed animals. Through that process, the children became open for healing their own trauma. Whatever happened in their brains, we do not know, but with the 17-year old, it was observed, and we believe, that going back and "being six years old" again for some minutes made it possible for his brain and feelings to integrate the trauma he experienced, and his behaviour changed and became enormously positive after this process. For 5-year-old Nancy, the "going back" had the qualities of a projective and parallel process for the healing of the toy, and for her own healing.

In concluding this section about how to treat children of different ages with Brainspotting, the following hint might be helpful for you as a reader. During a Brainspotting session with a young client it is good to forget almost everything that you have learned from developmental psychology! "I know that I know nothing" means trusting the child or adolescent to show you what state they are in, and how they want to be treated. In this way the access point for each child's unique Brainspotting process can be found, and opened.

Creativity using Brainspotting

In one of the "Brainspotting with kids" seminars the participants were asked what type of play they enjoyed most when they were younger. The answers included nearly everything that children always love to do: role play, creative arts, forms of moving, sports, outdoor activities, board games, constructing houses (safe places), music, etc. In the ongoing conversation with the participants they discussed how they could bring their own most loved children's activity into their working areas and offer Brainspotting with it.

Some ideas were:

- The pointer could be a toy, a piece of sports equipment – like a football, the bow of a violin, a paint brush, finger toys on top of the pointer – actually everything used during therapy.
- Brainspotting could be done outdoors.
- Playing board games often allows children to talk, and so the game situation could be transformed into a Brainspotting session. A gaming piece or token can replace the pointer. Eg: "Which of the play figures reminds you most of your anxiety ...?" Then the token can either be already on the right place or the place for the access point can be sought anywhere in the room. Board games often only allow the conversation about the traumatic situation and while playing, a gazespot can be found and, depending on the child's concentration, used for a longer Brainspotting process or a "stepping in – stepping out" process, which hyperactive children often do. In these cases, the board game can also help to stay focused.
- The use of gazespotting outside and inside of the therapy office.
- Constructing something can also be used to make processing possible – children can construct something and then walk around and see from which place they are physically most affected.

In short, almost anything in a child's world can be used to help the child orient to her/his unique activation and resource brainspots. We encourage the reader to think about his/her most loved "playing situations" and how the reader's favourites could be included into Brainspotting therapy.

Case Example 5 (mb)

Entering the children's home a little girl ran all the way along the courtyard, jumped up to the therapist and asked her, in a cheeky way: "Can you treat me today, please, please can you treat me today?" The therapist actually had just a few minutes and knew that 30 meters ahead a lot of children, trauma work, and responsibilities were waiting. Still they found themselves some seconds later sitting in the grass, talking about the girl's nightmares and her body's feelings about them. The therapist used a blade of grass as a pointer and the girl went through a short period of processing. Suddenly she jumped up and suggested that she would think of this little blade of grass and sleep better the upcoming night.

Creativity in Brainspotting has no limits, and in the authors' forthcoming book many examples and great ways of finding an access to children will be explained. From this chapter, we hope that readers will be motivated to try whatever suits the given situation, and will allow themselves and their young clients to remember that the Brainspotting process can grow out of any creative activity like games, testing, talking, painting, moving, etc. etc.

One technical example, which really works well, is the "double- side effect." Anything that has two sides (paper, wooden spoons, stones, wood pieces, cartoons, buttons, etc.) can become a pointer, to hold the child's orientation to a brainspot. When the point of activation access is first found, the child can be asked, which symbol would represent their post traumatic disorder like aggression, being anxious, being unable to concentrate, etc. Identifying this, and painting the symbol on one side of the "pointer," the actual Brainspotting process can be started with this symbol. As soon as the point of access turns more and more into a resource point, the other side of the item can be painted with a "resource symbol". The Brainspotting Process, then, can be finished with the resource brainspot. Giving this "double-sided symbol" to the child to take home as a present can further enhance the effect of the session.

The "double-side effect" allows children to realise that any bad feeling can turn into a good feeling, and that anything that we call "post traumatic disorder" is of importance. The "double-side effect" also allows access to well-being as a normal brain response. This technique promotes the understanding that there is no "bad part" of the child – just "wounded parts" – and that each trauma reaction is an important reaction. How lost would we be without any anxiety; how vulnerable would we be without ways of defending ourselves. In its simplicity, this creative tool explains the whole of trauma theory, and is worth trying.

Working with children and adolescents is an ongoing therapeutic self-discovery. The ideas can grow out of the therapeutic situations and are unlimited. Processing is possible with many creative tools and creative ways of accessing, as long as the basics of Brainspotting are followed.

What fascinates both of the authors in using Brainspotting with children, is the deep intuitive knowledge that even very young children have about themselves, and what their brains need in order for them to heal. Adults have this too, but with children, sometimes it's *all* that they – and we – have for guidance.

In accompanying David Grand to provide humanitarian service in the larger community where the Sandy Hook school shooting occurred, one of the authors (mj) discovered that most of the children of Sandy Hook didn't like or want to talk about the tragedy that happened at their school, and in their community. In fact, to the children, the "tragedy," as it is called, happened "a long time ago." Yet, two to four years after the event, some of their parents brought them for 1-session Brainspotting consultations. Some of the children had developed "worries" or "bad dreams;" others had difficulty transitioning to new, larger schools as they grew older. Most of the children knew at least some of the children and teachers who died, as of course, did their parents. Many of the children, themselves, were survivors from the school.

Case Example 6 (mj)

It happened by accident one day, that David was scheduled to work with the parent of my client. The therapy rooms shared a wall, and even with both parent and child listening to biolateral sound through headphones, the deep wailing of the parent could be heard in my room. My child client noticed it, but didn't seem overly concerned about it. "That's my dad, isn't it?" "Yes – he's working with Dr. David while you're here working with me." "Oh...Ok."

The sessions both continued. When father and child were reunited both noticed immediately that the other "looked better." After those sessions, we tried to schedule parents and children with same-time appointments, and each time we saw the same parent-child response. Each seemed to "know" that the other was receiving the help they each needed in that moment, and that, as David Grand says, although they were traumatized alone, they were healing together.

Conclusion

As co-authors, the clinical effects we have both witnessed in our work lead us to wonder about and continue studying how neurodevelopment in childhood might be protected as well as repaired, by Brainspotting. And we want to keep learning what other Brainspotters around the world have discovered in their work with children.

In finishing this chapter, it can only be said that there is so much more that could be shared about the theory and practice of using Brainspotting with children and adolescents! In the very beginning of Brainspotting development, its founder, Dr. David Grand says he was asked about working with Brainspotting and children. He answered that there were good initial practical results with it, and that he encouraged everyone who learned Brainspotting and has the chance to work with children, to try it, and see what happens. This was the authors' intention and as you could read briefly, we both "tried" it and came to the conclusion that it works extremely well, – so well that we are honoured to share our knowledge and experience with you. We now encourage you, the reader, to follow and stay in the tail of the littlest comets, and "try it," too!

Literatur

Grabe, H.J., Spitzer, C.,: Traumata, "Frühe Brandmale" in Spektrum der Wissenschaft 2.2017, pp. 6-11.

Daniel Siegel's works here are considered to be exemplary.

1Newton-Sandy Hook Community Foundation, INc., "Report of Findings from the Community Survey September 2016", can also be read on the following home pages: www.brainspottingaustria.com, www.brainspotting.pro

2Baumann, M., Bonn, MJ, Gos, M., Grixti, M., Jacob, P., Jacobi, M.: „Tief berührt...oder Brainspotting mit Kindern und Jugendlichen" , www.brainspottingaustria.com , 2012

Grand, D. (2014): Brainspotting – Wie Sie Probleme, Traumata und emotionale Belastungen gezielt auflösen. VAK-Verlag, Kirchzarten bei Freiburg

Louis Cozolino: *The Neuroscience of Human Relationships: Attachment and the Developing Social Brain,* 2nd ed. (New York : W. W. Norton, 2013), xviii.

Attachment-Focussed Brainspotting with Children and Young People

Mark Grixti

Paradigm Shifts

As a clinical psychologist based in the United Kingdom I have had the privilege of receiving many diverse trainings and learning opportunities over many years. My clients range right across the age-span, but the majority of my work has been in child and adolescent mental health, both within the National Health Service as well as in private practice. Much of my work has been with children and young people who have been adopted or are in foster care and have experienced the most challenging start to life. This complexity has shaped all aspects of their lives, not least their relationships. Therein lies the challenge for a psychologist working with this client group; how do you reach the children that are so wounded that they cannot risk entering what could be another damaging relationship?

Although I considered that I was often having some good results with my more complex child clients and their families, I was aware that despite my trainings, it was difficult to deliver some of these wonderful approaches to this client group. It was the open and inclusive nature of Brainspotting therapy that really facilitated the enhancement and incorporation of my experiences as I re-learned how to improve the interpersonal attunement in my work alongside the powerful impact of the neurobiological attunement central to deep body-brain processing. In this chapter I hope to share this experience with you through exploring attachment-focussed Brainspotting with children and young people. Brainspotting has been described in detail in other chapters of this volume, but as a reminder here are the basic core concepts.

Brainspotting therapy (BSP) is a body-brain-based relational psychotherapy discovered by Dr David Grand in 2003. The model is based upon the dual attunement framework of neurobiological and interpersonal attunement. Neurobiological attunement harnesses the body activation experienced in relation to a traumatic event through a resonating spot in the visual field (eye position). This is called a brainspot and by holding the attention on this brainspot the person can process the traumatic event towards resolving the body activation and emotional distress. This neurobiological attunement between the client and therapist is dependent on the all-important profound relational attunement, as the therapist tracks the client's experience attending to the verbal, somatic, and unconscious interpersonal interactions. Brainspotting gives us a tool within this clinical relationship, to neurobiologically locate, focus, process, and release experiences and symptoms that are typically out of reach of the conscious mind and its cognitive and linguistic capacity (Grand, 2013).

Empowerment through attunement

In a supervision session recently with an experienced and creative psychologist, we were discussing an issue that she was having whilst working with a teenage client. She told me all about the young person's history of complex developmental trauma and an extensive list of concerns and risks which were met with a long list of professional recommendations. The young person was overweight, had specific learning disabilities, was wetting and defecating in all the wrong places, and was often extremely violent to his dedicated, hardworking, loving, yet exhausted adoptive parents. He was out of education, without much hope and soon to be back into the looked-after system as his parents were desperate and their own health was diminishing fast. Most of the recommendations for therapy had been tried, with limited progress, and my supervisee was the final option. Despite her decades of experience, she felt the pressure of being this family's 'last hope' and was doing everything within her power to make a difference.

She reported through moistened eyes that in the previous session with the family she had failed in her efforts and then described what had happened. The teenage boy had sat on the floor, on his mother's lap, ignoring all the therapeutic toys and art materials that she had prepared. He was clearly agitated and tense in his body. Despite the psychologist's best efforts, the boy fell into the usual pattern of ignoring her and he fiddled with his mother's hair and broach. This time, partly out of submission, the psychologist said nothing and just let him. She recalled thinking at that point that a boy with this complex history, with these challenging issues, and a battery of assessments and fruitless recommendations just could not be reached.

The boy continued to sit, quite still on his mother's lap as the psychologist sat opposite just observing. He gently fiddled with his mother's cardigan as his large frame slid further down into her lap, looking up at her in a quiet, peaceful way. The three of them maintained this position for much of the session and at the end when it was time to go, he hugged the psychologist, and said, "see you next week". This was first time he had made a physical connection with the psychologist, addressed her directly, and expressed any intent to return. His mother raised her eyebrows inquisitively to the psychologist and they said goodbye.

Due to the risks around this child, the psychologist was uncomfortable with the session. She said that she had left the treatment plan, she had just sat there and given up on targeting this boy's trauma and behaviour. She reported feeling guilty of neglecting her duties, de-skilled, ineffective and responsible for not getting the boy and his family to achieve the goals of their care plan. She explained how she was also feeling inadequate as she had trained in many approaches and was constantly reading and hearing about amazing success stories; this felt a long way off!

The reader may recognise some of these feelings as a therapist. Despite our trainings and supervision, the human need to succeed when confronted by trauma and tragedy can become overwhelming. At such times, the therapist finds that feelings of guilt and fear can be more influential in organising them to be interventionist and dependant on a model, protocol, or technique. Diversions from the 'plan' can engender feelings of betrayal to the model and stimulate shame, inadequacy, and worthlessness.

Returning to the session outlined above, it was through such feelings that the psychologist actually harnessed something very important. She stepped back and let the mother and son take control of their session. She dropped her interventions and held the space whilst the boy was liberated to 'process' in the safety of this mother's arms and in the presence of his therapist. She realigned the power dynamic and let the boy be in control, to find his healing, in a way that only he can do. She was holding the space, attuned in her openness, aware of difficult physical feelings rising up from within her; she created an open context for the boy's body and brain to work in the safety and attunement of mother and therapist.

When I shared these reflections with my supervisee, she spontaneously burst into tears. She spoke of the relief in being 'allowed' to make this fundamental human connection in the session without agenda or expectation. She said that from this session onwards, she had allowed herself to 'return' to being truly present with the client and in doing so it had transformed her sessions entirely. She had returned to the values that she had always held as sacred in therapy, as indeed she did in motherhood, prioritising the young person over any other interference. As this divide between how she thought she should practice and how she felt she wanted to be had collapsed, her work reached new levels and she noticed how her own potential and that of her clients seemed to unlock, leading to some tough, but extremely fulfilling work for all parties involved.

I was interested in this idea that she had 'returned' to her deeply held values and beliefs. These jewels of her personal and professional identity had become somewhat jaded or compromised over time. We could postulate that her internal and interrelational emotional connection had been somewhat masked by service demands, as well as others. A possible imbalance as the rational thinking brain overpowers the role of the emotional brain. As Schiepek (2015) asserts, this is where the therapist loses authenticity and the client gets lost.

The 'return' as she described it gives us another opportunity to explore the importance of addressing the divide which so often limits our development. Through supervision, she was not presented with anything that she did not already know, or was not aware of at some level. My inclination is that if this was the case, then my comments would not have been attuned and would not have had such meaning for her at an emotional level. Rather than create something for our supervisees, or indeed our clients, just like the artist, poet, scientist or writer, we provide an opportunity to *re-present* them in such a way that can be expansive.

Attachment Theory Re-presented

The field of child psychology has often been the poor relative to adult work, and this has been reflected in the funding made available to research and mental health services. In the United Kingdom, the Independent Newspaper (November 2017), reported that despite the government's promise to substantially invest in child and adolescent mental health services, children's mental health has received less than 1% of the overall health budget. The need to invest in our young people, not only for them but for the health of society is abundantly clear. Those that work with young people appreciate this more and more with an improved understanding of the significance of brain development and how it is so strongly sculpted within early attachment relationships. Indeed, innovative recent developments from researchers, clinicians, and writers including Bessel van der Kolk, Dan Siegel, Alan Schore, Stephen Porges, Onno van der Hart, and Bonnie Badenoch have not only furthered our understanding of these relationships, but also led towards a radical shift in the emphasis on attachment as a central focus of our clinical work with people right across the age range.

An integration between child and adult approaches to emotional health and healing is augmenting important developments in the field of trauma, attachment, and neuroscience. Alan Schore has commented on how this has *re-presented* the importance of the early founders of psychoanalysis, with a strong resurgence in attachment theory over the last decade. In this chapter we will further explore how Brainspotting with children has advanced these principles in an exciting and pioneering way to contribute to attachment repair, trauma recovery, self-regulation, and possible permanent neuroplastic change. A more practical exploration of Brainspotting with children will be outlined later in this chapter after an exploration of the fundamental child-focussed attachment theory which is integral to its understanding and application.

John Bowlby's original attachment theory (1969) set out how the early stages in life influence the way in which people are shaped, though the lifespan, across all emotional and social functions. Advances in neurobiology over the past decade extend a deeper understanding of the early influence of life on the developing brain and contributed to an evolution in psychotherapeutic approaches.

This development is based on a biopsychosocial perspective, consistent with early attachment theory but extended to a greater emphasis on the relationship between the brain, mind, and body and the intersubjective or interpersonal matrix. That is, the relationship between the brain, mind, and body of both the infant and its carer are inextricably influenced, within the context of their environment contributing to a supportive, or restricting and damaging trajectory.

The developing dialogue between disciplines has profoundly influenced psychotherapy. An interdisciplinary approach has developed across fields including psychology, neuroscience, body-based work, traumatology, psychoanalysis, and systemic approaches. These developments have emphasised that after decades of the dominance of cognitive approaches, the prominence has moved strongly towards the emotional and social aspects of early human development. The links between attachment theory and brain development have indicated that the right-lateralised emotional brain is integral to body based sensations and the autonomic nervous system (ANS) and has a distinctly different anatomy and biochemistry to the left hemisphere which forms further along the developmental timeline (Schore, 2012).

At this point I would like to share a personal experience that indicated to me the power of right brain to right-brain, body-based communication. Some years ago, as an eager and expectant father to be, after a long and challenging labour, I held my newborn son in my arms. A matter of minutes later, not knowing what to say or do, he gazed square into my eyes, I found myself giving into an irresistible urge to poke my tongue out at him. To my amazement he instantly stuck out his little purple tongue right back at me!

This lovely moment of communication between us when my son was only a few minutes old could be understood as a moment of pure neurophysiological father/son attunement. A right-brain to right-brain intersubjective transaction whereby cues of social engagement were initiated and responded to in affective resonance. This spontaneous observation could be linked to one well-documented opportunistic moment in 1994 whilst Italian neuroscientists Rizzolatti and Craighero discovered what came to be known as mirror neurons. These special neurons implicitly transfer imitation, empathy, emotions, and intentions between people that are in synchrony with each other. This theory is interesting but remains controversial (Hickok, 2014) as other theorists state that that there is far more of the brain and body involved in this unconscious transfer of interpersonal experience and information. Such processes have been likened to a kind of neural Wi-Fi (Goleman, 2007), whereby high speed inter-connections are made between people through a 'wireless' medium.

The relevance of the right-brain body bias can be understood further as we observe how in the first year of life, the infant begins to learn to regulate affective states, pleasant or distressing, through dyadic regulation with the mother and/or the father. Through psychobiological attunement the caregiver and infant spend long periods with eyes locked in a non-verbal communication, prosodic vocalisations, and shared body gestures (Trevarthen, 1990) as together they experience body-based states of internal and autonomic arousal. Alan Schore (2012, pp32) advances the importance of this dialogic process as the carer and the infant attune and engage through various states of arousal, experiencing both relational rupture and repair:

"...the more she attends to his reinitiating cues for engagement, the more synchronised their interaction...the pair are in affective resonance...and a positive state occurs...in moments of interactive repair the "good enough" caregiver who has mis-attuned can regulate the infant's negative state by accurately retuning in a timely manner".

Through the process of attunement, mis-attunement, and re-attunement the preverbal infant develops a secure attachment and the beginning of a sense of self. As this is extended, the infant gradually moves from the reliance on the mother/father to regulate, to developing the increasing ability to be able to interactively regulate with others, or auto-regulate when alone (Schore, 2012). Neuroscience studies indicate that this emotional development and the infant's developing sense of self are largely dependent on the early evolving right lateralised system (Devinsky, 2000).

Conversely, where the mother/father are not attuned and repeatedly fail to re-attune, then the right-brain to right-brain communication system may be compromised, the implicit regulatory system is complicated, and the resultant attachment style is more insecure. Dan Siegel (Bryson & Siegel, 2012) describes how repeated missed opportunities to make this right-brain to right-brain connection between parent and child can result in changes to the physical structure of the brain. Siegel reports that there are one hundred billion neurons (brain cells) in the brain, each with around ten thousand connections to other neurons. The architecture of the developing brain is dependent on these early interpersonal interactions, neurons firing together and wiring together in the establishment of neurological pathways. Early critical periods of insecure attachment are of great significance as internal working models of inter-relationships and affect regulation are imprinted psychologically and neurologically at implicit, non-conscious levels (Schore, 2012). Children with a history of abuse and neglect are confronted by a complex paradoxical situation as they will try to fulfil their natural desire to socially engage; yet interpersonal relationships are often extremely complicated. "Phobia of attachment is often paradoxically accompanied by an equally intense phobia of attachment loss" (van der Hart, 2006). These children find that they cannot self-regulate satisfactorily and often find maladaptive or harmful solutions in an attempt to regulate affect. This cycle of abuse and distress can serve to strengthen the implicit internal working model of insecure attachment.

Attachment, attunement and psychotherapy

The internal working models that are developed in the infant's early years form a template within which the person relies upon throughout the lifespan through implicit awareness for relational communications between persons. Such interrelational transactions are usually reliant on extremely rapid implicit processes that are too fast to be tracked consciously and commented on verbally (Lyons-Ruth 2000).

When these processes of relating are then applied to the therapeutic context, we can appreciate how the implicit right- brain to right-brain of the therapist and the client are communicating at a rapid speed, non-verbally huge amounts of information at levels beneath awareness. The flow of communications at this level may include intonation and volume of the voice, expressions, body posture and movement, the speed of communication, eye contact, as well as interoceptive information.

Schore (2012) asserts how important it is to acknowledge that "all of these implicit non-conscious, right-brain, mind-body, nonverbal communications are bidirectional and thereby intersubjective". That is, BOTH the client and the therapists are influenced by the other in the relational matrix. This is a key point as experienced therapists can use their internal sensory awareness to assist a client non-verbally in somatic affect regulation. Indeed, Leston Havens (1979) asserts that, "perhaps the most striking evidence of successful therapy is the occurrence in our bodies of sensations that the patient has described in his or hers". This is clearly comparable to the process whereby parents attune to the infant, through mirror neurons, get a felt sense (interoception/nociception) of what is happening to their child emotionally and physically, stay with this experience as over time they reach interactive regulation. For this reason, the intersubjective relational connections are key to stabilisation, self-regulation, and trauma resolution through attachment repair in psychotherapy.

It can be a somewhat sophisticated process for a therapist to be aware of these dynamics, internal and inter-relational, whilst also engaging at a verbal level and conscious level with a client. Later in his chapter I will discuss how this can be managed more effectively with Brainspotting therapy, which has been developed with these aspects in mind. However, first I will give an illustration of a clinical experience that I encountered personally to show how implicit right-brain to right-brain intersubjective transactions can work – or not!

As I mentioned in the introduction, I am a clinical psychologist with a range of integrated trainings. Some years ago, newly qualified in eye movement desensitisation reprocessing (EMDR), I was working with a very distressed adult client around the child sexual abuse that she encountered from a 'family friend' when she was a young 5-year-old girl. I had been specialising in abuse for some time so this work was not unusual for me and the client, and I had quickly developed a good and trusting relationship. However, I was not experienced in EMDR and the power that it can have in accessing abuse at a deeper embodied right-brain level. In one transformational session with this client she felt, at a visceral level, all of the guilt, shame, blame, pain, and freeze energy dissipate. I enjoyed seeing her delight and surprise at the power of the process, and we closed the session and scheduled in one for the following week.

Over next 2 days I was confused and somewhat alarmed by the extreme feelings that were embodied in me. Feelings that I clearly could not truly recognise as my own were weighing very heavily as I felt nauseous, heavy-headed, dark in mood, and carried an inexplicable sense of defeat. As I explained this to my own therapist at the time, it reminded me of a story that I had read recently called The Green Mile (King, 1996). In this story a prisoner called John Coffey has the power to heal and even manages to heal the wife of the prison warden from a brain tumour. After the cure is realised, Coffey the healer is doubled up in extreme pain and a swarm of black creatures rise from deep within him and take exit through his mouth. It was indeed quite horrible!

Perhaps my reaction to what proved to be a very successful healing session was not entirely dissimilar to Coffey's experience. As I developed a more sophisticated understanding of the power of deep mind-body-brain processing in the intersubjective matrix, this *re-presented* to me its power and in doing so how it needed to be understood and used therapeutically. Indeed, this needs to be integrated into all supplementary trainings, as well as core training. Otherwise, it can be harmful both to the therapists through vicarious or unresolved trauma, or to the client as the emotional dysregulation may continue to be mirrored without resolution. Considering client complexity and the regularity of the therapist's exposure to the client's deep emotional world, good trainings and supervision are essential learning to recognise this mind-body-brain limbic countertransference within and after client contact.

This is alluded to by Shaw (2004) who states:

Psychotherapy is an inherently embodied process. If psychotherapy is an investigation into the intersubjective space between client and therapists, then as a profession we need to take our bodily reactions much more seriously than we have so far because ... the body is "the very basis of human subjectivity" (P271).

The body-brain connection

Over the past ten years there has been a shift in the understanding of mental health issues and the use of psychotherapy. The divide between specialties in this field has collapsed as what were separate and discreet approaches are now in alliance. The result has been a groundswell in energy in the understanding of emotional issues, and the field has enjoyed huge developmental leaps. As neuroscience, psychotherapy, and body-based workers integrate their resources, it is very exciting to see what could be achieved. Time and progress have also shown those in the field where we have been over-reliant on certain theories and approaches, coerced into ever more manualised and protocol-driven approaches, misguided by an over-reliance on simplified and unsophisticated notions of evidence-based practice, and dismissive of the wealth of evidence that we are surrounded by in our clinical practices and in our own felt sense.

The imbalance of how we have been culturally and politically organised is expressed powerfully in T*he master and his emissary* by McGilchrist (2009) in terms of the left/right brain division. He sets out his argument that the left brain, has taken over human functioning and is valued as superior in contemporary culture for its ability to prioritise rational, focused, logical, and analytic thinking. In mental health as well as education, the conscious, fixed, static, isolated, disembodied qualities of the left brain have taken priority over those of the emotional, changing, evolving, interconnected qualities of the right hemisphere. McGilchrist goes on to make the essential point that it is because the left brain is language dominant that it can access and articulate its own attributes. However language is inadequate to access the depth, speed, and emotional complexity of the right brain. To this end, he asserts that the left brain is akin to the master's emissary, often taking a superior role to its right-brain master, compromising the balance of the 'whole', often with harmful results. Is this right/left brain imbalance what we have seen in terms of priorities in mental health provision, manualised therapeutic approaches, in the education system, and with the explosion in the medicalisation of mental illness?

The recent move toward redressing this imbalance has seen more and more therapists and healers turn toward body-focused models in addressing trauma and other mental health issues. Peter Levine (2010) the founder and developer of somatic experiencing has done much to redress the left/right brain balance in his recognition of the necessity of addressing the body and nervous system to heal emotional wounds. Indeed, in a reflection on our historic relationship with trauma, Levine attends to the way in which the terminology has changed over time. In the wake of World War I, the extreme suffering of soldiers was called 'shell shock', which conveys some of the gravity and horror of their experience. A typically more left-brain cognitive conceptualisation replaced this graphic and emotive phrase, and it shifted by World War II to 'battle fatigue', 'war neurosis' and for the Iraq war the term 'combat operational exhaustion' was applied. Levine comments on how these 'objectified terms' continued and how following on from the Vietnam War, the current term posttraumatic stress disorder (PTSD) became fully sanitised as a medical disorder. This conceptualisation is said to serve the dispassionate nature of science, informs objectified constructs of suffering, and serves to establish a divide between the patient and the doctor. This divide offers another example of the potential detachment of the emotional connection between the client and the healer, as there is a missed opportunity to collaborate, attune, and access deep right-brain to right-brain emotional healing.

A deep and empathic right-brain connection with the client is central to Levine's approach to healing trauma. The client is believed to be locked in deep primal defences, akin to our amphibian or reptilian evolutionary predecessors. It may be the external environmental, exteroceptive information which has caused such horrendous damage to the person; however it is the integration of this information with the internal, interoceptive information from the body and somatic markers which is key to healing trauma and dissociation. Levine then seeks to access the 'unspoken voice' (2010) by focusing on the body to transform the injuries into healing. This focus on the body in therapy, including work with children, is central to Brainspotting as the body could be conceptualised as the organ of egoless wisdom.

Embracing uncertainty in Brainspotting

An interesting thing happened this morning as I began to settle into my rhythm to write this paper. An unmistakeable part of me, one that Richard Schwartz's internal family systems model (2001) might call a frightened protector, took over and got me feeling that I cannot write this chapter as I have nothing new or of great interest to share. As I listened to this part a little more closely, it was concerned that I would expose myself as an imposter, as I do not have all the answers, techniques, and solutions to offer in a bite-size downloadable protocol-style format. For example, what do you do if your child is wetting, stealing, having sleep problems, is anxious or depressed, absconding from school, has suffered abuse and is traumatised, is behaving in a dangerous way, or is dealing with significant loss? I could feel this overwhelm closing me down!

I decided to listen to this part though and tried to be compassionate in understanding it. From there I could acknowledge its attempts to look after me but let it know that in closing down this opportunity to explore as I write, I was getting further away from my skilled, thoughtful self that has acquired much experience over the years. In this compassionate attachment between self and the protector, I felt an easing in my body, and a playfulness returned to my work. Furthermore, I was refreshed by the relationship between the self and protector as I felt gratitude to the frightened part for its guidance, reminding me to hold onto some insecurity, a feeling that is so often an important part in clinical work. This insecurity, when nurtured, can be an essential part of the therapist's not knowing position – a core value in Brainspotting and in recognising the uncertainty principle.

As David Grand (2013) explained, the 'uncertainty principle' is a fundamental to successful therapy. Originally introduced by the physicist Werner Heisenberg (1927), Brainspotting translates this principle in the appreciation that we cannot know for sure what is happening between 2 molecules, let alone within the interrelationship between people, internal parts, and not between the billions of neurons and synapses. Our understanding of the power of the limbic system in processing strongly indicates how the conscious, thinking brain cannot efficiently access the deeper subcortex easily. Brainspotting strongly values maximising the efficiency of the subcortex through suspending belief, judgement and certainty and holding a position of uncertainty. Instead the role of the therapist is to allow the client to be the head of the comet and the role of the therapist is to blend into the tail of the comet and follow the head wherever it might go (Grand, 2013). This way the attuned therapist can provide the essential relational, interpersonal connection without obstructing the healing. The primary thing that therapy has to offer is the space for the client to self-heal as the brain processes and self-organises toward resolution (Damir del Monte – Brazil BSP International conference, 2016).

I would like to stay with the theme of uncertainty a little more. As therapists we are confronted with clients who have often experienced some of the greatest challenges in life. It is understandable that they have parts that can be hostile, submissive, controlling, and avoidant. I have already laid out the argument for amplified attunement in the session, as the therapist engages in a deep right-brain implicit intersubjective relationship with the client to enhance and make reparations to early attachment trauma. The therapist in Brainspotting is open and follows the client to wherever they need to go. This takes some confidence as the therapist with experience and sophistication learns to trust in this process, to depart from any protocol, guidelines, and procedures that, although well intended, can impede attunement, obstruct healing, and exacerbate feelings of helplessness on both sides. The truly attuned therapist is something of an advocate of improvisation, allowing oneself to follow whatever unfolds without impeding the flow or reverting to predetermined scripts or actions.

Initially, I would like to set out one of my Brainspotting therapy outtakes for the interested reader, as to when I have got it quite wrong! As with improvisation, we learn through our mistakes, but more importantly, we do not deny ourselves the opportunity to leave our comfort zone in our attempt to truly follow the client.

Charlie was an 11-year-old boy and had been in a loving and stable foster placement for 3 years when our work began. However, his early history was very traumatising as for the first 5 years of life he was systematically sexually abused, starved, and physically beaten by his birth parents and various other visitors to the house. From age 5 to 8 years the trauma continued intermittently through various short-term episodes of abusive foster care.

Around a year into our work, Charlie and I had built a good working relationship and, considering his past, there was adequate level of trust and stabilisation, and we had been working on the early life trauma. His foster carer attended all of the sessions with us to assist in his feelings of security and also to minimise potential issues of risk. Charlie said that Brainspotting was hard work as he got in touch with old and very difficult feelings; however he liked that he didn't have to articulate anything at all if he did not want to. In one session Charlie had said that he needed some extra help if he was going to begin to address the core of his early trauma. I suggested that we try a type of 'Double Brainspotting', which works directly with brainspots for the activation spot AND the resource spot at the same time. I have found that this approach has been very effective when working with highly dissociative children. The child can work up to and around the edges of the window of tolerance whilst feeling more in control in titrating and modulating arousal and affect regulation.

In Charlie's Double Brainspotting, an activation spot was located with the pointer at the point where he was connecting with the strong feelings around the abuse. Charlie chose a red tipped pointer which he said had an angry feel to it. A second pointer, which he topped with a small figure of a cute rubber cat was used to find his resource spot, which Charlie said would be his favourite characters from Peter Pan. Charlie, chose to begin on the activation spot, saying that his level of activation (SUDs) was a 9 and he felt 'funny' in his whole body. I silently observed him looking tense as twitches flicked momentarily across his otherwise very still, slightly reddened face. I could observe his pronounced swallow reflux and indeed felt an increased fluttering tension in my own chest which I imagine was an attunement with his own. After several minutes Charlie's gaze moved to his left toward the other pointer with the cat on top. After a while he said his first words of the process.

"I can see Peter Pan."

I remained attentive but silent.

"He's got his sword and is fighting them" (a reference to his abusers), he continued.

Charlie remained silent but in deep concentration for some minutes before saying to me,

"Can I go back to the other pointer now?"

"Yes, of course, as you wish" I replied, as he returned to the activation spot.

Again, after some minutes Charlie's face offered up a momentary smirk. I said nothing and just noticed my own deeper breath which was immediately mirrored by him. Charlie moved between the pointers at his own pace, often for a few minutes at a time. I was aware that my mind was trying to figure out what might be happening for him, but I let it return to a mindful state and just noticed.

"It's us", Charlie explained with eyes still on the red pointer, "Peter Pan, Tinkerbell, Wendy, and all his friends are me and my good family beating up the old horrible family". Charlie continued to process this on the red pointer for some time and I asked,

"What does it feel like to be Peter Pan in this battle?"

Charlie's face and demeanour shifted in a way that indicated to me that he was transitioning out of his process to attend to my intervention.

"No it's not that," he said. "My foster dad is Peter Pan. I'm Wendy!"

This was certainly not what I had expected and this is where, I realised, I had broken attunement to meddle with something that was working well and did not need my interjection and assumptions. I had let my interest and intrigue get the better of me and in doing so had obstructed Charlie's natural process. With the knowledge that the brain is very adept at self-healing under the right conditions, I would have preferred it if I had stayed out of the way and let Charlie/Wendy complete the process further. For the next part of the session Charlie was then out of that zone. As can happen with a dream, on waking the dreamer may wish to return to it but the process was unique and on waking is changed. From this session of Brainspotting I learned a lesson that has been employed in many sessions since to the benefit of my clients – stay out of the way! Thank you, Charlie and Wendy, for this.

Brainspotting with children and young people

As there is relatively little published on Brainspotting with children, understandably families were curious when I introduced this as an idea. Sure enough, there is nothing like trying something to understand how it feels and indeed if it works; however trust and confidence are so important in this field that families often needed a little more information. As I learned this from more and more clients, as well as child therapists, it was clearly time to make a gentle and informative family friendly picture book to explain Brainspotting. With the assistance of a few young clients who were pretty knowledgeable about Brainspotting and with the skill and dedication of my friend and artist, Rosanna Dean, we published a book for this very purpose: Brainspotting with young people: An adventure into the mind (Grixti & Dean 2015). The teaching material was extended by Grixti in 2018, with a sketch animation exploring a more theoretical explanation of Brainspotting through YouTube (https://www.youtube.com/watch?v=7FO_udVWkqA&t=58s).

Each family has its own unique set of dynamics and relates to its concerns in various ways. The therapist will always be absorbing this information and attuning to the family with this in mind. Much information is shared at this early point in therapy as to how issues are communicated, held, and experienced. The therapist will be reading these cues, as the framework for the therapy is being set through this complex interrelational matrix. At a certain point, depending on the trust and attunement that is developing, the therapist will be judging what seems to be the best point of access into working with the most important issues. When the time is right to incorporate Brainspotting, a 'least resistance approach' is important to uphold as the client continues to lead the therapeutic process and the flow and fluidity are maintained. For this reason, the set-up part of the Brainspotting session is not over-complicated or laden with a check-list of questions. As usual with this approach, you follow the client and take as much or as little time as is required to find the client's activation. Going back a far as Breuer and Freud (1893, cited in Van der Kolk 2014) finding the activation, or as they called it the "energetic reaction" to the traumatic event was deemed as essential to discharge the emotion so that it is no longer attached to the memory. With Brainspotting the activation that is held in the body at that point in time is considered the only reality that one can work with, contrary to some approaches that seek to lead a client into processing something on demand or assume residual emotions from a previous session. The client is then asked where this activation is located in their body. This line of enquiry is not always straightforward, especially to children, even though children regularly experience their emotions in their bodies, such as nervous tummy aches. Many clients may also have learned to dissociate off from their bodies, sometimes as a response to sexual abuse or traumatic surgical procedures. So in the attunement the therapist is constantly accessing important information on the client's relationship with the body, a place where the emotion or 'energetic reaction', is embodied. Many children will not consciously focus into their bodies to find emotional information, so interoception can be a challenge when asking them for a body sensation. However, it is so important considering that:

"...the only way we can consciously access the emotional brain is through self-awareness. i.e. by activating the medial prefrontal cortex, the part of the brain that notices what is going on inside us and this allows us to feel what we're feeling ... Neuroscience research shows that the only way we can change the way we feel is by becoming aware of our inner experience and learn to befriend what is going on inside", Van der Kolk (2014).

In my practice I have found that children often lose their blank, dissociated stare when they are asked if they feel any sensations in their bodies, and locate it swiftly and accurately if they are asked to place a toy or rubber ball where they feel the feeling in their body. This strategy can also be used later in the session to refresh the interoception or to help gauge its progress.

Brainspotting can be used very effectively in combination with parts approaches, such as ego state therapy (Watkins and Watkins, 1997) and internal family systems, (Richard Schwartz 2001). The therapist-client attachment is of course key to these approaches, and at another level this relationship will facilitate the all-important internal attachment repair between the clients compassionate loving self, injured parts, and subsequent protectors. Whether parts are referred to explicitly or more implicitly, Brainspotting gives the opportunity to use a brainspot that corresponds with a particular part and then process this to facilitate integration and promote inner compassion and harmony. I will give an example of how I have used this approach in my work to illustrate how complex parts formulations can be worked in a manner that appears to allow the child to access the deeper emotional parts of the subcortical brain.

John was a 6 year old boy who was brought to me by his mother as he was terrified at night. They told me at the first meeting how for the past year he could not sleep alone, he feared demons under his bed, often felt sick at night, and he had begun to reject the parties and sports clubs that he had previously enjoyed. The family had travelled widely over the course of John's young life but he had always adapted well and made good friends up until a year ago. He was the member of a small, but close, loving family and had one younger sister of 4 years old.

In session John appeared to be timid but he was also interested in exploring his worries with me and was fascinated when I told him how we might find Brainspotting helpful. He went on to explain to me that his biggest fear was a demon that he called Fluggers and he drew and then cut out this character. To my untrained eyes, the character looked a lot like a typical 6-year olds drawing of a simple, small human figure, but in John's description it was terrifying. John told me that even looking at the cut out of Fluggers now he felt sick and scared. The same feelings that he described as having at night at home. I moved Fluggers across John's eye line to see if I could locate the activation brainspot. This technique is called outside window as the therapist follows the client's reflexive cues. As Fluggers reached just left of centre of John's eye line he swallowed heavily, eyes exhibited a micro twitch and his chest expanded with a deep breath. Also aware of my own body sensations, at this point, in the attunement, I had a felt sense of 'worry' in my upper chest. I held Fluggers at this spot and silently waited to see where the processing would go.

John was silent for a short while and then told me about a 'friend' called Darren that he used to be nice to because the boy wore glasses. He told me how Darren had stolen his place in the football team and then teased and taunted him. John began to show a little more anger and shouted, "I hate him!", then said he wished that he had not been kind to Darren and let him get close. Tears welled up in John's eyes as he looked at Fluggers and he cried a little. Between sobs, John shared some other thoughts that were coming up, some of which I could try to understand but mostly I just listened, also tuning into my own somatic process as I gradually felt it ease and soften. At this point John shifted his eyes to mine, smiled and said, "I'm done!" We spoke for a while and he asked if he could draw again. John drew five characters, this time Fluggers was joined by four friends who all had awesome superpowers. John explained that Fluggers and the rest of the "Night Gang" were his friends and each one had a special skill and he spoke affectionately about them all. John said he was excited to tell his mum about the gang and also to share it with Darren. I found out the next week that he had indeed done this, the boys had enjoyed playing together, the night fears were minimal, and he was sleeping in his own bed again with his picture of the Night Gang mounted on his wall.

One could make many interpretations of what might have been happening here in terms of parts work. This is natural and often part of the intellectual fascination of our work. The important thing was that, unlike with Charlie who I presented earlier, I did not let my agenda interfere with John's processing and resolution. We found a part called Fluggers that represented fear and vulnerability for him, then trusted the process to allow John's brain to do the self-organisation required, in the safety of the attuned therapist. John moved from fear, through anger, to generating an extremely resourceful gang giving him strength, playfulness and compassion. The brainspot that was scary and activating became the resource spot. What a transformation!

Reading books and articles where the author describes a session that goes exceptionally well, as with the case of John, can irritate me at times. Perhaps the irritation is there to protect me from feeling ineffective at the times when my work is not going as well. I notice that I can become suspicious that the authors are being over-selective with the choice of their case studies to promote their interests and own esteem as mine is plummeting! I would like to give some insight to the reality of working in my consulting room, mostly with very complex clients whose internal protectors are doing a great job at not letting an untrusted adult near their vulnerability.

Shaneen – This 15-year-old girl was trafficked to the UK from an international war zone. Eventually after a series of traumatic events she came into the care system and was referred to my practice. The social worker had heard about my work and was optimistic that I could be helpful. In the first session Shaneen said not one word but wrote on her arm in perfect English, "I fucking hate you!". Next session, she actually spoke to me, only to enquire, "Why does your hair look like a girl's you loser?". A few sessions down the line, with me doing little more than holding the space, she softened a little and informed me that, "You're not quite as bad as some of those wankers!". Attachment repair in motion?

David – This 8-year-old boy was a looked-after child from age 3 after a history of emotional and physical abuse. In our first session he told me that he didn't want to be here because he was missing maths at school. I asked him if he liked this subject and he replied coldly, "No I fucking hate it!" He had made it crystal clear to me how much I needed to work with both rupture and repair in our attachment focussed approach.

Helen – This 17-year-old girl was brought up in a home with extreme domestic violence and drug and alcohol abuse. She was hearing voices constantly telling her to take her life and wanted these to stop. I was hopeful from my experience that we could make some good progress on this using Brainspotting and after some gentle psychoeducation, suggested that we move forward with this. The 'protective part' that was present in her auditory hallucinations was not impressed that its power might be compromised and turned its attentions to me. The voice told Helen, in no uncertain terms, that I was dangerous and tried to convince her to end therapy and banish any ideas of Brainspotting. Eventually, we managed to agree that our work could continue if plenty of room was made for the voice to be heard and processed.

As challenging as these situations are for any therapist, Brainspotting has been very helpful to maintain the focus of the work. As I discussed in the early part of this chapter, the client's internal working model of attachment that was developed as an infant is going to be re-enacted in therapy. Indeed, Van der Kolk (2014) states that if you lack a deep memory of feeling loved then the relevant brain receptors simply fail to develop, so the child will not easily be able to feel calm and grounded in their body. This point is important to hold as it is simply unfair to the client and the therapist to further propagate the myth that 'all children process quickly'.

In working with complex clients we recognise and work with the early relational templates in the transference and countertransference to facilitate a new experience of attachment repair through attunement, mis-attunement, and re-attunement. This becomes easier when the dual attunement framework is upheld despite the challenges. The client is conceptualised as the comet and the challenge for the therapists is to hold this in mind whilst working to join the tail of the comet. With these three more complex clients above, there was no way that, at this point, transitioning to doing Brainspotting with a pointer would have been accepted or attuned. Patience and timing are important.

With Shaneen, her caution was understood as a healthy defence considering the abuse that she had suffered. I followed her verbalisations and acknowledged the strength of feeling that she was having. I also followed my own bodily response to her anger to begin to make this more tolerable and regulated in the right-brain implicit intersubjective connection. David's angriness needed to be heard and shared too by someone that could tolerate this so it could begin to move from rupture to repair.

In the case of Helen, a similar opportunity arose whereby the voice, her protector, could be truly heard and validated. Helen had a history of domestic violence and in a disorganised attachment way had learned that those she went to for help were the same ones that she was running from out of fear. Only when the angry destructive voice could be heard could she begin to unblend from it as her ultimate protector. In time, the voice agreed to take centre stage and let Helen do a Brainspotting session so that it could be heard and understood without the interruption of anyone or anything else. We found a brainspot for this voice, as it gave me clear instruction using inside window, whereby the client (or their part) lets you know where they want the pointer to be to get the strongest connection. Again, emphasising that the client is the comet and the therapist is in the tail, the emotion that was associated with the auditory hallucination could begin to be processed in alliance, rather than in obstruction. When the activated part refuses to do Brainspotting altogether, it is interesting to see how the client will often unconsciously naturally find a relevant eye position, or gazespot. This unconscious recognition that a client is accessing a brainspot also informs the therapist in understanding how the processing is still happening, allowing them to step back and maintain attunement.

Summary

We know that in child psychotherapy, a systemic approach is important to appreciate the attachment patterns that hold the child in respect to their significant relationships, past, present, and future. This is extended in attachment-focussed Brainspotting as interpersonal attunement is profound as the therapist attends to the client at both explicit and implicit levels, tracking the verbal, somatic, and unconscious interpersonal interactions. The embodied therapist seeks to match the rhythmic crescendos and decrescendos of the client's regulated and dysregulated autonomic nervous system (ANS). With this relational framework in position, there is the opportunity to use eye positions, accessing neurobiological attunement, to identify, target, and process a brainspot and unresolved trauma.

The systemic approach also acknowledges that there is a frame within a frame within a frame. The young person's intrapsychic, neurobiological, and somatic experiences are always understood in context of not just being part of the therapeutic relationship, but also all other relationships past and present. Successful child therapy is continually oscillating between the relationship with the therapist, alongside those with family members, carers, friends school children, teachers and all other significant relationships. The complexity of holding an appropriate systemic frame for the therapy can at times be quite overwhelming for the therapist, yet important in working towards optimum efficiency in expanding the child's safety, resources, and potential for processing.

This chapter has attended to the importance of the dual attunement framework that is the core of child psychotherapy. In the identification and enhancement of affect resonance the therapists use their presence to help the child resource and regulate through the work. The body-aware therapist notices what arises in them physically and can regulate this to help the child regulate in parallel. An immense and authentic resource in processing trauma that can address and contribute to the repair of old attachment wounds.

The second part of the dual attunement framework is the neurobiological attunement, the use of an eye position to identify and process through a brainspot. Although a child may be intrigued by this in the early sessions, often the appeal to work with an explicit brainspot diminishes over time. This is where playfulness and creativity can assist as the therapist can use play, art, and role play to locate a brainspot for processing. For example, the child might have drawn a picture of an incident that is activating and then the therapist can hold up this picture moving it across the x-axis to identify the brainspot. Alternatively, a natural gazespot might be observed when a child is drawing or playing in a sand tray. The child's excitement can also be harnessed and liberated as s/he identifies resource spots or 'powerspots' through play, which can then be used and integrated into the processing.

A recap of some of the more explicit approaches that enhance the value of Brainspotting with children can be summarised here. Children have their own agenda and this playfulness and creativity can remind the Brainspotting therapist to embrace uncertainty and not impose a model or intervention. We have all had times when we have noticed ourselves becoming more directive and observed how the interpersonal relationship is altered. This is not a failing, but appropriate reflection through supervision can assist the process of repair following the rupture – essential attachment-focussed work. As the child's power is re-established in the therapy, in collaboration with the therapist, the child feels resourced and more secure and more likely to be able to express themselves though play, speech, or exploration.

The information that children will not put into words, perhaps due to the on-going development of the neo-cortex, will still be evident in the therapeutic relationship. This lens into the child's historic attachment style is an absolute gift for the therapists to be able to recognise what could not be ascertained verbally. Whether using Brainspotting in a more traditional way, or more implicitly, the core values of holding, uncertainty, acceptance, playfulness, curiosity, and empathy are the values that inform all good child psychotherapy approaches. This comes as no surprise to experienced therapists; however the Brainspotting framework can be fruitful to remind and refresh the therapists when they may have become caught up in the work and feel that their practice is compromised.

Therapists working with children will often report that there is a powerful avoidant part of the child. The child did not drive to therapy, pay for therapy, and often did not ask for therapy. The conditions of engagement and attunement are therefore different with this population. Avoidance is a somewhat healthy way to cope with overwhelm. So, this protector part of the child must be valued so that it can be worked with to overcome potential therapy blocks. Also, children will often use immediate scenarios to access past incidents and traumas. As these re-enactments happen in the consulting room, it can be conceptualised that the child is setting the frame through deep subcortical processing. The Brainspotting therapists would remind themselves at this point to value being in the tail of the child's comet.

Perhaps unlike many Brainspotting sessions with an adult, the child's process is often observed to be less linear and can appear chaotic and inconsistent. For example, the child may begin by drawing an incident with a bully, go out of the room to the toilet 3 times, play hide and seek with you, and crash out on their mum's lap and shed a few tears before receiving her cuddles. In Brainspotting we do not perceive this as a disrupted or incomplete session. Instead we value that this is all happening within 'the frame' and understand these actions as an important part of the process.

Children are often hyperaware of actions and reactions. This is important as some children have had to develop this skill as if their life depended on it. Sadly, with some children, it did. With Brainspotting the therapist can obtain 'permission' to playfully relate to the child whilst holding a position of genuine authenticity. This enhances trust and the capacity for the child to continually move through cycles of rupture and repair as they process early attachment wounds.

Finally, with playfulness and improvisation come 'mistakes'. If we can be authentic about our mistakes, our learning is enhanced at an exponential rate. Our child clients can also benefit immensely as they move from experiences of secrecy and shame to a more open acceptance of human limitations and extended experiences of taking appropriate risks without incurring harmful consequences. This is the foundation of trust, attunement, and healing as well as an essential factor in learning and education across the board. Some of the best discoveries have come from mistakes and with Brainspotting the therapist continually makes space for this as we are learning from children and young people ad infinitum.

References

Bowlby, J., (1969): *Attachment and Loss, Vol. 1: Attachment.* Basic Books.

Bryson, P. T. and Siegel, J., (2012): *The Whole-Brain Child.* Robinson Publishing.

Devinsky, O., (2000): Right cerebral hemisphere dominance for a sense of corporeal and emotional self. *Epilepsy and Behaviour,* 1(1), p.60-73.

Dubicka, B., (Wednesday 22nd November 2017): The Tories said they cared about child mental health – but the Budget implies the exact opposite. *Independent,* http://www.independent. co.uk/voices/young-people-mental-health-philip-hammond-budget-camhs-services-children-a8070431.html.

Grand, D., (2013): Brainspotting: The Revolutionary New Therapy for Rapid and Effective Change. Sounds True Inc.

Goleman, D. (2007): Social Intelligence: The New Science of Human Relationships. Arrow.

Grixti, M, (2018): Brainspotting Therapy – Developed by David Grand (PhD) – YouTube https://www.youtube.com/watch?v=7FO_udVWkqA&t=58s

Grixti, M. and Dean, R. (2015): Brainspotting with Young People: An adventure into the mind. Sattva.

Hart, d. v. O., Nijenhuis, S. R. and Steele, (2006): The Haunted Self. W. W. Norton & Company.

Havens, L. (1988): Making Contact: Uses of Language in Psychotherapy. Harvard University Press.

Heisenberg, W. (1927): Über den anschaulichen Inhalt der quantentheoretischen Kinematik und Mechanik, *Zeitschrift für Physik* (in German), 43 (3–4): 172–198,

Hickok, G., (2014): *The Myth of Mirror Neurons.* W W Norton & Company Incorporated.

King, S., (1996): *The Green Mile.* US: Signet Books.

Kolk, d. V. A. B., (2015): *The Body Keeps the Score.* Penguin.

Levine, A. P., (2010): *In an Unspoken Voice.* North Atlantic Books.

Lyons-Ruth, K., (2000) "I sense that you sense that I sense...": Sander's recognition process and the specificity of relational moves in the psychotherapeutic setting. *Infant Mental Health Journal,* 21(1), p.85-98.

McGilchrist, I., (2012): T*he Master and His Emissary.* Yale University Press.

Monte, d. D., (2016): Neurobiology for trauma therapists. *The International Conference for Brainspotting.* Brazil.

Shaw, R., (2004): The embodied psychotherapist: An exploration of the therapists' somatic phenomena within the therapeutic encounter. *Psychotherapy Research,* 14(3), p.271-288.

Schiepek, G., Eckert, Aas, Kravanja, Wallot and Wallot, (2015): *Integrative Psychotherapy.* Hogrefe & Huber Pub.

Schore, N. A., (2012): *The Science of the Art of Psychotherapy (Norton Series on Interpersonal Neurobiology).* W. W. Norton & Company.

Schwartz, C. R., (2001): *Introduction to the Internal Family Systems Model.* Trailheads.

Trevarthen, C., (1990): *Growth and education of the hemispheres. In C. Trevarthen (Ed.), Brain circuits and function of the mind.* Cambridge: Cambridge University Press. p.334-363.

Watkins, G. J. and Watkins, H., (1997): *Ego States.* W. W. Norton.

BrainSpotting, qEEG, Biofeedback and Neuro-feedback: Towards an Integrative Approach to Trauma Healing and Regulation

Santiago Brand Ortiz

Most (if not all) of us have been exposed or will be exposed to at least one traumatic event in our lifetimes. The American Psychological Association (APA) defines trauma as an emotional response to a terrible event like an accident, rape, or natural disaster. Immediately after the event, shock and denial are typical. Longer term reactions include unpredictable emotions, flashbacks, strained relationships, and even physical symptoms like headaches or nausea. While these feelings are normal, some people have difficulty moving on with their lives. Psychologists can help these individuals find constructive ways of managing their emotions. One of the limitations with this definition is that it fails to include the distinction between what Dr. David Grand, author of Brainspotting (2013) calls macrotraumas and microtraumas. Sexual assault, natural disasters, death of a loved one are known as macrotraumas, big events that we hear or read about in the news or have probably witnessed ourselves. While these are more "popular" or "main-stream", microtraumas can also cause a great deal of damage in a person's internal and/or external environment. On the other hand, microtraumas, such as economic loss, physical injuries, witnessing others grieving, minor surgeries or medical procedures, are usually events that people never associate with the conventional definition of trauma or think could be the cause of their physical, emotional, and psychological problems. Still, microtraumas can cause an equal or more aggressive trauma response than that of macrotraumas.

When it comes to trauma intervention and treatment of both macro- and microtraumas, psychologists and other mental health professionals can face several challenges. One of the most common ones is the social stigma created around trauma and the expectation that healing should be automatic or fast. Many of the clients I work with delayed seeking help for many years because their friends, relatives, and loved ones told them to "snap out of it" or "get over it" because "it happened a long time ago" or "because the same happened to me and I am not traumatized". Shame is a strong form of re-traumatization which causes the individual to withdraw or suppress even further to the point of making things worse. Moreover, lack of understanding the association between "trivial", "small", or "insignificant" events and the trauma response can lead people to believe that there is nothing wrong with them, that their reactions a figment of their imaginations, that they will simply outgrow them, or that they will just fade away using wishful thinking. To add insult to injury, the popular belief that there is no cure or effective treatment for trauma or that it takes years of therapy to see changes creates a recipe for disaster that can keep people from seeking the help they need.

In order to utilize an integrative approach to trauma, it is important to understand that the response to trauma is subjective; it varies from individual to individual. While two or more people might be exposed to the same event, they will all react in different ways and some of them might not be traumatized at all. Why? In his book "Waking the Tiger: Healing Trauma" Peter Levine (1998) cites a series of dynamics and factors that play a crucial role in identifying why some people are more resilient than others and respond more effectively to dangerous situations.

- The event itself: the duration, intensity, frequency, and level of threat make all the difference. Events that are continuous and intense are more challenging to the individual and their organism.
- The context of the person's life at the time of the traumatizing event: Whether there is support or lack thereof, the individual´s health and lifestyle will in part determine the physical, emotional, and psychological consequences of being exposed to a traumatic event.
- The individual's physical characteristics: "Zombieland" (2009), a film about a zombie apocalypse starring Woody Harrelson and Jesse Eisenberg, starts with one of the main characters, Columbus (played by Eisenberg), describing a series of rules for surviving Zombieland. Rule number one is cardio. The opening scene shows a zombie giving chase to a heavy-set young man on a football field; as the zombie catches up to this unfortunate fella, Columbus utters the words "when the virus struck, for obvious reasons, the first ones to go, were the fatties". While some may find this line funny or even offensive, the fact is that an individual's endurance level, strength, and speed could play a vital and decisive role in their survival before, during, and after the event.
- A person's learned abilities: Self efficacy, training, and even previous experiences can provide an individual with the tools necessary nor only for survival but also for being more resistant to traumatization. Individuals who act quickly and skillfully are more likely to be better off in the long run. As I often tell my clients, "expect the best, but be prepared for the worst."
- Internal and external resources: self-efficacy, self-confidence psychological attitude, cognitions, and beliefs can modify the way a person reacts to and is subsequently affected by a traumatic event.

- History of success and failure: whether or not the person has successfully dealt with similar situations in the past.

There are four components that will be present to some degree in someone who was exposed to a traumatic event and was not successful in either fleeing or fighting: Hyperarousal, constriction, dissociation, and freezing (1). When the energy from a traumatic response has remained encapsulated and not released for a long time, the central nervous system will become hyperaroused. Hyperarousal manifests as the combination of both physical (somatic) and cognitive (thinking) symptoms. Physical symptoms include excessive sweating, increased heartbeat, hyperventilation, low peripheral temperature, tense muscles, and dry mouth among others. At the cognitive level, rumination, fretting, poor executive functioning, and low cognitive flexibility are observed in traumatized individuals. Constriction is a tool implemented in order to find homeostasis and allostasis, a way of coping with menacing events in an attempt to deal with the threat. The problem for most is that constriction becomes a form of what David Grand calls maladaptive homeostasis; the person gets stuck in the stress response creating a damaging and vicious circle responding to threats that most of the time are neither present nor real. When someone has been traumatized and they space out or drift away into their own world or an alternate dimension, they are exhibiting the symptoms of what is known as dissociation. While the organism uses dissociation to thwart physical, psychological, and emotional pain, it also becomes a form of maladaptive homeostasis. Dissociation constitutes a disruption of the person's felt sense as well as a distortion of time, space, and perception. The more the trauma is repeated and prolonged, the more easily and readily an individual will dissociate. (2). Some of the symptoms and signs of dissociation include: flat affect, empathy, disconnection from the world, depersonalization, and disruption of the mirror neuron system (3). As mentioned above, when a person faces a threatening situation, the first option is to escape and when this is no longer a possibility, fighting for your life comes next. Nevertheless, for many people neither is an option either because of physical, chronological (age) or psychological disadvantages. If this is the case, these individuals will experience helplessness (freezing), a learned response or way of accepting that nothing can be done, that there is no escape or solution. As gloomy as it may seem, helplessness, or more specifically freezing, could potentially, in certain circumstances, allow someone to escape the threat or survive. It is that state of helplessness or freezing that will cause the person to remain traumatized and unable to move forward, living a happy, productive, and adaptive life. The reason? Our neocortex, where as other members of the animal kingdom (zebras, cats, deer, etc.), use and rely on their mammalian and reptilian brains to successfully escape dangerous situations and dodge the effects of the trauma response (4). If you have ever seen the Discovery Channel or National Geographic, you probably have come across a familiar picture. A deer, zebra or gazelle is enjoying some time off work and eating with its coworkers. All of a sudden a predator (cheetah, lion) comes out of hiding and a chase ensues, which now is literally a matter of life and death for both prey (not being eaten) and predator (eating the prey or going hungry and not feeding the kids). Three possible scenarios will emerge from this picture: One, the potential prey will escape the situation and only a few minutes later will go back to eating and back to the office to tell its coworkers about what an experience that was, but will not go home carrying the burden of that near death experience and take it out on its wife and children. Two, the unfortunate animal will be caught by the predator who will sink its teeth on the trachea in order to suffocate it; as it happens the prey will become immobilized as if it were giving up, activating that primitive mechanism kindly installed by mother nature millions of years ago, the freezing response. It is this very mechanism which ensures that as death seems imminent, there will be no pain or agony for the victim; the pain response shuts down; there is no "higher order" processing such as, "ah, this is not good; as I die here now Larry is going to take my place at the office" or any other kind of processing for that matter. The unfortunate prey, victim of mother nature's ways, lies there in a catatonic state just waiting for what now seems inevitable. But wait! Do not give up hope for that cute deer just yet! There is scenario number three; as it turns out the lion or cheetah is not the only hungry predator in the corporate ladder; along comes the freeloader, hiding in plain sight just waiting for someone else to do all the hard work to then steal it and claim credit for it, the psychopath of the African Savannah. As the unsuspecting lion is preparing to enjoy the spoils of war, along comes this moocher in the form of a hyena or even another lion. The predator lets go of its hard-earned meal for a second, hard worker and lazy scavenger stare at each other, hands at holster, spaghetti western music playing in the background, and as all of this is happening, the prey seizes the opportunity, quickly gets up, violently and beautifully shakes for a fraction of a second and makes a break for it while the other two just start playing the blame game, success!

What Bambi did in that split second, was to successfully activate the ability to self-heal, to let go, and "forget about it", something that mother nature provided every mammal (even human beings) with a very, very, very long time ago. After it is all over, the almost victim goes back to the office as it nothing had happened, notices Larry staring at him jealously, and then goes home to what is a very common situation: "Hi honey, how was your day", "Just another day at the office, What's for dinner, eh?" Nonhuman animals have a distinct advantage over human animals (not fair) when it comes to life-threatening situations and the trauma response. While animals react instinctively (they dash without thinking about it), human beings will often attempt to make sense of the situation, to think about it, to analyze it, to understand it, and that is when we pay the price. Our neocortex is the most advanced of all the species; it allows us to build rockets that take astronauts to the moon, create those hilarious Super Bowl commercials, speak to each other, cure disease, and do all the wonderful things our species has accomplished; it is nothing short of miraculous. Yet, when it comes to dangerous situations, it also causes us to overthink and rationalize, creating new dangerous situations every day. As ironic as it is, human beings, the most "advanced" species in the universe (until aliens land on the White House lawn and we get definite proof we are not alone) are at the same time the most and perhaps the only stressed and traumatized beings inhabiting this planet. Zebras, cats, dogs, dolphins do not threat each other with nuclear annihilation, do not kidnap and murder their own, do not fire each other from work after 20 plus years of giving the company everything, do not pay mortgages on the caves where they hibernate, do not max out their credit cards to send their offspring to college; they do not have a human neocortex.

That is what precisely the problem for human beings is. When they face a traumatic event, they will, more often than not, try rationalize it. On September 11, 2001, when the first plane struck the north tower of the World Trade Center, most people thought it was just a plane crash. People in the south tower were evacuated, but were soon allowed to return to their offices. The neocortex went into action and caused people to rationalize the event and come up with a simple conclusion without evaluating other possibilities. It was only when the second plane hit the other building that it became obvious that it was a terrorist attack. The same modus operandi applies for many other tragic occurrences in world history where thinking and not acting leads to long-term trauma. That is enough of the bad news; the good news is that human beings were bestowed with that same capacity for self-healing and the same ability to "shake off" the event and prevent traumatization and its dire consequences in the long run. More good news, our neocortex, the same one that can trick us into thinking all is well, has also allowed us to come up with solutions to our problems and generate creative, efficient ways to help each other heal. Not everything is doom and gloom. Our endless sense of curiosity has lead us, in spite of the world's troubles, into always looking for and finding ways to make life better, safer, more enjoyable. In the movie "K-Pax" (2001) the protagonist is an alien named "Prot" who comes from the planet K-Pax. He strikes up a friendship with a psychiatrist, Dr. Mark Powell. During one of the most salient scenes in the movie Dr. Powell asks the alien visitor, "Prot, why have you come to our planet?" To which he replies, "Well, I've been here many times before. But what brought me here first? I don't know. Pure curiosity, I guess. I'd never been to a Class BA-3 planet before."

Dr. Powell then asks, "Class BA-3?" Prot answers, "Early stage of evolution. Future uncertain, sometimes it's hard to imagine how you've made it this far." Well, had Prot studied us a little further he would have understood that we have made it this far because of our brain and its neocortex. It has provided us with one of the most precious gifts: resilience, which is how we have made it this far and is a skill that must be cultivated, practiced, and honed.

We have learned more about the human brain in the past decade than we have in the last fifty or sixty years. Our brain is nothing short of magnificent, the product of millions of years of evolution, the most complex organ in the known universe. We now have a clearer understanding of all the magnificent things we can do thanks to our brain, and one of those is to help others heal. To me, one of the greatest talents and gifts I have is that of helping others find "their way back home." I have come across, by happenstance or otherwise (depending on what you believe) three wonderful techniques that I love and implement in my mission to make this world a better place: Brainspotting, biofeedback and neurofeedback. In combination, I have seen miracles occur in front of my very own eyes, not only for me, but for others as well. The aim of this chapter is to explain how each works individually, how they can be implemented together, and why they are not mutually exclusive. In my personal and professional opinion, integration is the key to healing; the more tools one can provide one's clients with, the better. We are the byproduct of our life experiences, what happened when mommy was pregnant with us, when we were born, and every single event up to this point in time will help determine who we are and how we navigate this uncertainty called life. The purpose of this chapter is to show the reader why integrative interventions – those that combine different elements, such as BrainSpotting, qEEG (Brain Mapping), biofeedback, neurofeedback, functional medicine, and nutrition – could be more beneficial for clients who have suffered trauma and other conditions that affect their health, quality of life, performance, and happiness, and also be more effective alternatives to conventional approaches such as pharmacotherapy. The objective is not to favor one approach over the other or determine which one is better. Rather, the aim is to explain how such a cohesion could strengthen our ability to help people heal.

"Where you look affects how you feel" is the premise of Brainspotting, a technique discovered and developed by Dr. David Grand. His initial hypothesis is that the visual field is a reflection of the ongoing processes held in the brain and felt in the body (5). Therefore, wherever an individual looks and fixes their eyes is the place in the brain where a particular memory is held; which is known as a brainspot. The technique of Brainspotting involves locating and understanding these areas, because where we choose to look will activate certain reflexes, but is also key in triggering the healing process (6).

How Brainspotting actually works and the exact mechanisms at play are not currently known. Nonetheless, at the time of writing, the author was in collaboration with Dr. Sue Pinco and Deborah Antinori in the development of a pilot study that aims to answer these questions. The initial study took place in February of 2018 where the electroencephalogram (EEG) and peripheral psychophysiological measures of 10 participants were recorded before, during and after a Brainspotting session.

When trauma is not renegotiated and the energy has not been released, it gets encapsulated in the brain, wreaking havoc in a person's life. This energy Levine mentions manifests itself in the form of physical, emotional, psychological, and behavioral symptoms that act like a closed circuit, hindering an individual's wellbeing in all of the aforementioned dimensions. Brainspotting utilizes several different approaches such as outside window, inside window, gazespotting, partsspotting among others (7). When a brainspot is located, the client will exhibit a series of reflexes that implement the processing of the traumatic memory and lead to healing. Eye wobbles, twitching, crying, or hyperventilating are just some of those reflexes and reactions. By recording, observing, and analyzing the neuro- and psychophysiological processes, we can one, gain a deeper understanding of Brainspotting's exquisite and intricate processes and two, explore how we can implement other techniques such as heart rate variability biofeedback (HRV), not during the session because we do not want to interfere with it, but in between sessions so as to fortify the power Brainspotting.

The EEG is the recording of the amplified electrical activity or electric fields generated by the neurons. It is recorded by placing individual sensors or specially designed caps on the individual's scalp. An amplifier magnifies the electrical activity of the brain so it can be displayed on a computer screen. The activity is then shown in the form of brain waves, which in turn are the byproduct of how neurons talk to each other. (8). In essence, the waves produced by the brain are the result of complex and elaborate electrochemical processes and also the interaction of the cortex and subcortical (deep brain) regions. What the brain waves also reveal is how we human beings operate and what makes us an interesting, yet complex species. In addition, those rising and falling electrical patterns and fields can provide a wealth of information about our thought processes, how we understand and process information, how we learn, how we feel, and ultimately how we act and react. Whether there is love or friendship, rage or envy, the brain is at the core of those elements. The same applies for trauma and its consequences, and so understanding the brain waves will help us understand how trauma is processed in the brain and eventually how and why Brainspotting is such an efficacious technique.

In the EEG recording, two types of brain waves can be observed: slow and fast. Slow and fast brain waves have two characteristics. Frequency, refers to the speed of the wave, which is measured in Hertz (Hz). Amplitude refers to the size of the wave from base to peak and it is measured in Microvolts (µV). The basic premise in order to understand this better is: the slower the speed (frequency) the higher the wave (amplitude) and the higher the speed the lower the wave. Frequency and amplitude are also related to an individual's arousal or activation/anxiety level, and also to the synchronization and desynchronization of neuronal networks, meaning, turning specific brain regions on and off, depending on the activity (reading, learning a new language, memorizing etc.) (9). When I interpret the EEG, I practice what I like to call neurological archeology. The client's brain wants to tell us a story and a big part of that story lies within the brainwaves, the neurological patterns, and their biological components. Depending on what types of brainwaves are present and where in the brain they are present, we can understand and to a certain degree discern an individual's thought patterns, brain processing speed, mood states, regulatory skills, cognitive abilities, and other characteristics without the person telling us beforehand; is a form of scientific "mind reading".

What is being theorized based on some of the findings from the pilot study is that Brainspotting could be responsible for generating new neurons (neurogenesis) and neuroplasticity ⊠ i.e. the ability for the brain to change itself via activation or deactivation of neuronal networks believed to be tied to specific brainspots. Hence, when clients are processing their trauma, they are tapping into those networks and turning them on and/or off depending on the desired result. Changes were also observed in the peripheral physiological responses (body temperature, muscle tension, etc.), which lead us to hypothesize that Brainspotting also effects changes in physiology and psychophysiological responses (i.e. mind-body processes).

To further understand this, a brief explanation of the different brainwaves and the peripheral psychological variables is warranted. So we can understand things more easily, names were assigned to those waves. Delta, theta, alpha, sensory motor rhythm (SMR), µ (mu), beta, high beta, and gamma are the Greek word designations given to this electrical patterns. Delta brainwaves are the slowest in frequency and highest in amplitude of the brainwaves (0.5-4 Hz). They are related to deep, restorative sleep, but are also observed in traumatic brain injuries (TBI), dementia, learning disabilities, neuropathies such as fibromyalgia, and could also signal the presence of a brain tumor. Theta brainwaves (4-8Hz) can be seen in deep meditative states and are also beneficial for learning and memory consolidation; on the other hand, they are also present in attention deficit disorder (ADD), attention deficit hyperactivity disorder (ADHD), obsessive compulsive disorder (OCD), memory impairment, inattention, impulse control deficits, among other conditions. Alpha (8-12 Hz) represents an idling state of the brain where there is no metabolic processing (resting and energy optimization). It also has been observed in relaxation and meditative states, ADD/ADHD, anxiety, cognitive deficits, excessive marijuana consumption, brain fog, and low IQ. Mu (μ) (10-12 Hz) is recorded in the motor cortex and has been observed in some 30-40 % of people in the autistic spectrum disorder. μ has also been recorded in the EEGs of adopted children and victims of sustained and systematic trauma. Clients who present with μ in their EEGs tend to dissociate and depersonalize quite often; it marks a dysregulation in the mirror neuron system and a shutdown or disengagement of the pre-frontal cortex. (10). Based on my multiple EEG recordings of individuals in the aforementioned populations, it is my hypothesis that μ represents a defense mechanism that helps the client dissociate in order to escape from the physical, emotional, and psychological consequences of trauma. Since it also corresponds to an offline mirror neuron system and pre-frontal cortex, clients with μ often exhibit flat affect, pedantic language, reduced empathy for others, poor socialization skills, withdrawal, and are mistrusting of others. Conversely, μ has a positive aspect in that it has been observed in the EEGs of peak performance individuals (athletes, CEOs, surgeons, actors, musicians, and performers in general). ** (ask for literature) In this population μ rhythm is a performance enhancer, as it facilitates a positive dissociation allowing the athlete to isolate distractions, get in the zone, or achieve what sport psychologist Roland Carlstedt (11) calls repressive coping. Thus, μ needs to either be reduced to counteract its dissociative qualities in trauma sufferers or enhanced for peak performance purposes. Sensory motor rhythm (SMR, 12-15 Hz) is also observed in the motor cortex and correlates with positive neutral perfusion (blood flow). It is augmented and has been used successfully in treatment of migraines, epilepsy, sleep disorders anxiety, and ADD/ADHS. Beta (13-21 Hz) and high beta (21-35 Hz) help the brain consume and use energy in an optimal way that keeps us energized and engaged in the task at hand for long enough. On its dark side, beta has been observed in anxiety disorders, insomnia, OCD, rumination, fretting, and also in alcohol, cocaine, and heroin addicts. Gamma (35-100 Hz) has been seen in high order processing (i.e., math, calculations) and also has been observed in the EEGs of Tibetan monks who achieve deep levels of meditation and "feelings of blessings" (12).

There are several brain structures and networks involved or active in the trauma response. In the pilot study, we observed that the anterior cingulate cortex (ACC) is one of the most active areas before, during and after and BSP session. Part of the limbic system, the ACC regulates several functions such as mental and cognitive flexibility, ability to adapt to new environments, ability to shift from one thought or idea to the next, cooperation, going with the flow, and empathy. We observed excess theta, beta, and alpha in some of the baseline (10 minutes resting state, eyes open) recordings. In one participant a reduction in the activity of the ACC was observed in the recording following the BSP session (see images). It is the author's hypothesis that by locating the brainspot corresponding to the ACC and its surrounding networks, processing of the trauma will take place, therefore allowing that structure to function more optimally, resulting in a reduction in fretting, rumination, and anxiety and a rise in empathy, flexibility, openness, and the like.

A deactivation of the ACC (theta) and motor cortex (μ) was observed in another participant during the session as she went subcortical and started processing. The author also theorizes that Brainspotting could serve as a mediating mechanism in activation and deactivation of neuronal networks where trauma events remained dormant either as a direct consequence of trauma or as a byproduct of it. This and other hypotheses remain to be confirmed as more research with more repeated measures is necessary. Nonetheless, these initial findings are pointing trauma therapists in the right direction about the inner workings of BSP. What also needs to be taken into account is that everyone's EEG is different, as are their experiences, biological, physiological, and the way trauma affects them. Therefore, this uniqueness and this individuality need to be factored in for future research. One of the foreseeable advantages of using qEEG (brain mapping) technology and more specifically LORETA software is that it helps visualize the problematical subcortical Brodmann areas (areas of the brain that handle specific functions). Consequently, this software can potentially help being more specific in finding certain brainspots and processing traumatic memories. Also, research comparing different BSP modalities needs to be developed. Analyzing the way inside window, outside window, Z- axis, partsspotting, or gazespotting influences brain activity could lead to determine whether any of these modalities better suits certain clients or types of trauma. The changes observed in EEG activity immediately after a BSP session in some of the participants also lead the researchers to believe that a disengagement of sympathetic tone (activation) is at play while the person is processing and once it is completed. Another factor that warrants further exploration is studying how different brainwave patterns respond to Brainspotting and any of its modalities. As mentioned above, people's brains react differently to trauma; in some EEGs, fast beta and high beta waves might be dominant, signaling hyperarousal and excessive limbic output (high anxiety). Others show excess fast alpha wave activity which correlates with anxiety and depression while others will have visible μ or delta or theta waves which could be possible markers for dissociation and depersonalization, as well as a disruption of social interaction processes (flat affect, withdrawal, low empathy). Other recordings will show a combination of both slow and fast brainwave activity signaling a battle between the sympathetic and parasympathetic branches for real-state control in the brain. Additionally, the structures of a person's brain affected by trauma vary from individual to individual. Some recordings reveal excessive activity by the ACC (Brodmann areas 24, 25, 32 and 33), while others will reveal a disconnection of the mirror neuron system (Brodmann areas 1, 2, 3, 4 ,5 & 6), hippocampus (Brodmann area 28), executive network (Brodmann areas 39 & 40) and prefrontal or frontal cortex (Brodmann areas 8, 9 &10) (13).

Psychophysiological or peripheral measures could also offer a potential window of access into the efficacy of BSP. The body and the brain do not operate as separate entities, and what happens in the brain (or mind) will flow through the body and vice versa. If a trauma or traumas have not been successfully renegotiated, the encapsulated energy will generate a chaotic series of events that will wreak havoc in the organism's chemical, physiological and psychological processes. It will trigger or exacerbate chronic inflammatory stress, disease, and even death (14). For the pilot study, different physiological responses were recorded, each of the utmost importance for the mind-body relationship and processing and renegotiation of trauma. During the study, respiration rate, heart rate, heart rate variability (HRV), peripheral temperature, and galvanic skin response were recorded to track and measure psychophysiological changes before, during, and after a BSP session and at a one week follow up. The key element in respiration is gas exchange; every time a breathing cycle takes place (inhalation and exhalation) oxygen (O_2) and carbon dioxide (CO_2) are exchanged. CO_2 is the most important element in our breathing. The medulla (located in the brain stem) contains chemoreceptors that respond to changes in CO_2 levels. Every time we exhale, finishing the breathing cycle, those chemoreceptors signal us so that we start yet another breathing cycle and stay alive. Trauma and the trauma response will more often than not cause hyperventilation or over-breathing. When the average adult respires at a rate of 15 breaths per minute (ideal respiration rate 5-7 breaths per minute), it creates an imbalance in CO_2 levels (expelling an excess of CO_2) causing the individual to feel anxious or hypervigilant. One of the interesting phenomena observed during the BSP sessions was a reduction in the respiration rate in some of the participants. This is encouraging as it could indicate that Brainspotting contributes to the reduction of sympathetic tone via the vagus nerve and a balance of carbon dioxide levels, therefore regulating blood PH (more alkaline) and other health benefits (15). This, of course, is a claim that needs to be researched further. Heart rate (HR) records the number of times the heart beats per minute; in some traumatized individuals it can be increased above its healthy range because of the hyperarousal and sympathetic over-activation that trigger the release of adrenaline and cortisol. Heart rate variability (HRV) refers to the rhythmicity of the heart rate. Think of HR as the music and HRV as the dancer who can either dance or not dance to the rhythm of the music. HRV is the interplay between the sympathetic (SNS) and parasympathetic (PNS) nervous systems. When we inhale, HR increases because we are acti-

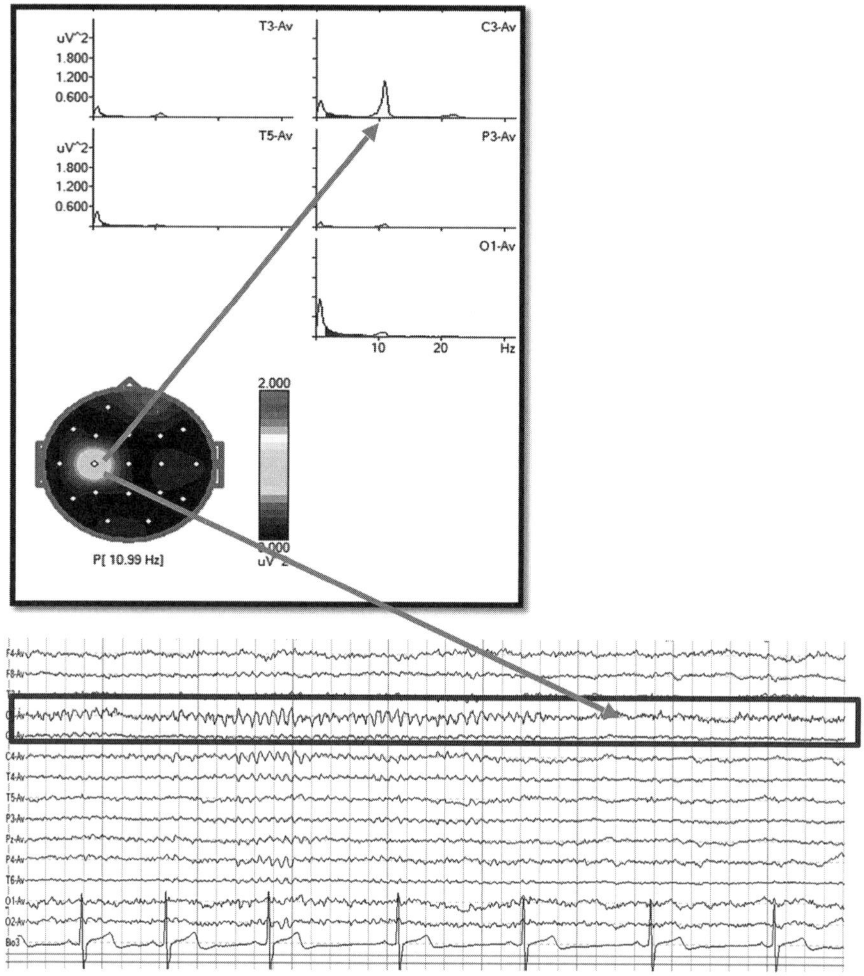

Figure 1. Desynchronization of the μ Rhythm at C3 after 5 minutes of coherent breathing.

vating the SNS and as we exhale, HR decreases because the PNS activates (16). In a traumatized individual three events can occur. One, there is sympathetic tone (hyperarousal), characterized by anxiety, hypervigilance, aggressiveness, and constriction. Two, parasympathetic tone (hypoarousal) where constriction, dissociation, helplessness, and depression are common. Or three, an interplay of hyper- and hypoarousal, the individual shifts states going from aggressive to depressed, from alert to helpless. Poor HRV caused by post traumatic stress disorder (PTSD) puts individuals at risk for many diseases or even premature or sudden death (17). The communication between the heart and the brain is 95% afferent (goes from the heart to the brain) and it is mediated by the vagus nerve through its innervations of various key brain structures such as the brain stem, the medulla (chemoreceptors), the amygdala, prefrontal cortex, and neocortex. By consciously and positively altering heart rhythmicity, brain states can also be positively altered, achieving autonomic balance resulting in a happier, healthier, more resilient individual. HRV biofeedback can be an adjunct intervention to Brainspotting in order to strengthen processing and healing. It would not be used during a session, as we do not want to interfere with its essence; however, HRV training can be taught to and used by the client between BSP sessions. To get an idea of how HRV modifies brain activity, look at figure 1. It is an EEG recording of a male client with a history of trauma. Rhythmic μ can be seen in the recording at C3 and C4 (motor cortex) signaling a dysregulation of the mirror neuron system and the prefrontal cortex. Among the symptoms reported by the client are flat affect and dissociation. The client was then coached on HRV breathing biofeedback and asked to breathe in a specific pattern. After a few seconds, a clear desynchronization (dissapearance) of the μ rhythm was observed in the EEG trace, signaling an activation of the frontal cortex and a disruption of the dissociative process (the client reported feeling more grounded and present). This after only 5 minutes of coherent breathing. Teaching clients HRV biofeedback and asking them to practice in between sessions can further alter brain activity in a helpful manner, thus reinforcing the gains obtained with Brainspotting. That way, both approaches become mutually inclusive and integrative. Peripheral temperature is the recording of blood flow to the periphery of the body, namely fingertips and toes. The activity of blood vessels in the fingers is influenced only by sympathetic innervations and it is mediated by adrenaline and nitric oxide, which affect the α-adrenergic receptors of the blood vessels (18). In traumatized individuals, hyperarousal and chronic activation of the hypothalamic pituitary adrenal (HPA) axis triggers the release of adrenaline, which will bind to the α receptor causing vasoconstriction; the blood will flow away from the periphery and the brain, a sign of sympathetic tone or high arousal. On the other hand, constriction, suppression, and dissociation can also cause vasoconstriction, which generally correlates with parasympathetic tone (helplessness, depression). In the pilot study, changes in peripheral blood flow and temperature were observed in some participants before, during and after Brainspotting. Most participants exhibited low peripheral temperature during baseline recordings. An increase in temperature was evident during and after BSP. Those participants who processed more or went subcortical had a higher increase in peripheral blood flow (they were more relaxed). Since the only way to increase peripheral temperature is to reduce sympathetic tone, it is hypothesized by the researchers that Brainspotting reduces sympathetic activity and helps with the suppression of adrenaline and cortisol, favoring production of nitric oxide with vasodilation as a result (better blood flow). Additionally, training clients in temperature biofeedback between BSP sessions can further favor the healing process by virtue of achieving higher relaxation. Further research is essential to better substantiate these findings. An individual's galvanic skin response (GSR) records changes in diaphoresis (sweating) in the palm of the hands. The sweat glands are exclusively innervated by the sympathetic nervous system. Hyperarousal and sympathetic tone will cause an increase in the sweating response (diaphoresis). Conversely, PTSD, constriction, dissociation, and helplessness can also cause a reduction or no visible activity in GSR recordings. Therefore, traumatized individuals can either sweat profusely or not sweat at all. The brain regions that influence GSR include the ventromedial prefrontal cortex, anterior cingulate, parietal lobe, insula, amygdala, and dorsolateral prefrontal cortex (19). Changes in skin diaphoresis (sweating) and skin resistance (dryness) were observed during and after Brainspotting, again leading to the hypothesis that the brain areas or brainspots influencing sympathetic activation are being either circumvented or deactivated the more the participants went subcortical and processed more material. Once more, the inclusion of GSR biofeedback training between BSP sessions could bring additional benefits at the physical, emotional, and psychological level. The neuropsychophysiological changes observed so far have led the author to believe in the existence of specific brainspots for specific EEG activity, psychophysiological responses, and that those spots can be found using different modalities such as outside window, inside window, vergence, rollerspotting, gazespotting or even partspotting. Future studies will hopefully shed more light on these pressing issues.

Brainspotting is a powerful, effective technique; the ever-growing number of professionals incorporating it in their intervention arsenal presents a strong case for its efficacy. Increasing media exposure is also spreading the word, and the changes seen in the people who have been through several traumatic events are helping to fortify its popularity. One clear obstacle faced by the BSP community is the lack of scientific evidence as to why it works so well and so fast. Thankfully, ongoing research conducted by the author, Deborah Antinori, Sue Pinco, Damir Del Monte, Steve Sawyer, and others not only will provide this much-needed evidence, but will also continue positioning Brainspotting as an effective and efficacious evidence-based therapy. EEG recordings have provided initial evidence of changes in brain activity, and the sustainability of those changes needs to be further demonstrated. Changes in psychophysiological measures have also indicated that there may be physiological and biochemical changes during a session that in turn generate physical, emotional, and psychological gains. These are exciting times as the field of psychology is favorably evolving towards the discovery and development of practical yet highly effective approaches. Moreover, the integration of said approaches could prove key to people's sustained healing. Training a person´s brainwave activity via neurofeedback could solidify the initial neuroplasticity generated by Brainspotting or perhaps help hone the mental health professional's skills and talents. Training clients in respiration techniques and HRV biofeedback could further enhance heart-brain communication and interaction deepening on an individual's processing and renegotiation. Peripheral temperature and GSR biofeedback could also expand the clients' awareness of their own self-healing abilities as well as the understanding of their own subcortical processes. Being the powerful intervention that it is, Brainspotting paves the way for other approaches such as qEEG (brain mapping), neurofeedback or biofeedback to help the client go from dysregulation to (self) regulation and to ultimately attain that ever-elusive yet highly coveted victory within.

References

1,2,4: Levine, Peter, *Waking the Tiger: Healing Trauma.* (North Atlantic Books, Berkley, California, 1997).

3, 9, 10: Kropotov, Juri D., Functional *Neuromarkers for Psychiatry: Applications for Diagnosis and Treatment.* (Academic Press, London, 2016).

5,6,7: Grand, David, *Brainspotting: The Revolutionary New Therapy for Rapid and Effective Change.* (Sounds True, INC, Boulder, 2013).

8: Steriade, M., Gloor, P., Llinás, R.R., Lopes da Silva, F.H., Mesulam, M.M.: *Basic Mechanisms of Cerebral Rhythmic Activities.* Electroencephalography and Clinical Neurophysiology, 1990, 76: 481-508.

11: Carlstedt, Roland A., *Critical Moments During Competition: A Mind-Body Model of Sport Performance When It Counts the Most.* (Psychology Press, New York, 2004).

12: Swingle, Paul G., *Biofeedback for the Brain: How Neurotherapy Effectively Treats Depression, ADHD, Autism, and More.* (Rutgers University Press, New Jersey, 2008).

13: Thompson, Michael., Thompson, Lynda., *Functional Neuroanatomy.* (ADD Centers, Ltd., Toronto, 2015).

14: Nakazawa, Jackson Donna., *Childhood Disrupted: How your Biography Becomes Your Biology, and How You Can Heal.* (Atria, New York, 2015).

15: Khazan, Inna., *The Clinical Handbook of Biofeedback: A Step-by-Step Guide for Training and Practice with Mindfulness.* (John Wiley and sons, Ltd., Malden, 2013).

16, 17: Moss, Donald., Shaffer, Fred., *Psychophysiology & General Health Heart Rate Variability* (HRV). (AAPB, 2007).

18: Romanovsky, A.A., *Skin temperature: Its Role in Thermoregulation.* Acta Physiologica, 2014, 210: 498-507.

19: Norman, R., Mendolicchio, L., Mordeniz, C., Pierangeli, E., Pannarale, P., Orsucci, F., Conte, E., *Galvanic Skin Response & Its Neurological Correlates.* Journal of Consciousness Exploration & Research, 7: 553-572.

The Yips Reconceptualized as Conversion Disorder: The Dynamic Brainspotting Treatment of Athletes

Calder W. Kaufman

Summary

This chapter presents the case for a puzzling sports phenomenon, the yips, as conversion disorder based on the constellation of symptoms observed in many athletes. Conversion disorder is a relatively rare psychiatric condition in which a patient suffers from Change to: an ostensibly physical condition in the absence of identifiable medical etiology. It is suggested that sports psychology fails to account for clinical considerations in the conceptualization and intervention of the yips, thus limiting effective treatment. This is compounded by the vast prominence of cognitive-behavioral therapy, a paradigm increasingly considered only on par with or even inferior to others based on large meta-analytic studies. Brainspotting is outlined as a therapeutic approach worthy of treating conversion conditions manifesting as the yips in athletics.

Introduction

Conversion disorders are a subdivision of the larger category of somatic symptom disorders and are frequently associated with a history of trauma. These conditions are known as *psychogenic* as opposed to *organic* since they mimic a general medical condition, but a medical diagnosis cannot be determined with usual diagnostic procedures such as blood work or imaging. They are often accompanied by *la belle indifference* which is a "puzzling emotional minimization of the seriousness of [disabling] conditions." (PDM Task Force, 2006, pg. 115) What is minimized by some patients is just as often described as quite troubling by others. Clinical presentations of conversion disorder are mystifying for both mental health and medical practitioners alike.

Those referred to psychotherapists for these conditions often come from puzzled (or rather astute) physicians who have patients with undifferentiated complaints such as dystonic (abnormal) movements, fatigue, numbness, diffuse pain, or gastrointestinal complaints, among many others. When no discernible medical etiology can be identified, psychotherapy or psychiatry is the treatment of choice. My assertion is that contemporary sports psychology does not typically utilize clinical knowledge readily at the disposal of trained clinicians and most certainly does not incorporate conversion disorder, or similar ideas, into its assessment of sports performance problems. *The fact that bona fide psychiatric condition emerges in an athlete makes it no less clinical than if it occurred in the general population.*

To understand conversion disorders in athletes one must understand dissociation, which is intricately linked with trauma and is perhaps the most salient symptom, or constellation of symptoms, of the post-traumatic stress disorder (PTSD) (Scaer, 2001; van der Hart, 2005). *Structural dissociation* is a term used in the study of complex PTSD and has implications for a wider range of conditions, including those of conversion disorder. These symptoms can present with somatoform or psychoform features. Somatoform dissociation can be medically characterized as a dystonia, or a condition involving involuntary contraction of muscles which are comprised of abnormal movements, pain, or numbness, among other symptoms (Nijenhuis & van der Hart, 2011). Dystonias can be focal when impacting one specific body part (the arm), or segmental, by afflicting two or more body areas (the trunk, forearms, and hands) (Mayo Clinic, 2018). It is well-recognized that dystonias worsen with high levels of emotional distress, and there is a high degree of co-morbidity between conversion conditions and more common diagnoses such as anxiety or depressive disorders.

Psychoform levels of dissociation are characterized by psychological symptoms emerging with either negative features, such as amnesia or apathy, alexithymia (the inability to identify and express emotions), or positive, as in intrusive thoughts, hypermnesia (enhancement of memory), or hallucinations in highly disturbed patients (Nijenhuis & van der Hart, 2011). Structural dissociation should be differentiated from adaptive dissociation, the latter of which promotes a person's health and vitality. Adaptive dissociation can eventually become maladaptive if overutilized or if it overextends beyond the presence of the original stressor. In other words, an adaptation to a threat in the environment is only pathological if it persists beyond the existence of the threat and causes secondary impairment.

As described by Scaer (2001), trauma is a *disorder of time* and based in specific types of implicit memory, called procedural memory. When combined with a threatening event, conditioned motor movements and salient emotions are stored concretely in the brain and form the basis for PTSD symptoms, particularly reexperiencing. The trauma, then, is experienced as happening in the here-and-now, rather than as a past, completed event. Scaer (2014) states, "procedural memories of a traumatic event...are linked to the visual perceptual space" and "procedural memories could also be linked to the precise position of the eyes at the moment of the trauma" (p. 175). This idea is fortified by psychologist Lisa Feldman Barret: "Your brain is organized in such a way as to [make] anticipatory guesses about what is going to happen next. And this is happening entirely outside of your awareness. You have past experiences, and those experiences become wired into your brain, and then your brain uses those past experiences to make guesses about the immediate future" (The Making of Emotions, 2018).

The term *the yips* has become a colloquialism for any instance of diminished performance not attributable to something physical, like a knee injury. The term is applied to whatever is assessed to be "mental" as opposed to residing in the pure biomechanics of the body. This attitude wrongly assumes the processes of the central nervous system, including the thinking and emotional parts of the brain, are somehow separate from the movement of the trunk and extremities. Such Cartesian splits are pervasive in society and most certainly in athletics. In many circumstances, rather than fostering a productive means of understanding the yips, the opposite occurs by limiting the "why" and "how" these problems emerge.

Another consequence is that struggling athletes are likely to be regarded with criticism or derision based on the common insinuation they are inherently lacking something fundamental in character or thinking, especially if their body is deemed healthy. It is decided the athlete must simply "get her head right" via basic attitude adjustment, or that she is failing to perform based on lack of effort. In most cases, the yips remain a relative mystery due in part to pervasive Cartesian dualism. The same is true for conversion disorders in the general population as the term psychogenic assumes a fundamental separation from the rest of a patient's physiology. This is simply psychologically inaccurate and physiologically impossible.

Conscious mental processes of the left pre-frontal cortex have little to do with previously learned motor actions which are controlled by more posterior brain areas and deeper structures like the cerebellum near the brainstem which are mediated by the midbrain. Further, the idea of "overthinking," which can intrude upon natural, reactive body movements, is a symptom of anxiety housed in the right midbrain, not solely in the left neocortex. Worried thoughts are largely representative of anxious activation of the limbic system, not a precursor to it, and attitudes of the athlete are of minor consequence. Beliefs and attitudes are most aptly reflective of the ingrained implicit self of the right hemisphere of the brain (Schore, 1994).

In athletics, a major problem with assessing the yips as simply "mental" is that the yip movement in question always involves a motor movement, typically a highly practiced maneuver such as a baseball player's throwing motion, a golfer's putting, or free throw shooting in basketball. These movements are mostly unconscious and procedural in nature and heavily influenced by the athlete's trauma history. In my experience, not only do conscious mental experiences not exist in a vacuum independent of the body, psychoform dissociative symptoms ebb and flow with somatoform based on the basal root of the individual's unique brand of trauma. These are interconnected, inextricably linked processes.

Brainspotting (BSP) is thought to have direct access to the midbrain processes implicated in trauma-based procedural memories. BSP is a "hook," of sorts, to these structures along with salient emotions and memories, as well as the dystonic, procedural memory-based motor functions expressed in yips symptoms (Corrigan & Grand, 2013). Brainspots are a focused access point in healing conversion conditions in athletes: "[T]he visual field is a reflection of the ongoing processes in the brain and felt in the body" (Grand, 2013, p. 91). The body is the instrument of the athlete and incorporation of bodily and psychic damage incurred by the athlete, and often resulting in dissociative-based conversion symptoms, is essential in the treatment of the yips.

Where Are Conversion Disorders in Athletics?

I have not personally examined any of the subsequently referenced individuals and am making gross conjectures based on distant observation to provide general context and example. None of the following is intended to reflect formal assessment or diagnosis.

Conceivably, conversion disorder is anywhere you can find the yips. For example, if you closely watch the throwing motion of a star Major League Baseball (MLB) pitcher when he attempts a routine throw to first base, it is as if his arm is trying to pass through a vat of butter. The quick, powerful throwing motion he makes towards home plate to deliver a fastball is not present. In slow motion, his arm is stiff, the arc of motion forward and backward truncated, and the movement of his upper body mechanical. This pitcher's throws to first base have often sailed far high, wide, or straight into the ground and advance the runner to second base. He once went two years without throwing to first base; a maneuver commonly accomplished by a pitcher at least several times a game. Theoretically, there is a procedural memory, manifesting as a somatoform-based dystonic movement greatly inhibiting the All Star pitcher's ability to perform an extremely simple athletic maneuver, while confusingly allowing him to perform more complex ones with precision.

I have worked with many baseball pitchers with yips-like symptoms. All of them reported some form of somatic and perceptual abnormalities. Commonly, the pitcher's felt sense of the baseball and his hand is altered. The ball will feel too small ("like a golf ball") or too large ("like a beachball"), and the pitching hand will be described as numb, paralyzed, or even absent. Further, perception of distance to the throwing target is abnormal: the first baseman appears "miles away" or "inches in front of my face," or the catcher's mitt is perceived as "the size of a button." Note that baseball fields are uniform in dimension, the distance from the pitcher's mound to is 60 feet, six inches, and bases are exactly 90 feet apart. Also, catcher's mitts do not vary in size more than an inch or two. Variations of these experiences are ubiquitous in sports performance problems and possess obvious dissociative characteristics. In adaptive dissociative moments, the pitcher can perceive the catcher's mitt as larger and closer than it objectively is, which prompts feelings of confidence and control.

Another example is Mackey Sasser, a former New York Mets catcher (Grand & Goldberg, 2011). His arm would simply freeze when throwing back to the pitcher and it would take several tries to override the frozen state as he would "pump" his throwing arm several times, sometimes with a throw ending up directly in the ground or over the pitcher's head. Tossing a baseball back to the pitcher is recognized as an incredibly routine maneuver requiring far less physiological arousal and biomechanical complexity than throwing to second or third base, which Sasser performed with ease.

A related example from another sport is "alligator arms" in National Football League (NFL) wide receivers. Rather than extending fully towards the football, receivers' arms freeze and stop significantly short of the thrown ball. Even Hall of Fame-caliber receivers have been accused of suffering from alligator arms (Foster, 2018). Also in football is the phenomenon of quarterbacks going into a premature "turtle" position despite having time to throw a pass and when there was otherwise no reason to do so. Collapsing and covering the most sensitive of internal organs is an involuntary response to sudden threat (Levine, 1994). These phenomena occur despite these athletes' best intentions, attempts, and attitudes to perform an athletic maneuver they have successfully completed thousands of times.

The phenomenon of alligator arms or turtling can also have elements of the psychoform dissociation. The wide receiver "blanks out," forgets his route, and exhibits a negative somatoform symptom in which his arms fail to extend from his body. Quarterbacks can fail to see a rushing defensive end or forget the play he called. Similarly, ballet dancers can suddenly and mysteriously forget their routine and "hear" jeers from the audience that are not heard by others. In either case these are examples of the athlete experiencing a trauma-based disorder resulting in the disruption of often simple, well-practiced muscle movements, or well-rehearsed football plays. Clinically, these are examples of focal or segmental somatoform conditions with elements of psychoform dissociation: In short, athletic conversion disorders.

Whiplash is a phenomenon that occurs in most sports, but especially in contact sports such as football. Whiplash has been implicated in a range of neurological disorders and can explain some of the converted symptoms of sports trauma. BSP, or more accurately an individual brainspot, is hypothesized to represent the *boundary rupture* reflecting previous trauma to the body (Scaer, 2014). Akin to one who is in a car accident, the body of a football player comes to sudden stop on a routine basis, causing recurrent episodes of whiplash. Velocity accentuates the damage, and wide receivers who eventually develop alligator arms are often ones to run across the middle of the field, subjecting themselves to vicious hits by defenders. Frequently, wide receivers do not see the opposing player prior the hit and thus do not implement defensive maneuvers (e.g. tensing muscles against the impact, taking evasive action).

Finally, according to a superintendent of a well-known southern golf course, a member of the Professional Golfers Association (PGA) is a brilliant but noticeably flawed golfer: "[He] is probably the best golfer I can think of that is known for missing the putt when it matters. He finally broke through and won The Master's ... but you may be able to find numerous examples of missed putts in the final round when pressure mounted throughout his career." This golfer is widely regarded as one of the best overall performers in recent memory yet has lost matches on putts widely considered to be a simple "gimme." Putting yips have been identified as a focal dystonia, likened to a disorder of movement such as Parkinson's disease, but such research did not provided comprehensive theories about etiology (Adler, 2013). This chapter, however, does.

Sports Psychology & Cognitive-Behavioral Therapy: Appealing to the Lowest Common Denominator

I am not a certified sports psychologist and have no formal sports psychology training endorsed by the American Psychological Association. I am a former collegiate baseball pitcher and high school football and basketball player who is now a psychologist. My impressions of sports psychology are limited to reading literature associated with the discipline and speaking with athletes who have been treated by sports psychologists prior to working with me. Admittedly, this may obscure my view of how sports psychology is practiced in vivo.

Still, my impressions of contemporary sports psychology are that it exists as a subclinical amalgamation of the coaching and medical staff. Based on my reading of research articles and practitioners' websites, it appears to provide shallow conceptualizations and overly-simplified interventions to complicated and poorly understood conditions such as the yips. There are few distinctive characteristics differentiating sports psychology from unsophisticated coach-speak and "mental training." The yips are etiologically conceptualized by the sports psychology community as rooted in "beliefs, attitudes, and mindsets" with treatment tailored to altering performance at that level (Association for Applied Sport Psychology, n.d.). I suggest this is a misguided approach addressing only a narrow sliver of psychological phenomena while ignoring the possibility of more comprehensive theories with more explanatory power.

Consider a scene from the baseball classic *Bull Durham* wherein Kevin Cosner's character Crash Davis imparts wisdom about talking to the media to the young Nuke LaLoosh, played by Tim Robbins: "This is a very simple game. You throw the ball; you catch the ball; you hit the ball. Sometimes you win; sometimes you lose; sometimes it rains." While brilliant in its poetic simplicity and function as a guide for navigating interviews, there is strikingly similarity to the main interventions I observe in contemporary sports psychology: slow down and "breathe," simplify, take it one game at a time, and so on (Rohan, September 30, 2015). If such banal interventions prove effective, they are probably subject to more plausible psychodynamic characteristics (Shedler, 2011), not unsophisticated platitudes mistaken to be agents of change.

These strategies reflect the practice of rigid adherents to cognitive-behavioral therapy (CBT). CBT arose as the cognitive sciences were expanding and melding with behavioral theories and techniques. This method of therapy was in part a reaction to the major tenets of psychoanalysis and other forms of so-called depth psychotherapy. It was also considered a shortcut to the often drawn out process of long-term psychoanalytic approaches. Originally well-intentioned, contemporary CBT has circumvented many of the interpersonal processes that make psychoanalysis effective and became a feeble caricature of what it was originally intended to be: a means of making psychoanalysis work in a faster, more focused manner. CBT is now tailored to address economic concerns by being significantly time-limited. Yet it fails to account for meta-analytic literature suggesting the inefficacy of isolating psychotherapeutic ingredients as one would a chemical medication, particularly in the treatment of trauma (Shedler, 2017).

CBT mimics the predominately linear thinking of the medical professions, and formal research has followed suit. In the vast majority of CBT literature, a sequence of specific and measurable hypotheses is tested via randomized control studies (RCTs) which assign participants to treatment or control groups. These typically pit one treatment against another, or a treatment against a placebo (a "dummy" treatment). CBT research is prolific yet frequently poorly done with significant methodological concerns and limited ability to generalize about real-world patient populations. Unfortunately, a consequence of CBT's large body of literature is that unsophisticated clinicians take the results literally and adhere inflexibly to therapeutic interventions resembling "coach-speak" platitudes. Sports psychology has followed the path worn by CBT in an even more narrow fashion.

Freud famously described psychology, and therefore psychotherapy, as occupying the middle space between philosophy and medicine. Medicine, on one end of the spectrum, aptly utilizes RCTs to compare the effectiveness of one medication to another or placebo, and to identify and document side effects. For example, it is rather clear cut to measure and assess the administration, prognosis, and response to treatment of a urinary tract infection with an antibiotic, based on graded doses in milligrams of the medication and measurements of the presence of unwanted bacteria. This is not to denigrate these types of studies or the artfulness required to detect and treat physical disease but differentiates the type of thinking required in medical versus psychological literature.

Psychology, on the other hand, does not typically encounter phenomena as immediately observable and alterable as bacteria. Philosophical thought can encompass anything available to the mind including the nature of existence, language, politics, or morality, among many others. Even medicine itself is steeped in philosophy; look no further than the theoretical divide between osteopathy and allopathy. Clearly, contemporary medicine is based on an array of philosophical ideals, yet there are clear distinctions in the theory and utilization of generally psychological versus generally medical approaches, especially in research methodology. Making these distinctions runs the risk of falling back into Cartesian dualism, yet my hope is that the reader can make reasonable connections and differentiations between the practice of medicine and psychology without reducing psychology to the study of "mind" and medicine of "body."

Many mental health practitioners harbor feelings of inferiority when they compare themselves to those in the medical field. These individuals have great difficulty accepting their position as medically adjacent, and to the detriment of psychology. This probably reflects fears of being unable to control a patient's symptoms, or that their clinical opinion will be minimized by more prominent health practitioners such as a medical doctor. It is calming for many of us to operate from a psychiatric diagnosis as the ultimate assessment of a patient's problems. Yet there is as much variability within say, a generalized anxiety diagnosis, as there is between diagnoses. I believe that sports psychology, as currently researched and practiced, is self-limiting and shallow based on its attempts to mimic CBT and the medical profession and is an example of the worst of professional inferiority complexes.

The mind and body are not at all separate, but part of an intricately interlinked and vast system subject to the laws of physics, chemistry, and biology. While only a small portion of these processes can be consciously understood, they can be intervened upon through predominately philosophical, psychological, or medical interventions, all of which can significantly adjust the physical, chemical, or biological structures of the human system. Psychologists and other psychotherapists must accept uncertainty as part of the therapeutic and research process, a construct embraced by BSP (Grand, 2013). Uncertainty is a stance which allows for the examination and intervention of athletic conversion conditions from a place of curiosity, flexibility, and expansive thought. Continual attempts to think and act like physicians (or coaches) are of great detriment to the field.

A BSP Trauma-Informed Biopsychosocial Model of Sports Performance Problems

David Grand and Allan Goldberg (2011) have already outlined a comprehensive argument for the yips as a trauma-based condition and present the use of BSP as an effective treatment for such conditions. When athletes seek psychological help for a performance problem, they nearly always enter with a litany of physical injuries. These range from relatively minor, as in the case of sprain and strains, to major in the form of spinal injuries, concussions, or compound fractures. Athletes are typically blasé about their physical injuries, even to the point of failing to recognize or recall many of them. This is a form of *la belle indifference* and in some cases is an example of psychoform dissociation.

Athletes are even more reticent to acknowledge or recall injuries of an emotional or psychological nature. These can encompass public failures or losses and verbal or physical abuse at the hands of coaches, parents, or teammates. All involved fail to regard this brand of injury as equal to physical ones in their potential to cause future performance problems, despite the neurological fact that physical wounds are inherently emotional as well (Grand & Goldberg, 2011). Further, conversion disorders are fundamentally resultant of psychological damage to one's physical or emotional self. Feelings of shame, self-criticism, and fear are emotional states which linger in the brain-body system and, when reaching a critical degree, cause psychophysiological turmoil in the athlete. BSP is a way to simultaneously uncover an athlete's trauma and treat it immediately.

Athletes frequently discover bad relationships with coaches have lasting negative consequences. Some coaches rely heavily on shame-based techniques as global means of interacting with their players. This is done through critical comments or physical punishment. Notably, there is significant difference between a "tough" coach saying things like "I need you to play better!" or prescribing pushups for a mental error, and outright abuse in the form of making a player run to the point of vomiting, choking players, or using global derogatory statements such as "you're worthless." The former is a relatively healthy means of coaching while the latter is rather sadistic.

In the case of the sadistic coach, inducing or exacerbating fear of humiliation is mistakenly viewed as positive punishment with the power to motivate the athlete to work harder, play smarter, and perform better. To a degree, there is truth here. By admonishing or humiliating a player for missing a shot, there is a spike in cortisol resulting from an emotionally threatening experience. For a short period of time, the player may conceivably be able to run faster, jump higher, or whatever is required of their sport by being put in a fight-or-flight state. Yet, there are long-term negative consequences of sadistic shame-inducing coaching tactics. This is particularly true and damaging if sadism and shame were present in the athlete's family of origin.

Karen Horney (1950) discusses the plight of the developing child when exposed to recurrent neuroses of the parent. Willingly or not, coaches fundamentally fill or mimic parental roles with their players. Parental attitudes toward the child involving resentment, criticism, or inattentiveness ultimately create pathological states of fearfulness and profound insecurity. A coach-player relationship is identical in many ways to the parent-child dyad and thus subject to the same complications of human attachment. Human psychophysiological development is promoted or impeded by the interpersonal exchanges between parent and child. The structural and psychic compositions of Shore's *implicit self* are subject to caregivers, be them parents, coaches, or psychotherapists.

To illustrate the damage, mammals should not be in a heightened state of fight-or-flight for more than a brief period. Longer, and there can be severely negative consequences on the body and most certainly on performance. Cortisol is a hormone allowing for quick access to glucose and energy but whose long-term presence in the system causes damage to the brain, muscles, heart, and other critical areas of the body. This speaks for itself in terms of the harmful effects on the finely tuned functioning of athletes at a basic physiological level, and on their body's basic ability to recover. Athletes identify a discernible difference between playing in a fearful state induced by a coach, and a more adaptive goal and growth-focused state supported by healthy coaching strategies. I do believe there is room for coaches to interact with athletes somewhat aggressively in a prosocial manner, but only in a relationship containing essential elements of trust, consistency, and affection.

Spikes in adrenaline can aid in athletes' gross motor movement but such intense physiological states impede *fine motor* functioning in the short and long-term. There is incredible biomechanical intricacy involved in throwing a baseball, hitting a golf ball, or shooting a basketball. Watch a baseball pitcher in slow motion: the movement of kinetic energy from the lower body to the trunk, and extending out to the arm, hand, and fingers is a beautifully complicated endeavor. Unfortunately, one hitch in that process can cause a one-millimeter error in the baseball leaving the hand of the pitcher, and result in literal feet differences in throwing accuracy, or a severe reduction in pitch velocity. Arousal based on abuse does not serve athletes well and will diminish performance at some point.

The case of a young gymnast patient illustrates shame-based coaching and its negative impacts not just on sports performance but on psychological development as well. This young man presented with the mysterious inability to do a back handspring, a very basic gymnastics maneuver. In preparation to do a back handspring he reported severe pain and constriction in his abdomen and numbness and disconnection the extremities. His body lacked the ability to guide him through a relatively simple and well-practiced movement. These problems occurred persistently and were accompanied by extreme anxiety, embarrassment, and impairments in his basic athletic, social, and academic functioning. Given this constellation of symptoms, he met criteria for a conversion disorder with weakness, paralysis, and abnormal movement as outlined by the DSM-5 (2013).

Upon exploration through the BSP process, recollections and felt sensations emerged related to chronic ankle and shoulder sprains: His body often felt inflamed and tender, which led to protective abnormal dystonic movements. In other words, he altered his body to protect against physical pain and "forgot" how to do movements, even simple ones like the back handspring, that caused pain. The fact that the back handspring is considered "simple" exacerbated the protective movements based on feelings of embarrassment and vulnerability. The pathogenic belief "when I do the back handspring, I feel bad" reflected ingrained physical and emotional trauma and resulted in conversion disorder symptoms.

This athlete's problems were immediately met with shame and rejection from coaches. He was told things like "you don't deserve to be on this team," and "you're embarrassing us," but the most painful response was being ignored and shunned by the coaches he yearned to impress. He wished for their attention yet was sequestered from other gymnasts until he could perform better. He began to self-harm cognitively through self-critical statements such as "I suck" and "I hate myself" and through dietary restriction, which caused loss of muscle mass and even further inhibited success. All of this occurred in the context of body-shaming inherent in gymnastics, which often results in problems of self-image and disordered eating (Smolak, Murnen, & Ruble, 2000). The gymnastics environment is a notorious breeding ground for one of the worst of physical and psychological traumas, sexual assault, as in the case of former USA gymnastics doctor Larry Nassar (Windsor, January 25, 2018).

BSP Considerations in the Treatment of Conversion Conditions

A major hurdle in properly conceptualizing and addressing these problems is to convince sports psychologists to operate clinically. It is foolish to regard an athlete's performance problems as somehow fundamentally different than those found in the general clinical population;, yet that is the state of the profession. Barriers to taking a clinical approach to athletes do not just exist within sports psychology but are systemic in athletics. Athletes do not want to be conceptualized as "head cases" or "weak" and often fail to seek psychological help until a problem is entirely entrenched. This is reinforcing of trauma since it limits the scope of available help by promoting isolation from resources. Furthermore, persistent conversion symptoms put the athlete at greater risk for injury because of things like muscle constriction or failure to pay adequate attention to their surroundings.

Common defensive structures of avoidance, minimization, and repression are also active on the individual athlete and systemic level, and in large organizations such as the NFL or USA gymnastics. The ways in which the NFL has ignored chronic traumatic encephalopathy and USA gymnastics sexual abuse proves the ingrained level of pathological defensiveness involved. Trauma experiences fundamental to sports are not within the scope of what is regularly recognized as negatively impacting athletes. Even within the clinical realm, CBT minimizes and denies more complex way of understanding psychopathology, missing the larger picture of the yips or diagnoses like conversion. Unconscious systemic processes of repression are evident in managed care organizations such as Blue Care Network or Value Options who restrict psychotherapists' interventions to highly over-simplified cognitive therapies, and refuse to reimburse, as an example, psychodynamic therapy. This is a self-reinforcing cycle of denial.

BSP can be viewed as a conduit for athletes to be afforded the same level of thorough psychological attention as they would medical, and an opportunity to break through many of the systemic barriers preventing adequate treatment. BSP is an interventional paradigm entrenched in the language of physiology, which is a dialect to which athletes are acutely attuned. The sensory organs of the athlete are everything: The acute vision of an expert hitter like Bryce Harper, the raw power of Serena Williams's trunk muscles, the felt sense of quarterback Aaron Rogers shifting away from a defender in the pocket, or the precision of the wrists in Annika Sorenstam's short game. They understand their body better than anyone, and BSP speaks to them in this language.

Athletes and general clinical patients suffering from this type of condition commonly enter my office with a few things: (a) confusion, (b) frustration, and (c) a mysterious symptom. They have undergone a litany of tests including needle pokes, hours in a magnetic resonance imaging (MRI) tube, arduous physical therapy, and other terribly unpleasant but required experiences. Their conditions involve recurrent feelings of embarrassment, self-doubt, and fear. I have found a few rules of thumb to abide by when initially interacting with conversion disorders, especially in the case of athletes:

1. These individuals have undergone enough assessment. Immediate attention should be paid to their basic sense of suffering without knowing why, which is clinically significant in itself. Assessment tools such as symptom measures or personality inventories are counterproductive at the outset of treatment. In many ways, diagnosis is secondary unless it adds immediately to intervention.
2. Most people, particularly athletes and regardless of diagnosis, enter with some narrative based Cartesian dualism. It is beneficial to slowly introduce ideas that dispel the disconnection between "mind and body." Most people need time to assimilate this information in a way that works for them, yet many intuitively comprehend more dynamic ways of understanding relatedness between their psychology and physiology.
3. The physical symptom is a starting point and representation of the overall struggle of the athlete. Often, what is generalized becomes localized and what is specific becomes diffuse. Despite indifference or fixation on a symptom, it is important not to reduce the patient's pain to simply the focal complaint nor to attend only to defensive strategies such as *la belle indifference* (a dissociative symptom).
4. The functional or physical symptom nearly always, if not entirely always, relates to an emotional or physical wound incurred at some point in an original pathogenic relationship or situation. These are most damaging at critical stages of development and exacerbated by similar relationships or situations. Subsequent interactions with coaches or sports executives mimicking earlier wounds potentiate the original physical or emotional trauma.
5. Rapport must be attained between therapist and patient around the presenting symptom. BSP allows for this to be achieved deeply and meaningfully via the dual attunement to a brainspot, and historical data will present itself naturally. De-emphasis on rapport for the sake of technique is incredibly inhibitive to treatment, and BSP attunement to physiological processes is imperative.

Customarily, the therapist gathers a great deal of information during an "intake" and formulates the diagnosis and treatment plan after the initial clinical interview, sometimes with the aid of formal psychological testing. A BSP approach does not require an exhaustive history to render effective, targeted treatment. In fact, the treatment itself is what leads to explicit background information of implicitly held trauma and is a dual form of diagnosis and treatment (Grand, 2013). BSP is a highly relational, inherently psychodynamic treatment uniquely suited to treat these conditions (Kaufman, 2015). The conversion symptom itself is enough to begin psychotherapy and is an immediate access point to be linked with a brainspot.

The population of athletes is large enough to be representative of large swaths of society in terms of personality makeup and associated ways of thinking, feeling, and relating to others. This is important to acknowledge as to avoid inflexible assumptions which can inhibit therapy. Still, it is also beneficial to know that athletes, particularly collegiate, professional, and Olympic-level individuals, are subject to unique and pervasive stressors. These can be imparted on them by parents, coaches, and large bodies such as the National Collegiate Athletic Association (NCAA), or are simply a ramification of the physically and emotionally taxing reality of athletics.

High-level athletes are frequently regarded by fans, coaches, and executives as commodities. There are dehumanizing stances that distance third-parties from athletes' individual ways of experiencing the world and limit awareness of their potential suffering. The NCAA, for example, gives lip service to the idea of the "student-athlete" via largely ignoring abuses of power by authority figures and the health and long-term financial and social stability of the athlete. Look no further than Penn State University and the actions of Jerry Sandusky and Joe Paterno. Universities, essentially massive corporations, derive millions of annual dollars from tickets and merchandising sales based on the free labor of the "student" athlete. Very frequently, those in positions of power and executive privilege are white, affluent males and the athletes are minorities born in poverty. Abuses occur in many ways from minor to major, including transgressions up to and including outright sexual assault of children are ignored.

Power dynamics based on race, gender, and socioeconomic status have implications for understanding yips conditions and why many do not have access to more evolved treatments like BSP, and less like CBT. It is common for some to label a struggling black athlete as "lazy" or "weak" while his white teammate is considered something far more benign. Shame-based sadism of coaches allows for blame to be assessed on the basis of flaws in thought or attitude. Minority athletes bear the brunt of this bias unwittingly supported by CBT which assigns blame to the patient for not "learning the skills" when treatment fails. These patterns occur on the field of play and in the therapy office.

Assumptions such as these are not based in neurobiology, nor do they account for the psychodynamic complexity of conversion disorders. However, BSP does, and its basic tenets of neurobiological attunement are therapeutic grounds for the restoration of humanizing regard for the athlete. Failure of treatment must not be blamed on the failure of the patient to properly incorporate the intervention, but on the intervention for improperly accounting for the dynamic complexity of the patient.

Many patients enter therapy with intractable symptoms, even after years of psychotherapy and pharmacological treatments. In the case of many athletes, their career simply ends but the emotional and physical suffering does not. Even after working with some sports psychologists, their struggle continues. When I ask them about their personal relationship (the therapeutic alliance) with the psychologist, a well-documented and fundamental aspect of treatment, they often do not recognize that one existed. The sports psychologists treating these athletes engaged with their patients as sports psychology markets itself: Providers of advice and prescribers of techniques to manage their symptoms. Sports psychologists do not operate as the highly trained clinicians they are and ignore a wealth of knowledge of the most current psychological and neurological literature.

Rather than dispensing transiently placating mental strategies, BSP practitioners attune to the psychophysiology of the athlete. They are taught to observe unconscious phenomena such as eye blinks, subtle shifts of the head, alterations in breathing rate, and facial flushing as cues to unresolved trauma held in the brain-body system. The conversion disorder is a screaming orange forest fire of accumulated physical and emotional trauma, and a glaringly obvious clue for the treating therapist. The process of dual attunement is therapeutically humanizing and serves to undo the bad practice of previously failed attempts to help which can be re-traumatizing in and of themselves.

Athletes can truly be difficult patients and present with a high degree of confidence, even narcissism. These personality attributes are necessary components of their day-to-day existence and serve them well in their professions as adaptive personality traits. However, these patterns involve common ego defenses including minimization and isolation which are typical defenses implemented by many initially entering therapy. Instructive of parallels between the general clinical population and athletes is the case of a male physician. He is a well-respected practitioner of his trade and accomplished in procedures requiring intricate hand-eye coordination. Mysteriously, he began to experience painful muscle twitches in the face and neck, primarily during routine consultations and interactions with his staff.

Additionally, he forgot relatively straightforward material to tell patients during routine examinations. He was incredibly embarrassed and resorted to obscuring his symptoms by wearing a surgical mask even during regular exchanges with patients and their families. He relied on nurses to fill in the gaps of knowledge that he had successfully relayed to patients for years. Through all this, his more difficult medical procedures were completed flawlessly and the deft and miniscule actions of his forearm, hands, and fingers remained unaffected. To draw a parallel, think of the previously described MLB pitcher unable to throw to first base while easily throwing to the catcher in the middle 90s per-hour perfectly and from a greater distance, over and over.

Consider also the example of golfer presenting with the putting yips in the "gimme" range of only a few feet. She assumes her problems are limited to the putting green, but upon examination they exist in more subtle ways: the slowing of her club when chipping, muscular tightness before teeing off, gastrointestinal problems before competition, and so on. Largely, however, she drives well and has a solid iron game. BSP is a means of recognizing, feeling, and discharging parallel experiences between all facets of this woman's golf game: A self-protective behavior emerging in overt and covert ways rooted in a trauma-based fear response, created and maintained by early shame-inducing experiences at the hands of parents or coaches and injuries to the body areas involved in her swing motion. This is a constellation of motor movements, affective experiences, and thought patterns associated with many athletes across a range of sports, ethnic backgrounds, and socioeconomic statuses.

It is not uncommon for highly trained and confident individuals, such as athletes or physicians, to experience their conversion symptoms as just a "small" hurdle to success occurring in "one" area of their life. It is initially difficult to admit how very troubling this issue is for them or to see its reflections or roots in other areas of their life. This is because an acknowledgement of their vulnerabilities or insecurities is poorly regarded by their peers, be them medical students or teammates. It also conveys, in their perception, weakness to patients who are suffering greatly or teammates who are battling by their side. A stoic invincibility is required equally in the cool confidence of a golfer on 18th green at Augusta National or the focused arrogance of a closing pitcher in the ninth inning of the World Series.

While easy to consider these as inhibitory factors in therapy, from a BSP perspective defensive strategies are anything but and an avenue to salient psychological and physiological cues to roots of the presenting problems. Feelings such as shame, immobilization, anger, or fear, and dissociative symptoms such as numbness, amnesia, or disconnection are not symptoms to be immediately eradicated, thought they often are with treatment, but somatoform and psychoform elements of trauma-based structural dissociation. These are not signs of a resistant patient or an uncommitted athlete but are symptoms in and of themselves, and ones to be treated as any other.

From a BSP perspective, it is counterproductive to seek to eradicate negative belief systems; rather these are fundamental starting points for the BSP process. Take the shame experienced by the golfer. Shame is a facet of her experience of being in therapy or having a problem deemed "mental." It is also an emotion felt when observed by other golfers and fans when failing to complete a supposedly easy putt. It may also be a feeling state relating to many life experiences dating back to early childhood. Shame is described by most people as a "heavy" emotion eliciting psychomotor retardation which is often observed upon mental status exam. It is clear how this somatosensory experience would inhibit the intricate nature of a golf putt especially when combined with physical injury history.

BSP intervention in this case necessitates a rather simple but targeted progression of intervention: Where does the athlete feels "shame" in their body? How intense is it? Where do they feel it the most, looking right, middle, or left, up, center, or down? Holding the patient's gaze in that direction, both therapist and patient watch what happens. A brainspot is considered a link to the midbrain and therefore trauma-related memories, feelings, and somatic sensations (Corrigan & Grand, 2013) and a localization of the athlete's presenting difficulties.

Hypothetically, assume the MLB pitcher unable to throw to first base were to enter BSP treatment for his throwing yips. Based on what can be observed when he throws to first base, there are several areas of abnormal movements and a theoretical conversion condition with somatoform and psychoform features: truncated extension of the arm backward, inhibited forward movement of the arm motion with non-rotation of the trunk, "forgetting" to throw to first or not being able to locate first base, and intrusive recollections of past bad throws to first. Respectively, these are symptoms of focal dystonia, segmental dystonia, negative psychoform dissociation (amnesia), and positive psychoform dissociation (hypermnesia). It is suggested this pitcher could be effectively treated if his problems were conceptualized as such.

Future Considerations

For sports psychology to be an effective discipline, it must operate clinically and incorporate the burgeoning evidence supporting BSP's ability to identify, process, and release physical and emotional traumas which underlie the yips. Understanding these conditions as conversion disorders with elements of somatoform and psychoform dissociation, combined with BSP's philosophical and practical framework, is a comprehensive means of conceptualization, diagnosis, and treatment for athletes. This is reflective of larger disconnections in the field of psychotherapy from limiting, economic-focused treatment such as CBT.

Mental health clinician's availability to athletes has only recently become more accepted and commonplace. Yet there are stark limitations in what sports psychologists are allowed, or willing, to provide to athletes. Simplistic anxiety reduction techniques are hardly beneficial in clinical settings except in the immediate outset of treatment. If they do have therapeutic value long-term, it is because they pull on intricate attachment systems of the brain and soothe based on an attuned therapeutic relationship. People do not get sustainably better only because of an isolated suggestion to "breathe." Further, therapeutic gain is not achieved simply by acknowledging that the athletes have "trauma" in their history but through the localized, sustained focus of a brainspot that targets procedural memories to the trauma and stores them differently in the brain. This comes only with attunement, flexible thought, and, often, time.

Far more often than the average person, athletes are subjected to recurrent physical damage. The athlete consciously considers this only an insignificant facet of the profession; yet unconscious threat response systems regard even minor injury as an assault on the vitality of the organism. Complicating matters is the emotional vulnerability of the athlete, experienced by the midbrain as similar, if not identical, to a physical wound. The recurrent dosages of these incidents leave a neurological imprint on the brain of the athlete which creates and maintains athletic conversion disorders.

The reasons for failing to understand the yips as a conversion disorder is wide ranging and will extend beyond this writing. Generally, psychotherapists and other health practitioners defend against their own unconscious fears of injury, death, or losing control, for example, by denying the same in others (consider the policies of MCOs as an example). It is palliative for the clinician to assume the yips exist only as a problem of thought or attitude because the clinician's own problems can then exist in the same realm. It is unconsciously protective for them as well as the athlete but incredibly inhibitory to treatment. This is akin to a physician treating a severe infection as just a dermatological condition while denying the presence of the malevolent bacteria underneath. It's also incredibly lazy and occasionally inhumane.

I suggest a few things: There should be thoughtful, more empirical research about conversion disorders in athletes. Conversion is complicated as evidenced even by how it is referred to in practice. The same constellation of symptoms can be defined as "conversion," "somatoform," "psychogenic," or "somatic symptom." These are all apt terms and not necessarily fundamental to treatment but each can have different connotations. Furthermore, the subdivision of levels of structural dissociation is complex and opaque to many. Research is required to delineate these issues as they exist in athletes not to mention the general population and should be disseminated thoroughly.

Sports teams, amateur and professional, should allocate resources to mental health at the level of medical services. This is a radical suggestion but a reasonable one. For example, a magnetic resonance imaging scan (MRI) costs over $2,000 to administer, but if BSP is effective in reducing conversion symptoms in athletes and therefore injury,

MRIs become less frequent. Federally, there is precedence for equality of mental and physical health coverage and reimbursement (Mental Health Parity and Addiction Equity Act; NAMI, 2018). I propose teams hire highly qualified clinicians with broad training in trauma and dissociation, specifically BSP. These teams will perform better and have reduced physical injury and diminished recovery time from injury by employing these treatments. Athletes should not be referred to a BSP performance specialist only when their plight is dire, and all other options have been exhausted. BSP should be an immediate first-line treatment for conversion disorders in athletes and the general population.

Bibliography

Adler, C. (2013): Parkinson's Disease and Movement Disorders Lab: Charles H. Adler – The Yips: A Focal, Task-Specific Dystonia. Retrieved March 02, 2018, from http://www.mayo.edu/research/labs/parkinsons-disease-movement-disorders/yips-focal-task-specific-dystonia

Association for Applied Sport Psychology (n.d.): Retrieved December 24, 2017, from http://www.appliedsportpsych.org/

Corrigan, F., & Grand, D. (2013): Brainspotting: Recruiting the midbrain for accessing and healing sensorimotor memories of traumatic activation. *Medical Hypotheses,80*(6), 759-766. *Diagnostic and statistical manual of mental disorders: DSM-5.* (2013). Washington, DC: American Psychiatric Publishing.

Dystonia. (2017, December 27): Retrieved January 08, 2018, from https://www.mayoclinic.org/diseases-conditions/dystonia/symptoms-causes/syc-20350480

Foster, T. (2018, February 06): The Lions claimed Randy Moss had alligator arms. Retrieved March 02, 2018, from https://terryfoster.blog/2018/02/06/the-lions-claimed-randy-moss-had-alligator-arms/

Grand, D. (2013): *Brainspotting: the revolutionary new therapy for rapid and effective change.* Boulder, CO: Sounds True.

Grand, D., & Goldberg, A. S. (2011): *This is your brain on sports: beating blocks, slumps and performance anxiety for good! Indianapolis,* IN: Dog Ear Publishing.

Horney, K. (1950): *Self analysis: neurosis and human growth.* New York: Norton.

Kaufman, C. (2015): A constructivist grounded theory approach to brainspotting. (Doctoral dissertation), from https://search.proquest.com/openview/95ba3efe9426e0fb20d748d6d328808a/1.pdf?pq-origsite=gscholar&cbl=18750&diss=y

Levine, P. A. (1997): *Waking the tiger: healing trauma.* Berkeley, Calif: North Atlantic Books.

NAMI. (n.d.): Retrieved February 08, 2018, from https://www.nami.org/Find-Support/Living-with-a-Mental-Health-Condition/Understanding-Health-Insurance/What-is-Mental-Health-Parity

Nijenhuis, E. R., & van der Hart, O. (2011): Dissociation in Trauma: A New Definition and Comparison with Previous Formulations. *Journal of Trauma & Dissociation,12*(4), 416-445.

Psychodynamic Diagnostic Manual (PDM). (2006). Silver Spring: Alliance of Psychoanalytic Organizations.

Rohan, T. (2015, September 30): Mets' Psychologist Helps Players Catch Their Breath. Retrieved December 17, 2017, from https://www.nytimes.com/2015/10/01/sports/baseball/mets-psychologist-helps-players-catch-their-breath.html

Scaer, R. (2014): *The body bears the burden: trauma, dissociation, and disease.* New York: Haworth Medical Press.

Scaer, R. (2001): *The body bears the burden: trauma, dissociation, and disease.* New York: Haworth Medical Press.

Schore, A. N. (1994): *Affect regulation and the origin of the self: the neurobiology of emotional development.* Hillsdale, NJ: L. Erlbaum.

Shedler, J. (November 19, 2017): Selling Bad Therapy to Trauma Victims. Retrieved January 28, 2018, from https://www.psychologytoday.com/blog/psychologically-minded/201711/selling-bad-therapy-trauma-victims

Shedler, J. (2011): The Efficacy of Psychodynamic Psychotherapy. *Psychodynamic Psychotherapy Research,* 9-25.

Smolak, L., Murnen, S. K., & Ruble, A. E. (2000): Female athletes and eating problems: A meta-analysis. *International Journal of Eating Disorders,27*(4), 371-380.

The Making Of Emotions. (2018): https://www.npr.org/sections/health-shots/2017/06/01/530103479/the-making-of-emotions-from-pleasurable-fear-to-bittersweet-relief

Van der Hart, O., Nijenhuis, E. R., & Steele, K. (2005): Dissociation: An insufficiently recognized major feature of complex posttraumatic stress disorder. *Journal of Traumatic Stress,18*(5), 413-423. doi:10.1002/jts.20049

Windsor, S. (2018, January 25): Larry Nassar tragedy is worse than Penn State – and we were complicit. Retrieved February 02, 2018, from https://www.freep.com/story/sports/college/michigan-state/2018/01/25/larry-nassar-tragedy-worse-than-penn-state-and-we-were-complicit/1063743001/

Brainspotting and Creative Performance

Christine Ranck

Brainspotting has an often astonishing and mysterious effectiveness with actors / performers in the process of creating a character and can profoundly enhance an artist's performance. The amazing results can perhaps be explained as a holographic process (every part contains the whole). 2) Clients may describe having strong intuitive feelings and actions in their lives. With the premise that intuition is the mind's creative process, you will learn how to work with the highly intuitive client to create quantum leaps of insight and enhanced self-esteem. 3) Highly creative clients may experience (and describe) their Brainspotting sessions with metaphoric imagery exclusively. You will learn how to work with this kind of metaphoric imagery by following the tail of the comet. 4) Using fascinating case examples, the specific techniques for character development and performance enhancement in all of the above contexts are discussed.

The artist is the antennae of the race.
(Ezra Pound)

If you ask me what I came to do in this world,
I, an artist, will answer you:
I am here to live out loud.
(Emile Zola)

"I can always be distracted by love, but eventually I get horny for my creativity."
(Gilda Radner)

Brainspotting with Performers

"My very first seizure," Othello cried, "came when I was 8. I was sitting on my horse in the courtyard. My convulsions were so severe that I lost control of the reins and fell to the ground. My father's enormous horse became frantic and nearly trampled me. Almost too late to save me, my father's men dismounted and gathered me up until I stopped convulsing."

Othello, the great Moorish warrior from the Shakespearean play by the same name, was weeping on the couch in my office.

Then, shaking uncontrollably, Othello slid down into the couch in what appeared to be a full-on seizure.

I was stunned (and a little worried).

Only moments before, I'd been mesmerized watching Dr. David Grand, Brainspotting's developer, prepare my friend and magnificent actor, David Toney, for the role of Othello in an upcoming professional performance. Seated before us, Toney was wearing headphones and listening to Biolateral sound (the Biolateral soundtracks used with Brainspotting that oscillate back and forth from one ear to the other, which David Grand developed).

Grand had asked Toney to begin the transformation into Othello by first performing one of Othello's monologues from the play. Then, using his BSP pointer, Grand guided Toney to locate the Inside Window "Othello brainspot" – the eye position where Toney had the strongest felt-sense of Othello (emotionally and in his body), whose words he had just spoken. Toney easily located the Othello brainspot in the upper left corner of his field of vision, and fixed his gaze on it.

Almost instantly I had the rather creepy – and very visceral – intuitive sense that Othello, himself, was now sitting on the couch speaking to us. The hair on the back of my neck stood straight up.

I had watched as Grand spoke *directly* to Othello who, according to Shakespeare's script, was plagued throughout his life with terrible epileptic seizures. Grand asked Othello to spontaneously recall any important incident from his childhood – whatever popped into his mind – as a way of continuing to deepen the development of the character. That was the moment when Othello instantly cried out, in great, passionate detail, the terrifying circumstances surrounding his first childhood seizure on his horse in the courtyard.

And then Othello had the seizure.

At this point I'd like to say that you haven't truly lived until you've experienced something like this in your office.

Thankfully, Othello did soon recover. Grand, having discovered that "when you take an actor so deeply into character, it is unwise to leave him there," then guided the actor to find the David Toney spot (his "self-spot"), the eye position where Toney felt most *himself,* so that he could process his way out of Othello and back into his own skin.

Wanting to hold onto what he had discovered about Othello's "essence" during the session, Toney asked if there was a way, using Brainspotting, to easily recover Othello upon demand. Grand asked Toney where he would like to hold Othello in his body, and Toney pointed to his heart. Together they found the Brainspot that coincided with that desire for connection, and processed it there. In the future, Toney would then only need to touch his heart to recapture the essence of Othello. That is, three spots were used in the process: The Othello Character Spot, then the Self Spot (for getting back out of character) and finally, the Connection Spot to facilitate future access to the character.

A skilled actor will attempt to integrate the character's past experiences holistically into that character's present. Our past experiences affect the way we behave in the present. On some level, those past events are still present now. David Grand states: "A character in a scene is both a person in a situation, and a person with a history that shapes their reactions to that situation. And the most formative aspects of a character's history, like the actor's, are the developmental stages of early life, and the profound life experiences that leave indelible imprints on the character's destiny" (D. Grand, 2001, p. 201).

Usually, an actor uses the script to inform him about a character's history, but playwrights often don't provide much history. So then the actor might fill in the gaps by making choices about *possible* historical events he could use to fuel the character's emotional life. Finally, by identifying with the character, the actor may use real memories from his own life that can help to activate him with the appropriate and authentic emotions for the character. For example, if the character's brother has died in the play, the actor may recall and use his own memory of grief at the loss of a loved one.

In Othello's case, I already knew that there was no specific incident in the play's script about Othello's childhood seizures. So in our later discussion, when Toney was back out of character, I was curious. I asked him, "Did you use a memory from your own childhood to emotionally evoke Othello's traumatic memory of a seizure in the courtyard? Did anything like that ever happen to you?" Toney was surprisingly adamant that NO, there was absolutely nothing even remotely similar in his own life, nor had he ever experienced seizures or anything like them.

But what was more extraordinary, Toney said, was that the emotional impact of Othello's "character memory" of convulsion and near-death by trampling – as well as the sensory details that accompanied it – felt completely "three-dimensional" and utterly real to him in the moment. Furthermore, Toney said, Othello's character memory had emerged instantly and spontaneously on its own, without any effort from Toney – *as if he was actually remembering it.*

Needless to say, we were all fascinated by this seemingly impossible development and pondered how this 3-D character memory might have been generated. Amazed by what I had seen and heard, I turned to my colleagues and spontaneously said, "Well, this reminds me of holograms." They both looked at me, mystified, and asked, "What do you mean?" I couldn't answer them at that time, because I didn't even know why I'd said it.

The eventual discovery of my own personal answer to this mystery was much more exciting than I could have ever imagined then. I will explain a little later.

Getting into Character

"Fundamentally, the actor explodes the myth of a single, unified human personality. Actors recognize and give expression to the variety of ego states and inner personalities that most of us ignore or repress. They change themselves physically, mentally, and emotionally. They trust their intuition and remove all the self-constraints of expression in their path to release all of this inner potential. The creation of a character is a process that draws on experiences from within, and completely engages their attention" (Bates, 1987, p 202).

Since the 1930s, many of the principal rules of acting theory have come from the writings and work of Konstantin Stanislavski. Stanislavski describes what it means to be an actor and what is required of the individual who chooses to "live out loud" through this intense level of artistry.

"Our type of creativeness is the conception and birth of a new being – the person in the part. It is a natural act similar to the birth of a human being. Actors are influenced by their parts, which affect their daily lives ... Laws regulate Nature, whether she is creating a new phenomenon biologically or imaginatively" (Stanislavski, 1961, p. 312-313).

Historically, shamans were the first actors, and for thousands of years every traditional society had head shaman / actors who were regarded as the guardians of wisdom. They had special abilities to communicate directly with the spirit world and lead their audiences in ritual journeys. But all shamanic actors had one consistent characteristic: a painful, isolated childhood and adolescence (Eliade, 1972, p. 36). The shaman's way to heal himself was to become a "magical actor" (Halifax, 182, p. 25). He was expected to risk life and death in performances, and acting was seen as the creative integration of a traumatic childhood with inner strength, a gift shared with the audience in creative, healing ways.

Today that artistry is still physically demanding and involves taking enormous personal and emotional risks ... Actors often commit so much energy to their work – it is so important to them – that acting literally puts them moment-to-moment into life-and-death situations. (Bates, 1987, p. 149) You can clearly see this from David Toney's Othello experience above.

The Americanized version of Stanislavski's basic teachings is called "The Method," and is often described as an "inside-out" approach. The actor bases her performances on her full identification with the character. She prepares for the role through a series of exercises using memory and imagination to access those emotions.

"Each and every moment must be saturated with a belief in the truthfulness of the emotion felt, and in the authenticity of action carried out by the actor" (Stanislavski, 1965, p. 129-130).

The actor's containment of powerful emotional experiences as he becomes one with the character is a kind of "possession" that most of us experience very rarely. The actor seeks to "encourage his inner impulses that are relevant to the role to emerge as dominant; and to *encourage the domination of the whole personality by one part."* (ref) (italics mine).

"You only need claim the events of your life to make yourself yours.
When you truly possess all you have been and done, you are fierce with reality."
(Florida Scott-Maxwell)

Parallel Processes

The parallels between the process of acting and the process of Brainspotting are striking. The actor works with deep structure on a felt-sense level, as personal experiences are recalled and intuitively fed into the development of a character. This is a symbolic, intuitive process without translating or filtering through logical, judgmental consciousness. This is also a perfect description of the deep-brain processing that occurs during Brainspotting – deep experience without words, in the language of metaphor and imagery. Brainspotting often evokes spontaneous, internal re-enactments of old memories that have been completely forgotten, along with all the feelings, senses, and people that were present during the actual event. These visualizations are a rebirth of experience, the reliving of a life.

"The fundamental aim of our art is the creation of the inner life of a human spirit and its expression in an artistic form. That is why we begin by thinking about... how to create its spiritual life through the help of the internal process of living the parts ... (C. Stanislavski, 1961, p. 14).

Combining these two powerfully symbolic mediums, acting with Brainspotting, can facilitate astonishing transformations of the actor into a fully-formed character through accelerated character development, while also eliciting "deeper relaxation, heightened focus, and a natural and fluid access to emotion." (Grand, 2001, p. 179) This synthesis truly becomes an art form, not just a technique.

Note: The Othello process, described above for an actor, works as well with singers, dancers, and performers in all contexts. Instead of using a monologue to begin getting into character, you can invite the artist to perform a song, a dance, or other creative medium. Together you can then look for the Brainspot that most captures either the felt-sense or essence of the medium (like the feeling, essence, or message intended in a song or dance, for example), or of the character that will be performing it.

The Hologram Mystery

Sometime after the remarkable session with Othello, and my statement that the session "reminded me of holograms," I recalled my utter fascination with holograms that had begun many years earlier in the 1980s. Simultaneously, I realized what had fascinated me in Toney's remarkable Brainspotting session. In it, I had observed the spontaneous creation of a complete, separate "entity," the character of Othello, who – most importantly – had his own "Othello memories" that emerged organically and belonged only to the character.

It was this entity's amazing emergence in the session that had seemed holographic to me.

Although holograms are somewhat familiar these days in films (famously, Princess Leia in Star Wars) or the tiny ones on our credit cards, viewing an actual life-size hologram is a rather mystical experience. And the secret contained within them is even more amazing.

During that distant time, I had loved visiting the shadowy halls of the Museum of Holography in New York City, sadly long-gone now. There on the walls in the cool darkness, all kinds of bizarre, three-dimensional images, called holograms, eerily poked their way out of the frames in which they lived. Near the entrance, illuminated in the darkness by some invisible light source, lived the winking lady, a life-sized, three-dimensional woman who grinned and winked at me each time I passed her. Further down the hall a ferocious Doberman lunged in the air over my head so realistically that the first, second, and third time I passed him I actually jumped. Both of these holograms were designed so that you could see all the way around to the back and the underneath of them – just as you would if you turned your head around any real object to look at it from all sides – *even though they each lived in flat picture frames on the wall.* To me this was absolutely extraordinary.

Deeper in the dark central gallery was the museum's tour de force, an enormous, twinkling pot of gold. It was lit from underneath, so you could walk all the way around the pot and get a close look at the treasure. But if you reached out to touch the gold, your hand sliced right through the air because, of course, there was absolutely nothing there.

The Museum of Holography was an utterly magical place.

Holograms are created with a single laser beam that is split into two separate beams. One is directed to reflect off an item – like Princess Leia ... or an elephant – and this beam then carries a jumble of scattered light waves that contain optical information about the object. The second beam is directed by mirrors to collide with the first beam, which creates a swirling interference pattern that is then recorded on a special emulsion film. In this way, a three-dimensional image (a "holograph") – of an elephant – is captured and encoded in the film. Finally, when a third laser beam is directed at the film, the swirls of information hidden in the film are decoded, and a very real-looking, life-size, 3-D elephant pops out into space!

But here is the real mystery of holograms. If you wanted to, you could break the holographic film of the elephant into a hundred small pieces. And, unlike regular photographic film (which would be totally destroyed if you cut it up), *every single piece of the holographic film would still contain the entire 3-D image of the whole elephant.* No matter how many shattered pieces there were, each and every piece of the hologram could still reproduce a 3-D elephant!

In other words, with holograms, every part contains the whole.

This is the science of quantum physics. And, reading this, if you are now thinking, like I did, that this is impossible (how *can* it be possible?), you are not alone, for even quantum physicists have the same awed puzzlement when they investigate holograms and the part-equals-whole concept.

It defies reason as we know it.

"Reality is not a fixed entity.
It is a contingent interlocking of moving events.
And events do not just happen to us.
We are an integral part of creating every event."
(unknown)

A Fascinating Possible Explanation for Brainspotting-Induced Character Memories

All science's past attempts to understand how the human brain stores information have been based on the assumption that it is a "localized" process – that is, every piece of information is stored in a specific (local) place in the brain, just like the books in a library, or the memory in a computer.

But there are so many problems with that idea! First, individual memories have never been successfully located in any particular place in the brain. And second, the removal of part of the brain doesn't necessarily remove a memory, or any specific part of one.

Quantum physicist Karl Pribram was inspired by the part-equals-whole feature of holograms because it finally showed how memories could possibly be *distributed, instead of "localized,"* in the brain (Talbot, M. 1991, p. 13).

Pribram postulated that if it is possible for every fragmented piece of holographic film to contain all the information necessary to create a whole image, then it could also be possible for every part of the brain to contain all the information necessary to recall a whole memory, along with all its sensory and interconnected data.

That is, memories may not be located in a "place." Instead, the energy of creating or storing a memory may be emitted and absorbed by the whole system, so that theoretically in *every* part of the brain there may exist the possibility of all memories, in a wave state. Just like the wavy information stored on the film of a hologram. The enfolded information reveals a 3-D object with just the right angle of a laser beam.

This could explain why you don't have to rewind back through every detail of the last ten years in order to remember something that happened ten years ago. Instead, the memory, along with all the sensory details of the time when it happened, is distributed everywhere in the system (non-local) and is instantly accessible, as soon as you look for it.

Computers have *nothing* on your brain!

Furthermore, as Pribram and other scientists have suggested, holograms may explain the brain's vast capacity to store so many memories in so little space (a staggering 2.8 x 10 (280,000,000,000,000,000,000) bits of information (McCrone, 2002, p. 12). According to physicist Stephen Hawkings, holograms have a fantastic capacity for storing information. "A one-inch-spare of holographic film can store the same amount of information contained in fifty Bibles" (Hawkings, 2001, p.181.).

As if that weren't enough, it is also possible to record multiple different images on the film surface of a hologram. Imagine, for example, storing the image of a cat, right on top of an octopus, on top of a peacock, just by changing the angle at which the laser beams strike the film. The 3-D cat, or octopus or peacock could each be viewed *sepa-*

rately, their image teased out by illuminating the film at exactly the same laser angle at which it was recorded. Or you could choose to view a composite image of *all* the animals at the same time by shining a laser beam directly through the film. The resulting weird image would probably look like a 3-D science fiction monster, with multiple arms, feathers and fur all akimbo ("limbs flung out widely and wildly")!

The individual images can be viewed separately, but they are also integral parts of a much larger whole.

Scientists say this suggests that our ability to remember something may be analogous to shining a laser beam at just the right angle on holographic film to access a particular memory. And when we *can't* remember something, it may resemble using the wrong laser angle for teasing out the specific image.

This brings us back to David Toney and Othello. Othello's character memories are separate from David Toney's memories, but equally powerful.

David Toney – the whole – contains Othello, the part. And Othello – the part – contains David Toney, the whole. And vice versa.

Three Frequent Outcomes with Actors

Below are three frequent results achieved from Brainspotting with actors that imply a holographic (part-contains-the-whole) process:

1. The power of Brainspotting is not just in the actor's ability to create a character, but in the actor's ability, with spontaneous character memory, to craft the character's full relationship with life. Character memory appears to be *memory that is created and remembered at the same time.* In a sense, Brainspotting brings forth a total incarnation of another person. The result is a "complete inner world, which allows a character to emerge organically, with real flesh-and-blood characteristics" (David Grand, personal communication). Actor David Toney says, "It is not acting, it is more a matter of being. Giving all of yourself to possession by this character, you are taken by this personality inside of you, even physically, so that there is literally no space left for you."
2. The actor's character can become so three-dimensional, organic, and authentic that the actor in character may be able to experience a felt-sense of his relationships with family members and others without having to consciously *think* about them. For example, the character's mother might enter a scene, and without even turning around to look at her, the character may sense her presence and their relationship – without making it conscious – in exactly the same way that we all know when our

mother has entered the room. This is working within a deep structure, without the necessity of translation into a language of consciousness. Logical, linear thought is not required. The process is deep-brain and holographic (part-equals-whole) in the fullness of the experience for the actor.

3. Once the actor is fully in character, the BSP practitioner is able to conduct a Brainspotting therapy session with the character.

As Othello's session progressed, Grand guided him through a Brainspotting therapy session related to his traumatic experience in the courtyard. Othello clearly had PTSD! He found his activation spot (a SUDs of 9) and processed it down to a 2. This deepened the authenticity and truthfulness of the Othello character. In effect, the character becomes more real as it is being healed. And the character heals as it becomes more real.

"There is no healing without creativity,
and there is no creativity without healing."
(David Grand)

A Holographic View

The parallel levels that are operating to achieve this kind of transformation can perhaps only be understood through a holographic paradigm. I visualize the process as if the character (the part) is a separate hologram with its own essence and memories, vibrating within the actor's hologram (the whole) containing all his aspects. They are separate entities, yet deeply connected by a common spirit, and the actor can move fully between them.

NOTE: As a Brainspotting acting coach, after the actor (singer/dancer/performer) is in character, consider conducting a Brainspotting session *with the character*. Your focus can be on the emotional issues that come up for the character in the play (or whatever the character wishes to focus on. Consider processing the script, song lyrics, or dance moves line by line to enhance the character's understanding of herself, the deepest meanings of the words/lyrics, even the intentions of the playwright/composer of the piece. Treat the character as the client, and conduct a BSP session exactly as you would with any other. Even character trauma has the potential to block full expression of the holographic entity and inhibit creativity. *Just remember to find a self-spot for the actor afterward, so that she can process her way out of character and back into her own life.*

When we look into a broken mirror, we see that each piece has its own view of us. We see the face of our selves – our parts, our identities, our consciousness – that is shattered into many pieces, each with a unique set of desires, beliefs, and expectations. We know, from trauma, that fragmentation is one of the psyche's defenses against soul-crushing pain and fear, which is parceled out to multiple "parts" who bear what would otherwise be unbearable for one. These fragmented ego states are not broken, jagged-edged shards, but may be a collection of smaller wholes, complete and self-sustaining but dissociated and out of synch with each other.

Holographic theory states that every piece of the psyche and the universe, no matter how it is sliced, contains the intelligence of the whole. That means that we, as individual beings, are not isolated and random. "Each of us is a microcosm that reflects and contains the macrocosm. If this is true," consciousness research Stanislav Grof says, "then we each hold the potential for having direct and immediate experiential access to virtually every aspect of the universe, extending our capacities well beyond the reach of our senses." (Grof, 1985, p. 173).

That is, *you are not in the universe. The universe is in you.*

"First he conceived from the depth of his being a something, neither mind nor matter, but rich in potentiality ... and yet the whole must be no other than the sum of all of its parts and each part an all-pervading determination of the whole. It was a cosmical substance in which any individual spirit must be, mysteriously, at once an absolute self and a mere figment of the whole"
(Stapledon, 2008, p. 25).

Brainspotting with Mirror Visualizations

The inexperienced actor or performer, or one who has not yet familiarized himself with a character, may need more assistance in a Brainspotting session before performing a monologue or finding a character brainspot, In such a case, you can also introduce the use of a mirror visualization to assist the actor's transformation into a holographic character incarnation. This technique can also be used with a singer or dancer, as they too become "characters" expressed through their creative medium. Below, substitute "actor" for any performance artist.

Described below is a guided visualization presented to the actor (who is wearing headphones with Biolateral sound) by the therapist.

Mirror Visualization

Below, Carol, the actor, is creating the character of Juliet.

BSP Therapist: "Carol, walk down a long hallway. On the right is a door with a golden doorknob. Open the door and flip on the light. You are entering a large room. You see an enormous mirror on the far wall. Walk over to the mirror and look at yourself in the reflection. Notice your face, your eyes, clothes, what it feels like to be you, looking at yourself. Now, slowly, as you are looking, you begin seeing the image of Juliet, the character you will become. Notice Juliet's face, what she's wearing, especially what is on her feet, and notice her contact with the ground. What are you feeling as you look at her? What is she feeling?

"Now Carol, imagine raising one arm and placing your hand on the mirror. You also notice as Juliet raises her corresponding hand, and your two hands meet on the mirror. Be aware of the felt sense of your hand and Juliet's hand connecting. Notice what you're feeling in your hand right now.

"Right now, as the mirror gently rotates all the way around so that now Carol is inside the mirror, and you are Juliet outside the mirror, notice as Carol looks back at you from inside the mirror. Juliet, gently lower your hand. Notice how Carol does also. Feel your body, your posture, your breathing.

"Juliet, when you are ready, watch in the mirror as Carol gently morphs into Juliet, and you are now Juliet looking at Juliet in the mirror. Notice the feel of your body as Juliet, and use all your senses. Raise your hand, as Juliet in the mirror raises hers. Feel your hands touching as they join at the mirror.

"In your own time, Juliet, turn and walk away from the mirror, walk to the door, turn the golden doorknob and open the door while turning out the light. Now walk out of the room, closing the door. Go down the hall, walk directly onto the stage and into the play, and begin your lines.

"From now on, I will speak to you as Juliet."

Take plenty of time with this process and encourage the actor/performer to notice and experience as much sensory detail as possible. Ask questions about the character's breathing, what the character is wearing, how the character is feeling as she sees herself in the mirror, and anything else that can assist in creating a full embodiment. At this point the actor will have a much deeper sense of the character, and perhaps can now recite lines or a monologue (or sing a song, perform a dance), and thus more easily locate the character spot.

When the session is coming to an end, the mirror process should be exactly reversed (so that the Juliet character goes back to the room, sees herself in the mirror, as the image gently morphs back into Carol when the mirror revolves). The return process is crucial, as mentioned earlier, for without it the actor/performer will continue to carry emotionally charged aspects of the character. The mirror process seems to allow the actor to step fully out of the character's hologram and back into her own essence.

Mirrors have always awed and perplexed us. They suggest that there is more than one way to observe and interpret reality, by both dividing and joining. The introduction of either a real or an imaginary mirror, as in the above exercise, instantly creates two separate worlds out of just one. And the act of removing a mirror causes integration, since the image in the mirror disappears right into the object.

"Our mind is a mirror of a universe that mirrors our mind."
(Pearce, 2002, p xiii)

Stanislavski told his students:" You must be very careful in the use of a mirror. It teaches an actor to watch the outside rather than the inside of his soul, both in himself and in his part" (Stanislavski, 1961, p. 126). However, with BSP, the mirror is the doorway that allows the actor to step right *into* the soul of his character, and travel through the looking glass into and out of a new hologram.

Performance Anxiety

It may be surprising to discover that many, if not most, performers have terrible fears about performing, suffering paralyzing stage fright, with panic, vomiting, fainting, and many other symptoms. Some of the most confident, famous, and gifted performers in the world experience these symptoms, which often then completely disappear once they are on stage. It is usually the anticipation of failure (in front of masses of people) and the specter of potential, horrifying shame that is the most debilitating. And for some, the suffering AFTER the perceived imperfect performance is also absolutely devastating. (It makes you wonder why they do it, in the face of such suffering. Most will say they do it because they have no choice – theirs is a calling, powerful like no other.) "There's no business like show business" can mean many different things to different artists, both positive and negative, while unaware audiences assume that performing is all about joy and creative freedom. As a Brainspotting therapist, it is paramount to understand that the choice to perform (or spiritually die) is challenging beyond imagination, and also how very vulnerable the performer must make him- or herself in order to do the required work discussed above, and show it to the world. Of course, the symptoms described above are most likely trauma-based, lending themselves to the many treatment options that Brainspotting provides.

That said, there are many other versions of performance anxiety besides those connected with walking onto a stage, whether they occur in the stresses of daily living, in school, or in corporate settings – wherever peak creative performance is expected and required. In the next pages are explorations of two cases in those other settings, to illuminate the creative process and all its demands in the context of Brainspotting treatment.

Intuition, the Mind's Creative Process

Farmer Haggett knew that little ideas that tickled and nagged and refused to go away should never be ignored, for in them lie the seeds of destiny.
(From the movie, Babe)

Intuition is our perception of the world in wholes, rather than parts to be analyzed. It is a creative process that does not ask; it just knows instantly. Most of us have countless experiences of intuitive understandings that imply an underlying connectedness to a greater source than is obvious.

Brainspotting and Creative "Blocks"

The soul should always stand ajar;
Ready to welcome the ecstatic experience.
(Emily Dickinson)

The A-ha! experience of creativity is that intuitive moment that, like a lightning bolt, crackles and pops with energy, then delivers some bold, formerly hidden truth or insight. Intuitions are unexplained feelings that something is true, even when there is no evidence or proof of it.

Below is a session in which a creative intuition saved a life.

Jason's Session

"Jason" and I were in for a shocking Eureka! surprise that day, one that neither of us was even remotely expecting.

Jason, a 28-year-old actor, had come to me for Brainspotting because he had already twice flunked his pharmacy exam (to become a pharmacist "for his day job"), and he only had one remaining chance. He hoped that for his third and final attempt, BSP would help him pass.

A moment of profound creativity and intuition probably saved Jason's life.

While he was riding his bike through a secluded park one day at age 10, Jason was knocked over by a large man, who dragged him into the woods. After forcing Jason to perform oral sex, while muttering over and over that he was going to kill the boy, the man was about to penetrate Jason anally when Jason turned around, looked at the man straight in the eyes, and said,

"My mother just died yesterday."

The man looked up with "wild, crazy eyes," as if suddenly frightened, then cursed profusely, shoved Jason to the ground, and ran off.

Since Jason's mother was alive and well at the time, Jason was mystified about the origin of those life-saving words.

Unfortunately, having told no one about what had happened to him, Jason had, over the next eighteen years, internalized the traumatic experience as confirmation of his weakness and stupidity: If he'd been "normal" he would have physically fought off his assailant, instead of "saying something really dumb and pathetic. I am such a wuss."

Below, during his second BSP session (of three), Jason begins to take credit for the power of his creative, intuitive action.

The frame of the session was Jason's frightening experience with the man. The focus was on the worst and most terrifying moment of his near-rape and murder. We used an Inside Window Brainspot for Jason's panic (body tense and visibly shaking), with a SUDs of 10+.

Jason: I'm feeling fearful and rushed [common feelings for Jason]. I'm thinking of my recurring nightmare: I'm in space and everything is really huge or really tiny. Distances are being obscured. It's dark, and there's something unknown. It's different from anything else, and I have no idea what it is.

Therapist: Just notice what you're feeling and see where it goes.

J: My father didn't like laziness and procrastination. Wow! I don't know where that just came from!

J: Any small efforts I made to do something never led anywhere. So I watched a lot of TV. I'm feeling kind of dumb and noncreative. People don't like me because I'm too intense.

J: People are always looking at me like I'm stupid. On the subway, I know they're thinking how pathetic and dumb I am. I can see their faces, like they're mystified, and they think I'm nuts.

J: That guy in the park gave me the exact same look. I had no power, so I said my mother died yesterday. So the guy dusts himself off and runs away. Why did I take it, and act so stupid like that?

[Long pause, quiet.]

J: Yuck! The man is like an animal devouring something. My chest just caved in! I want to grab him and throw him off. Beat the shit out of him! I'm doing it. Me and little Jason, we're killing him!

J: He's looking at me.

J: He looks disbelieving, like I'm challenging him in a way that he didn't expect.

Therapist: Just keep looking.

J: He looks hurt. That makes no sense at all.

[Another long pause.]

J: It looks like my father's face. My father had to control everything. He couldn't stand to be challenged. My older brother left home when he was really young, out of protest, and my father was heart-broken. I NEVER fought with my father. I didn't want to hurt him like my brother did.

J: Oh my GOD!

[Therapist is thinking, "Uh-oh, what is coming next", and assuming all kinds of theories about what all this was about. Thankfully, the therapist said NOTHING.] (Uncertainty Principle)

J: I just realized I was protecting that man from my rage, just like I protected my father.

J: Oh my God! Oh my GOD!!!

[Long pause, while therapist worries silently.]

J: That thing I said to that man. *I said it so I wouldn't hurt his feelings.* He wouldn't think I was challenging him, so I said something soft and sad, so then maybe he would just leave me alone.

J: That was *my power. I saw my father's face, and it saved me.*

Therapist: SUDs?

Jason: Zero.

- - -

The next week, during our third and final BSP session, Jason began to take full credit for the astonishing intuitive action he took that saved his life. Using a resource brainspot to expand and enhance his new awareness of his strengths, Jason now began to see and experience himself as smart, intuitive, and creative instead of pathetic and stupid. The lens through which he saw his world had changed.

"A change of world view can change the world viewed."
(Pearce, 2002, p. 4)

Jason soon took his third and final pharmacy test, passed with flying colors, and never returned.

The real voyage of discovery consists
not in seeking new landscapes
but in having new eyes.
(Marcel Proust)

Quantum Leaps of Creativity

The deepest recesses of ourselves are mute. The mid- and hind-brain do not speak using words, conceptualize what's happening, or try to reason their way through life. Instead they operate on instinct, reflexes, and ancient survival mechanisms. These parts of us just *are.* But they do communicate with us at the time through our dreams that exist without language, and our feelings and body sensations, which speak for themselves. When we don't understand these messages – when we are confounded by our feelings and confused by our dreams – we tend to experience them as blocks that are holding us back. But the resolution for the message is embedded in the block itself. In other words, the block is the message.

In the above Brainspotting session, Jason first identified the perceived "block" (his "stupidity," failing his exams), then gave it a voice, thus transmuting it into a gift of insight. His system spontaneously reframed his experience, so that he would never again see his intuitive, life-saving statement as anything but what it was: Brilliant. Blocks are often gateways to something else that is dissociated. *The answer was there all along, but hidden from Jason's awareness because he was looking elsewhere.* Trauma blocks us all, and its resolution give us access to a consciousness not previously available to us, as it begins to work its magic.

We know that ego state transformations are common with the use of BSP. Jason became his 10-year-old self and through his younger part's eyes, was able to understand first-hand why he followed the intuition that saved his life. The holographic concept of part-equals-whole helps to explain these transformations that defy reason: BSP holographic visualizations are often complete 3-D experiences that are systemically very real, in the same way character memories feel real to the character, as previously discussed. Jason was there. Seeing the truth that was there all along made it possible for him to integrate this information, as child and adult merged. The transition from a state of passivity into taking full responsibility for and power over your life is an A-ha! moment that means living in one world one minute, and living in a totally different one the next.

Beam Me Up, Scotty!

In science, moving to a different plane of existence without physically moving is called a quantum leap. When an electron jumps from one atomic orbit to another, it never travels through the space between orbits. Instead, it simply ceases to exist here and simultaneously appears over there. Right now, try to imagine jumping from a high curb to the street without passing through the space in between. This is what electrons do! It's like watching fireflies on a summer night. You see a sudden flash here and then a twinkle over there, but you have absolutely no idea where the firefly is between your observations. (I've tried to actually follow a firefly, and it is almost impossible!)

Just like watching fireflies, scientists cannot predict which orbit the electron will jump to, or when it is going to leap. They can only make good guesses, based on probability, but in the moment in between orbits, the possibilities for where the electron may show up are infinite. And in that very moment, a window of opportunity opens up for something new – true, cosmic creativity – when almost anything can happen. Poet Emily Dickinson wrote, "I dwell in Possibility." If an electron could talk, this is probably how it would describe itself! According to physicist Steven Hawking (1990), in a cosmos made up of leaping particles, the entire universe is constantly evolving in a state of possibility.

In Star Trek, the captain of the Enterprise says "Beam Me Up, Scotty," and those "energized" people travel through hyperspace to some place specific (they hope). When they get there and materialize back into ordinary space, nothing new has happened to them except their location. But Star Trek writers have apparently missed something quite wonderful, because what happens on an actual quantum leap is completely uncertain. Electrons, in between jumps, are in a state of transcendent "possibility waves" where probability and uncertainty reign, making room for something truly, unpredictably creative to happen.

That means that in reality the crew of the Enterprise, like atomic particles, could move without traveling through any space, but they could also land almost anywhere on their leap. In fact, they would probably have to wait a really, *really* long time to actually get to where they intended.

Quantum Creativity

As with Jason, quantum leaps can also be entirely internal. There is no distance between us and our transformation ... the only distance is in our ability to see it. By turning our attention inward to "look," change can sometimes be as effortless as getting up and moving into a different room. Our consciousness will slowly become integrated and in less conflict with its parts, and in the place of conflict we can discover certainty.

Jason already had all the answers inside him, he just couldn't "see" them. There was evidence all around him that he was not stupid, that in fact he was intelligent, intuitive, and highly creative. But his system was only "looking" for the evidence that reconfirmed what he believed. Our consciousness literally cannot focus on two things at the same time. "The brain is unable to deal with conflicting information unless it can be integrated, so it tends to pick one perspective and repress all the information that doesn't fit" (Medina, 2014, p. 231). As one experiences more and more of life through that limited perspective, fear and helplessness can eventually become almost the only lens through which your brain chooses to see anything.

Thankfully, revealing something that is actually already there, but just hidden from view, requires considerably less effort to discover because it already exists. For example, you no longer have to believe in the ocean once you've been there, seen it for yourself, and actually jumped in. When that happens, belief is replaced with something much more precious: direct knowledge of your own power. This power is the true source of creativity, and it is not something exclusive to artists or geniuses.

The artist often has a heightened sense of intuition. As with Jason's life-saving intuition, and his new appreciation for what he had actually done, creative, intuitive breakthroughs have the feeling of truth or wholeness, a sudden illumination that appears to be directly connected to the escalation of an event into consciousness .... the "A-ha!" moment. All that is required is attention to our own awareness. "Certain intuitions seem to penetrate beneath the visible reality ... when there is a solid sense of "knowing," enabling one to act with a precision and confidence unwarranted by the facts of the situation" (Goldberg, 1995, p. 19).

Our culture inhibits and discourages our capacity for intuition, our sense of connectedness, and our creative expression. We have gradually lost touch with our true nature. But the new sciences have begun to confirm the deep connectivity we share with the cosmos. Just as creative intuition is a temporary state of our whole mind (brain/nervous system), we are joined in that state by the whole universe.

...it takes time to understand humans because they don't understand themselves. They have been wearing clothes for so long. Metaphorical clothes ... That was the price of human civilization – to create it, they had to close the door on their true selves. And so they are lost, that is how I understand it. And that is why they invented art: books, music, films, plays, painting, sculpture.
They invented them as bridges back to themselves, back to who they are.
(Haig, 2013, p. 125)

Creativity on Demand

It was the eyes, on Earth, that mattered.
You saw the person, and the life inside them, if you saw the eyes.
(Haig, 2013, p. 166)

If the brain were so simple that we could understand it,
we would be so simple that we couldn't.
(Lyall Watson)

Working With Metaphoric Imagery and Brainspotting

In Brainspotting, creatively gifted clients may resolve a problem or an issue by spontaneously experiencing metaphoric imagery, sometimes exclusively. It can be quite fascinating for the therapist as well. The abstract nature of the imagery, in which there is often little or no identifiable connection to the stated issue, is conducted in a kind of cyberspace. This is symbolic, intuitive deep-brain language that requires no translation, and is not filtered through logical, judgmental consciousness. Here, the uncertainty principle becomes paramount, as we try not to interfere with this often magical creative process.

Below is the third BSP session with Beth, a corporate creative director who had a reasonably stable childhood, but suffers with bouts of low self-esteem, and, at 30, is fearful that she has missed her opportunity to find a life partner and have children. In this session, she is feeling a lot of anxiety about her performance at a new job and an upcoming conference, where she will be required to deliver "creative ideas on demand." She is fearful about not having access to her creative ideas when she needs them.

That day, Beth gave me the great privilege of riding with her on a fantastical trip! In this session, I chose to be slightly more verbally active than usual, as she seemed to need me to come along with her on her voyage of discovery.

Beth: My anxiety is coming back for the first time in five years. I feel I'm not meeting expectations for others or myself. When I feel like this, I forget all I have done. I only see myself as a failure.

Therapist: As you say that, what do you notice feeling in your body?

B: I feel tense and muddled. I feel it terribly in my stomach and chest.

[The SUDs was a 9, and we used inside window to find the brainspot.]

B: I just went into my brain. I need to polish my brain. It's a huge job, and I need help. I'll ask my family [tearful]

B: "Why is my brain all old and moldy and muddled? My boss is shaking his head because he thinks I'm behind.

Therapist: Ask him why he thinks that.

B: He says I need to have everything clean in order to be ready. I'm ashamed to show my boss the insides of my brain. I just need some time.

B: When I don't know what I want to *do,* I don't know who I *am.*

B: I would die for independence and truth and creativity. Kindness is important to me.

B: My brain has cleaned up a lot already! My sister and I are in there. The work section is glowing blue. The love section is red. My sister is saying, "Look how *big* it is and how many interests you have!" The natural design is incredible. I am going to sit in each section.

B: I'm sitting with my sister in the blue section of work. I see the red section (love). I'm not there right now, but it's a place I could go back to. It just feels kind of warm.

[Beth then visited the green section (her passions) where she played and turned somersaults, the yellow section (her friendships) where she received hugs and reassurance.]

Therapist: Is there anything you want to do in your brain?

B: I'm going to bring a big vacuum into the work section and clean up all the dust. My love section needs a little dusting too. I'm putting down a rug. I'll make it out of the dust. Now I've got a chair. I just made a little office. I've got a Lazy-Boy so I can lounge. Well, what do you know! There's a Dust Buster in a little closet. I just invited my family to come in. They're impressed!

Therapist: What about your boss?

B: I just kicked him out. He's nice but I just don't trust him. If I get laid off .... I've been burned before. Maybe later I'll have a cocktail party and invite him in with other people too. Even though I'm scared, it will make going back to work easier. A little social stuff to feel more myself.

B: In my brain, I feel very confident and comfortable and OK.

[Long pause. Beth then saw herself doing pull-ups to remind herself that she's strong. She went into the purple room, where she saw a garden of gorgeous flowers, reminding her of other parts of herself. Then she revisited her blue room of work.]

B: I'm practicing my presentation now in the blue room. Maybe I can bring the blue room with me to my office tomorrow. It's feeling much better. A big screen and equipment. I can laugh at it too. I'm drinking hot chocolate. It's sweet and warm. I can look at all this and laugh. It's not life or death. It's almost like I'm watching an old family film, watching myself as a comic character in a film reel.

B: My family is saying it's time to go. My sister says, "Where shall we visit next, your *KIDNEYS?* Your *SPLEEN* for a *really* good time?"

[At this point, Beth and I are both laughing.]

B: My father says, "See, your brain is already organized."

Therapist: Earlier you said, "When I don't know what I'm doing, I don't know who I am." How do those words feel right now?"

B: It's less true. I don't have to know where I'm going. There might be a better room that fits later, but this is OK for right now. I really am those values of independence, truth, creativity, and kindness. That can't be taken away from me when I leave this room.

B: I see a magic cape in the room with all these values layered into it. I can throw that on. The other values are me, but I'll also throw on intelligence – it's the thing that's most lacking in this room. That's what I really need there. Intelligence, confidence, decisiveness, patience, articulation. Ha! I'll have to *rent* that room! (laughing). I can do a 6-month lease!

B: The cape is more of a jacket. A black leather model I can wear whenever I want and no one will know what it *really* is. Confidence and intelligence radiate in the jacket. I'm keeping it on for this conference.

Therapist: Go back to where we started, feeling muddled and seeing yourself as a failure.

B: It feels much further away. I can connect to it, but it's only a 2. I do really feel that room! [smiling] And I feel much less scared and overwhelmed.

- - -

Beth seemed to have taken a shamanic journey, possibly for retrieving lost parts of herself. On such a journey, one often discovers what is needed to become a master in one's life. In this virtual, holographic cyberspace, Beth and I, on some level, crossed over the boundary separating self and universe.

The following week, Beth reported a wealth of new ideas, a successful presentation at the conference, and, with her team, and compliments from her boss. She redesigned her office to reflect her blue room, and began bringing in flowers. She said she felt confident and strong all week.

In our next session, Beth spontaneously explored her heart by swimming around in it with her sister, through all its chambers and arteries.

She was much relieved to discover that her heart was clear and open, and ready for love.

As a therapist, I wouldn't have missed that experience with Beth for the world! However, follow-up is important after a metaphoric session like this one, in order to assess the usefulness of this kind of processing. What has happened in between sessions? Based on the positive results reported the following week, Beth's Brainspotting session had in fact ignited beautiful metaphoric imagery that was directly related to her issue, from a deep-brain state in which anything is possible.

Most striking is that Beth resolved the issue with spontaneous creative imagery exclusively. The abstract (and sometimes entertaining) nature of this imagery, when combined with the often surprising results achieved, implies access to a direct line into absolute truth or essence, which Beth even mentioned discovering. Contact with essence, like a laser beam that illuminates an essential internal hologram, is a primary characteristic of Brainspotting and a universal dynamic of both human and cosmic creativity.

Our spiritual dimension has usually been called our spirit or soul, but in the context of Brainspotting, I like to call it *essence* based on my own personal experiences and those of my Brainspotting clients. I think that essence is a personal energy field or a core identity, a beingness that simply exists when we are able to be present and aware. (Actor David Toney also calls it *isness).* We just *are.* And in our state of essence, there is the potential for something new and unexpected to happen, and all we have to do is get out of the way so healing and creativity can get on with its natural process. Brainspotting is designed for just that.

"The art of a poet lies not only in her words; the art of a painter lies not only in his choice of colors; it lies in the ability of each to engage vitally with life in a way that draws a quality of soul out of each. Then an expansion of feeling and perception, of life and energy, takes place that transcends the form of the craft." (May Sarton)

The symbolic representation of Beth's issue (the part) was transformed into a freed-up energy she could actually use in her creative life (the whole). No other logical analysis was necessary for Beth to make some important shift. Instead, what she experienced was pure creative intuition and intention. Like Jason, she made a quantum leap.

Mental images like Beth's evoke the experience of seeing without any visual input from the eyes. Instead, they are acts of *creative seeing,* a truly remarkable feat of the brain. (I have often said to my clients, in an effort to explain why Brainspotting imagery is so effective, that "the brain doesn't know the difference between fantasy and reality. This is the same reason that nightmares, in the moment, can be so terrifyingly real").

Furthermore, the screen of the mind, upon which we "see" the imagery that appears, has never been located in the brain. ("So then, where is it?" I ask.) But mental images on our internal screens, "like the images in a mirror, are not in this sense imaginary at all. We *do* actually experience them and they are no more imaginary than sensations or feelings. Indeed, to those who experienced it, an image-world would be just as 'real' as the present world is..." (Epstein, 2000, p. 6).

The Holographic View

The holographic brain's almost endless capacity for memory storage and retrieval illustrates how Brainspotting imagery during processing can contain an entire constellation of information. A single image (even a metaphoric one) may contain complex data about attitudes, childhood trauma, ego-strengths and self-esteem, relationships, spiritual experience, and sensory information, all enfolded into the scene. The metaphoric image, as part, contains the whole, which unfolds with shifts in beliefs and profound spiritual experiences.

"Presence" is another universal element of creativity that is evoked in Brainspotting processing, as the performer's distracted consciousness is guided into full attentiveness to the present moment – to be aware of the flow of attention itself, being conscious of their consciousness. We follow the flow of energy and experience, wherever it goes, fully trusting that it will find its own way. Actor David Toney calls this "creative speed" in acting; that is, "reaching a point where nothing else matters."

"Many artists have said that when life itself becomes fully conscious, art as we know it will vanish. Art is only a stopgap, an imperfect effort to wrest meaning from an environment in which nearly everyone is sleepwalking. Pain is the aversion; the healing magic is attention. Properly attended to, pain can answer our most crucial questions. Conflict, pain, tension, fear, paradox...these are transformations trying to happen." (Ferguson, 1980, p. 156)

In my experience, Brainspotting artists (and other clients) often give the impression that finding the missing piece in some jigsaw puzzle was all they needed to seize the strength they'd had all along and finally use it to make new creative choices in their lives. Then, what follows is often a fascinating decision-making process while bringing their own special *essence* into the forefront.

Creativity, the Great Healer

The truth is, we become most alive when we are creative.
Our creative moments are the greatest moments of our life.
Amit Goswami

"What wound did heal but by degrees."
Othello

For small creatures such as we, the vastness is bearable only through love.
Carl Sagan

In the current worldview of modern physics, separation does not exist. We are connected in subtle and important ways with the universe. Like the electron in between quantum leaps, we have access to infinite creative possibilities.

And if this is so, then on some level we already have what we wish for. Like Dorothy in the Wizard of Oz, home really has been in our own back yard all along. In creativity, everything you need you already have. *You're already there.* This is the awareness we offer our Brainspotting clients as they make those leaps. Like the hidden images in a hologram, the holographic mind and universe are revealed by discovery of their enfolded processes. But when we get to look beneath the surface, where creativity flows freely, we begin to see the truth of who we are...and who we've always been.

What do they say in car adverts.
About the navigation system?
Comes as standard.
Everything you need to know about right and wrong is already there.
It comes as standard.
It's like music.
You just have to listen.
(Haig, M, 2017, p. 152).

The power of transformation is a shared experience, and it is probably never felt more profoundly than in the mutual process between the creatively gifted client and the Brainspotting practitioner. And if every part contains the whole, then when our beliefs are transformed, so, inevitably, is the world.

We have some power in us that knows its own ends.
It is that which drives us on to what we must finally become.
We have only to conceive of the possibility
and somehow the spirit works in us to make it actual.
This is the true meaning of transformation.
This is the real metamorphosis.
Our further selves are contained within us,
as the leaves and blossoms are in the tree.
We have only to find the spring and release it.
Have you found wings?
(Malouf, 1978, p. 54).

At the end of a very healing Brainspotting creativity session, my client, Aaron, a professional singer/songwriter, described how he had no memories of crying and being comforted by anyone as a child – and thus remained stoic into adulthood and afraid to show any feelings. His greatest emotions were only fully expressed in his music. As he spoke of this, a great sadness came up, and I invited him to sing something that expressed that sadness. He sang a beautiful song that he had composed himself. Together we located a Gazespot for the sadness, as Aaron spontaneously visualized returning to his childhood home.

Aaron: I could try to re-experience the pain, or maybe I could revisit that time and think of it differently

Therapist: Which do you want to do?

Aaron: [pause] I want to be with little Aaron, and let him feel safe. My parents are not at home. It is daytime. I'm taking him through each room in the house, holding his hand. There is an illumination filling each room, like liquid sunshine. As we walk around, it spills slowly into the next rooms. The whole house is filled with golden liquid sunshine. Now it's moving down the blocks of my old neighborhood. Everywhere it spills, it creates safety, so I'm letting it spread to all the places I knew. My school, the freeway. It's a new zone of safety. But it's not covering up anything. It's transforming what is there into a new peacefulness. I'm glad to have finally found it.

In seeking, we find what was never really lost. Through the healing, creative process of Brainspotting, we can finally remember what we've always known. We can at last have a grand reunion with our spirit, with our essence. We only have to respond to that invitation.

We must assume our existence as broadly as we can in any way we can;
Everything, even the unheard-of, must be possible in it.
That is at bottom the only courage that is demanded of us;
To have courage for the most extraordinary, the most singular
And the most inexplicable that we may encounter.
That mankind has in this sense been cowardly has done life endless harm
(Rainer Maria Rilke).

Love is the whole thing.
We are only pieces.
(Rumi)

\- - -

References

Bates, B. (1987): The way of the actor: A path to knowledge and power. Boston: Shambhala Publications.

Eliade, M. (1964): Shamanism: Archaic techniques of ecstasy, Bollingen Series, vol 76. New York: Pantheon Books.

Epstein, G. (2000): The imaginal, the right hemisphere of the brain, and the waking dream [on-line serial] 4 (14). Available E-mail: drjerry@drjerryepstein.org..

Ferguson, M. (1980): Aquarian conspiracy. Los Angeles: JP Tarcher Inc.

Goldberg, H. (1995): The intuitive edge. Los Angeles: JP Tarcher Inc.

Grand, D. (2013): Brainspotting: The revolutionary new therapy for rapid and effective change. Sounds True. p. 26

Grand, D. (2001): Emotional healing at warp speed: The power of EMDR. New York: Harmony Books.

Grof, S. (1985): Beyond the brain: Birth, death and transcendence in psychotherapy. State University of New York, Albany.

Haig, M. (2017): How to stop time. Penguin Random House LLC.

Haig, M. (2013). The Humans. Simon & Schuster Paperbacks.

Halifax, J. (1982): Shaman: The wounded healer. London: Thames and Hudson.

Hawkings, S. (2001). The universe in a nutshell. New York, Bantam Books.

Malouf, D. (1978): An imaginary life. New York: Random House.

McCrone, J. (2002): How the brain works: A beginner's guide to the mind and consciousness. New York: DK Publishing.

Medina, J. (2014): Brain rules. Pear Press.

Pearce, J. (2002): The crack in the cosmic egg. Rochester: Park Street Press.

Stanislavski, K. (1989): Building a character. Routledge.

Stanislavski, K. (1989): An actor prepares. Routledge.

Stapledon, O. (2008): Star Maker. Dover Publications.

Talbot, M. (1991): The Holographic Universe. HarperCollins Publishers

Authors

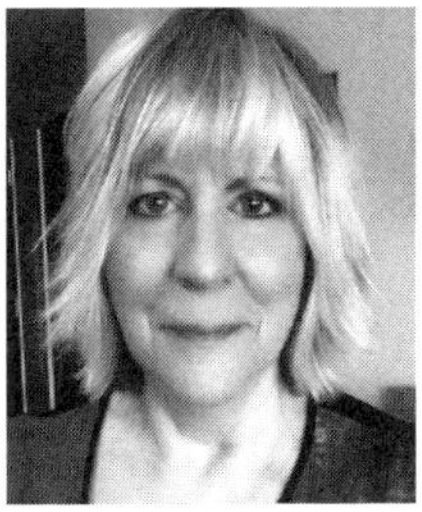

Deborah Antinori, MA, LPC, NCC, RDT, FT
Brainspotting trainer and certified consultant
Master of the Arts in Drama Therapy
Licensed professional counselor
National certified counselor
Registered drama therapist
Fellow in thanatology
Address:
77 Hudson St., #3606
Jersey City, NJ 07302
U.S.A.
dantinori@gmail.com

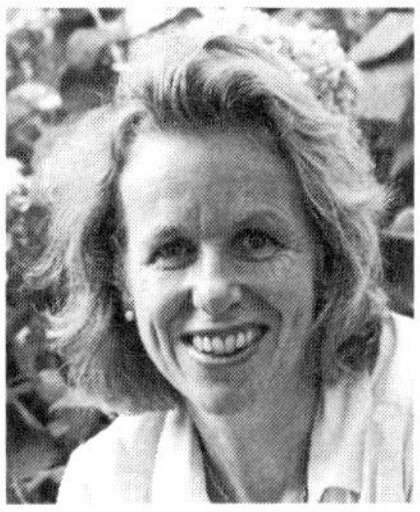

Monika Baumann, Mag., psychologist/psychotherapist/
Brainspotting trainer
Address:
Serravagasse 6/2
1140 Wien
+4367682877777
brainspottingaustria@gmail.com
www.brainspottingaustria.com

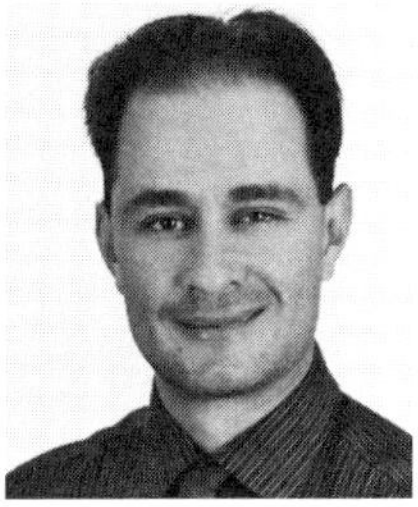

Santiago Brand
Clinical Director Brand Neurofeedback Faculty Member Brain Science International (2013-2015)
Brainspotting Therapist, Neurofeedback Therapist, Biofeedback Therapist
Address:
Calle 140 # 11-58, Bogotá, Colombia
Mobile: 57-321-455-9810
Office: 47-1-6151652
info@brandneurofeedback.net
www.cerebroysalud.com

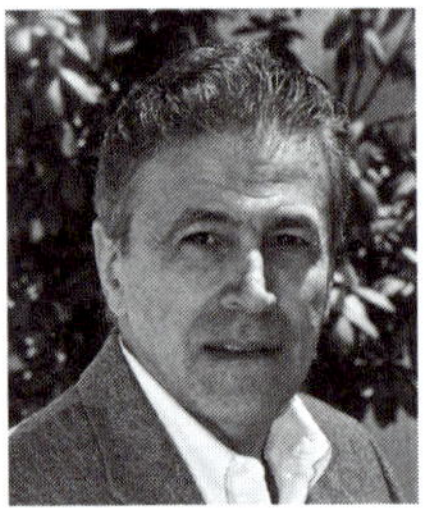

David Grand
Ph. D., Psychotherapist, Psychoanalyst, international expert in Trauma Therapy, writer, lecturer and performance coach, in private office in Manhatten and on Long Island, discoverer and developer of Brainspotting, Brainspotting Senior Master Trainer, also developer and producer of CDs for acustic biolateral stimulation (www.biolateral.com).
Address:
2415 Jerusalem Avenue, Suite 105, Bellmore, NY 11710
www.brainspotting.com

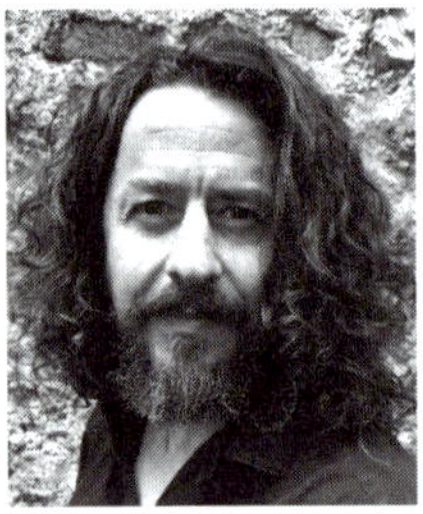

Dr Mark Grixti is a chartered clinical psychologist, obtaining his doctorate in clinical psychology in 2002 from the University of Surrey in England. Since then Mark has worked in NHS Child and Adolescent Mental Health Services, Tier 4 specialist service for children with sexually harmful/problematic behaviour, and Looked-After Children's Mental Health Services. Mark is the director of Specialist Psychology Services and for over 10 years has run private clinics in both London and Sussex specialising in trauma and attachment. Mark is the Brainspotting trainer in the UK (www.BSPUK.co.uk) and author of Brainspotting with young people: An adventure into the mind (2015). He teaches on psychology clinical doctorate training programs, presents at international conferences, trainings, and workshops.
Address:
40 Wilbury Road, Hove, East Sussex, UK
Email: info@bspuk.co.uk

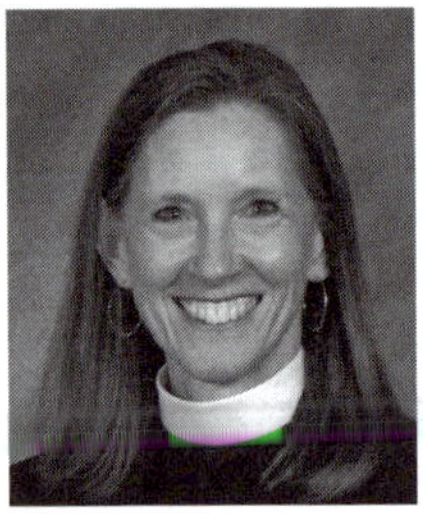

Martha S. Jacobi
Lutheran pastor/therapist/Brainspotting trainer
Address:
116 W 23rd Street, Suite 500, New York NY 10011,USA
+01 917-929-2562
BrainspottingHappens@gmail.com
www.brainspottinghappens-marthasjacobi.com

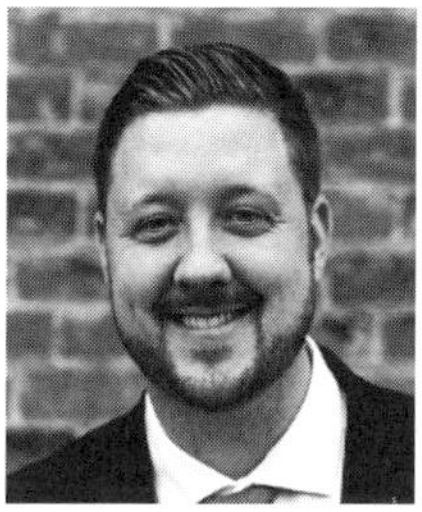

Calder W. Kaufman, PsyD
Clinical psychologist
Brainspotting trainer and consultant
Supervising psychologist & Director of the Center for Psychological Evaluation at the Birmingham Maple Clinic
Doctoral Dissertation: A Constructivist Grounded Theory Approach to Brainspotting
Address:
2507 Edison St.
Detroit, MI 48206
calderwkaufman@gmail.com

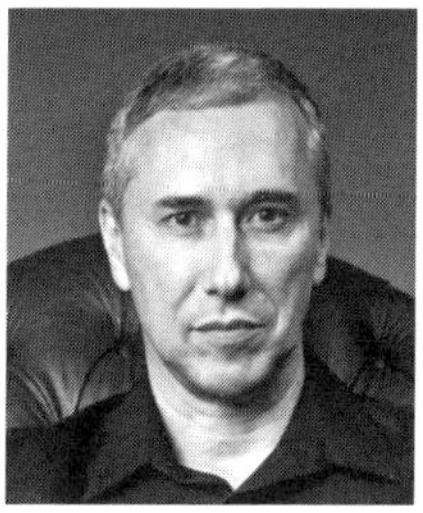

Dr. André Maurício Monteiro
Dr. André Maurício Monteiro, psychologist, MSc and Doctor in Psychology; EMDR facilitator and Trainer of Trainers (EMDR® Institute – USA), EMDR Ibero-América supervisor and trainer; EMDR-Europe approved consultant and trainer; Co-founder and 1st President of EMDR Brasil Association (2009–2012); Honorary member of the EMDR Association in Portugal; teaches Theory and Psychotherapy of Dissociative Disorders, and Transgenerational Transmission of Trauma in various cities in Brazil and in Portugal.
Professor and Supervisor in Psychodrama and Action Methods (Brazilian psychodrama Federation – Febrap); Brainspotting Expert, teaching the advanced module on Brainspotting and Dissociative Disorders.
Coordinator of the website: www.espacodamente.com, with online video courses on psychology, psychotherapy and neuroscience.
Address:
SQN 310 Bloco G apt 603
CEP - 70.756-070, Brasília - DF, Brasil
andre@espacodamente.com
FaceBook: Espaço da Mente

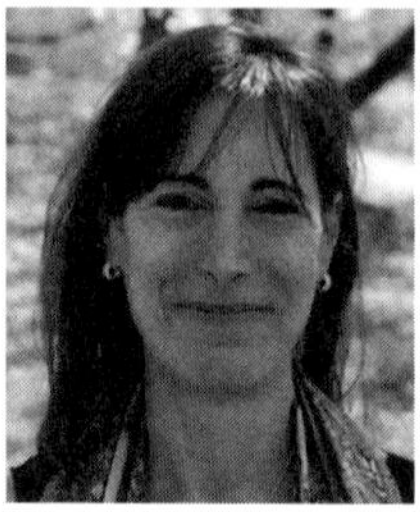

Susan Pinco, Ph.D., LCSW is in private practice in NYC and teaches internationally, offering courses in powerful, somatically-informed, treatment modalities that bridge the gap between mind and body. Susan is a certified BrainSpotting (BSP) consultant and trainer and has been using Brainspotting since its inception, having been a member of Dr. Grand's New York supervision group since 2001. She is also an EMDR certified consultant and an ASCH certified hypnotherapist/consultant and offers courses in Crisis Communication and Crisis Response and the Mandala of Being, a Multi-Modal Approach to Spiritual and Psychological Practice. She is currently working on a book that encourages therapists to utilize silence to facilitate integration and healing.

Address:
170 West End Avenue, Suite 1K, NYC, NY 10023
+1 (201) 747-6789
SusanPinco@Coherentself.com
www.coherentself.com

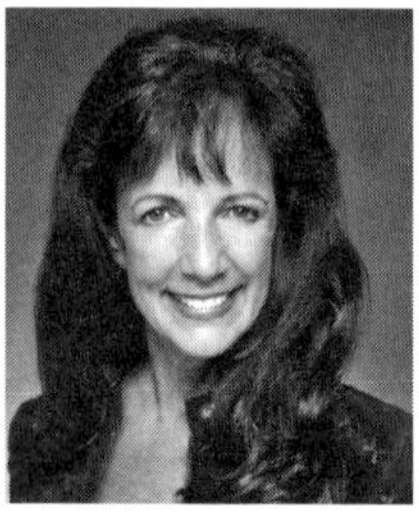

Christine Ranck, Ph.D., LCSW (licensed clinical social worker) is a Brainspotting trainer and psychotherapist in private practice in New York City. She is also a working professional singer/actress, and co-author of the best-selling book, "Ignite the Genius Within: Discover Your Full Potential."

Address:
116 W. 23rd St, 5th floor, #135
+01-917-353-4636
ChristineRanck@gmail.com
www.ChristineRanck.com

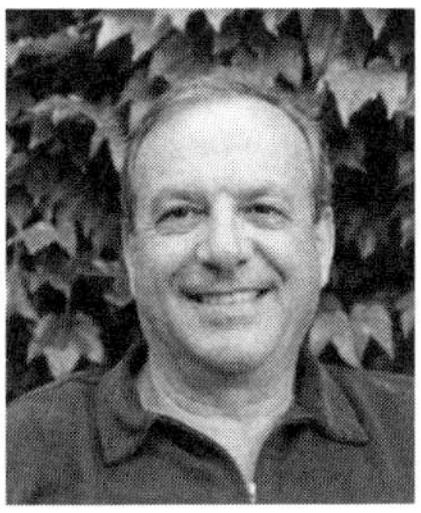

Mario C. Salvador
Clinial psychologist, a certified BrainspottingTrainer and Supervisor, EMDR practicioner/consultant, Integrative Psychotherapy Trainer and Supervisor from IIPA and Prov. Trainer and Supervisor Transactional Analyst by EAT-TAA. Director of ALECES, Institute for Integrative Psychotherapy and Brainspotting Spain, President of the Spanish Brainspotting Association. Author of the book: "Beyond the Ego; Finding our Essential Being Through the Healing of Trauma", international lecturer and trainer in Spain, Brasil, Slovenia, Italy, Austria, and Ecuador.
Address:
+34 669408069, 936759279
msalvador@aleces.com
www.aleces.com

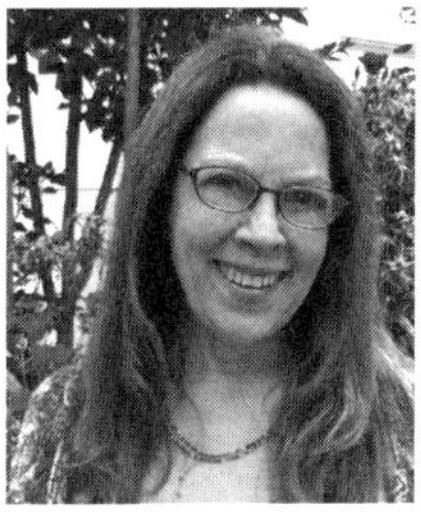

Cynthia Schwartzberg, LCSW, owner of Cynthasis, LLC, President of the Southeast Brainspotting Institute is a Brainspotting trainer, consultant and therapist, She has trained with David Grand at the highest of levels of Brainspotting since 2000, and continues to attend supervision group with him in NYC. Cynthia brings her experience in Brainspotting and mind/body therapy, which she has practiced and taught for over 30 years. She is committed to helping therapists gain skills to support their clients and to grow. She specializes in trauma PTSD, relationship issues, life patterns and transitions, performance enhancement and spiritual guidance.
Address:
455 East Paces Ferry Road, Suite 204, Atlanta, GA 30305
cynthia@cynthasis.com
www.cynthasis.com

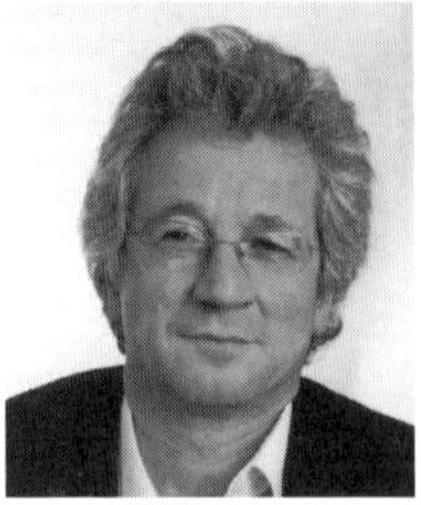

Gerhard Wolfrum, Dipl.-Psych.
Psychologischer Psychotherapeut, Psychoanalytiker,
Fach-Psychotherapeut für Traumatherapie, Gruppenpsychotherapeut
Lehr- und Kontrollanalytiker, Supervisor, BSP-Trainer
Address:
St. Wolfgangsplatz 9 c
D-81669 München
+49-89-537610
gerhard.wolfrum@gmx.net
www.gerhard-wolfrum.de www.brainspotting-germany.de